INTERPERSONAL ISSUES
IN HEALTH CARE

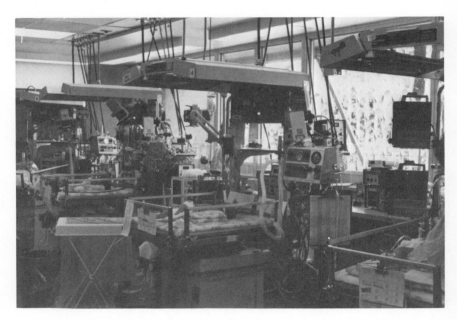

This picture of a newborn intensive care unit reveals the complexity and sophistication of the technical side of modern health care. This book concerns the other major influence on health and health care—namely, interpersonal relationships among practitioners and patients. (Photo by Howard S. Friedman. The cooperation of Kathy Wolff and the University of California, San Diego, Medical Center is appreciated.)

INTERPERSONAL ISSUES IN HEALTH CARE

Edited by

HOWARD S. FRIEDMAN
M. ROBIN DiMATTEO

Psychology Department
University of California
Riverside, California

1982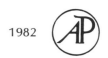

ACADEMIC PRESS
A Subsidiary of Harcourt Brace Jovanovich, Publishers
New York   London
Paris   San Diego   San Francisco   São Paulo   Sydney   Tokyo   Toronto

ACADEMIC PRESS, INC.
111 Fifth Avenue, New York, New York 10003

United Kingdom Edition published by
ACADEMIC PRESS, INC. (LONDON) LTD.
24/28 Oval Road, London NW1 7DX

Library of Congress Cataloging in Publication Data
Main entry under title:

Interpersonal issues in health care.

    Includes bibliographical references and index.
    Contents: Interpersonal issues in health care /
Howard S. Friedman and M. Robin DiMatteo -- Social
science and the art of medicine / M. Robin DiMatteo and
David D. DiNicola -- The social influence of physicians
and other health-care practitioners as agents of change /
Judith Rodin and Irving L. Janis -- [etc.]
    1. Medicine and psychology--Addresses, essays,
lectures. 2. Medical care--Psychological aspects--
Addresses, essays, lectures. 3. Interpersonal relations
--Addresses, essays, lectures. I. Friedman, Howard S.
II. DiMatteo, M. Robin. [DNLM: 1. Interpersonal
relations. 2. Social medicine. 3. Social sciences.
WA 31 I61]
R726.5.I6 1982   362.1'042   82-8681
ISBN 0-12-268340-4   AACR2

PRINTED IN THE UNITED STATES OF AMERICA

82 83 84 85   9 8 7 6 5 4 3 2 1

For Rhonda Bethie and Lucille Pal

CONTENTS

I

PERSPECTIVES ON SOCIAL INFLUENCE IN HEALTH CARE

1

2

3

The Social Influence of Physicians and Other Health Care Practitioners as Agents of Change 33

JUDITH RODIN

IRVING L. JANIS

4

Nonverbal Communication in Medical Interaction 51

HOWARD S. FRIEDMAN

II

RELATIONS WITH OTHERS, SOCIAL SUPPORT, AND THE HEALTH CARE SYSTEM

5

The Interpersonal Dynamics of Cancer: Problems in Social Relationships and Their Impact on the Patient 69

CHRISTINE DUNKEL-SCHETTER

CAMILLE B. WORTMAN

CONTRIBUTORS

Numbers in parentheses indicate the pages on which the authors' contributions begin.

NANCY E. ADLER (119), Graduate Group in Psychology, School of Medicine, University of California, San Francisco, San Francisco, California 94143

SONIA BLACKMAN (169), Department of Behavioral Sciences, California State University, Pomona, California 91768

M. ROBIN DiMATTEO (3, 9), Department of Psychology, University of California, Riverside, Riverside, California 92521

D. DANTE DiNICOLA (9), School of Medicine, University of California, Los Angeles, Los Angeles, California 90024

CHRISTINE DUNKEL-SCHETTER (69), Department of Psychology, University of California, Berkeley, Berkeley, California 94720

HOWARD S. FRIEDMAN (3, 51), Department of Psychology, University of California, Riverside, Riverside, California 92521

SHARON D. HERZBERGER (101), Department of Psychology, Trinity College, Hartford, Connecticut 06106

IRVING L. JANIS (33), Department of Psychology, Yale University, New Haven, Connecticut 06520

RUSSELL A. JONES (145), Department of Behavioral Science, University of Kentucky Medical Center, Lexington, Kentucky 40536-0084

ROBERT M. KAPLAN (187), Department of Psychology, San Diego State University, San Diego, California 92182, and Community and Family Medicine, University of California, San Diego, La Jolla, California 92093

ROBERT KASTENBAUM (233), Adult Development and Aging Program, Arizona State University, Tempe, Arizona 85284

DEBORAH A. POTTS (101), Department of Psychology, Northwestern University, Evanston, Illinois 60201

JUDITH RODIN (33), Department of Psychology, Yale University, New Haven, Connecticut 06520

SHELLEY E. TAYLOR (209), Department of Psychology, University of California, Los Angeles, Los Angeles, California 90024

CAMILLE B. WORTMAN (69), Department of Psychology, University of Michigan, Ann Arbor, Michigan 48104

FOREWORD

SPSSI, The Society for the Psychological Study of Social Issues, has as one of its major goals the encouragement of research on important social concerns of the times. One of the ways in which this goal has been implemented is through its publication program. Thus SPSSI has a tradition of sponsorship of social science volumes that are topical and sound. This book, *Interpersonal Issues in Health Care,* by Drs. Friedman and DiMatteo is another notable contribution to the genre. The issue of health care and its many aspects has become increasingly salient in the present economic and political climate. As our ability to pay for such care declines, it becomes ever more critical to define and evaluate its quality. Possibly the most important dimension to be included in such definition and evaluation is the interpersonal one. This book defines the problem, makes the issues explicit, and directs us to further exploration as well as to efforts to influence and advocate treatment changes. SPSSI is pleased that Friedman and DiMatteo, together with the chapter authors, have made it possible for SPSSI to publish this timely book.

MARTHA T. S. MEDNICK
SPSSI President

PREFACE

Although concern with interpersonal issues in health care is as old as the field of medicine, it is only in the last several years that such matters have emerged as an organized scientific discipline. Social psychologists have begun analyzing, integrating, and testing the collections of clinical impressions variously known as "the art of medicine," "humanistic or holistic health care," "the will to live," and "the warm, supportive health environment." It is exciting to witness the rapid emergence of a social scientific endeavor that holds such promise of societal benefits. It is also emotionally rewarding to work in a field in which there is such a thirst for knowledge by the field's professionals.

Several years ago, we coedited a volume of the *Journal of Social Issues* (published by the Society for the Psychological Study of Social Issues or SPSSI) entitled "Interpersonal Relations in Health Care" (vol. 35, no 1, 1979). That volume, produced under the guidance of *JSI* general editor Joe McGrath, was very well received. It generated hundreds of requests from people in various disciplines for reprints of articles and was even sometimes adopted as a textbook. Soon after, Alan Gross suggested that we consider expanding that journal issue into a book. This proposal was enthusiastically supported by the original contributors, by several potential new contributors, and by SPSSI's board and publication committee. All the previous material was extensively revised and updated, and several important new chapters were added. The result is a more comprehensive, readable, integrated, and, we hope, valuable contribution to the application of social science to health care.

This book is directed at the many professionals and paraprofessionals involved in the social science aspects of health care. These include clinical and counseling psychologists, primary care physicians, social workers, nurses, and educated volunteers involved in medical support groups (such as those for cancer patients, abortion patients, pain patients, and the terminally ill). This book is in no way a "how-to" manual, but rather presents current social psychological thinking on a number of basic health care issues, while keeping jargon to a minimum. It should also prove useful to graduate students in psychology and sociology, and to researchers new to the medical field. For those interested in using this volume as a course textbook, we have prepared a complementary course syllabus, which may be obtained by writing to the editors (Department of Psychology, University of California, Riverside, California 92521).

ACKNOWLEDGMENTS

We would especially like to thank the contributors to this volume. Most if not all have achieved considerable distinction in their field; yet they patiently revised chapters that had already been revised several times. In addition, most of the contributors provided comments on the chapters of other contributors.

Many of the editorial ideas reflected in this book were refined when the senior editor was a visiting professor at the medical school of the University of California, San Diego. Many of the medical students and physicians there were extremely helpful, especially Terence Davidson, Phillip Barrata, Doris Howell, Jon Wolff, Joel Snyder, Robert Kaplan, Lawrence Schneiderman, Paula Sundance, Zora Rogers, and Lydia Bartholomew. At the University of California, Riverside, among the many people who contributed to the development of this volume were Cari Baum, Deanna DiNicola, David Eckmann, Becky Halt, Monica Harris, and Ronald Riggio. We would also like to thank SPSSI's reviewers, Judith Hall and Bertram Raven, and SPSSI's publication committee, Jeffrey Rubin and Marilynn Brewer.

I

PERSPECTIVES ON SOCIAL INFLUENCE IN HEALTH CARE

1

Howard S. Friedman
M. Robin DiMatteo

Interpersonal Issues in Health Care: Healing as an Interpersonal Process

Modern health care is faced with two major but insufficiently recognized challenges to its ability to improve health. The first of these challenges concerns prevention. The past decade has seen a number of calls for intervention *before* disease occurs (e.g., Surgeon General, 1979). There is little doubt, for example, that a pediatrician who prevents an adolescent from smoking can be much more effective both medically and economically than the oncologist, thoracic surgeon, and radiation therapist who might otherwise deal with the patient 30 years hence. Similarly, the internist, nurse practitioner, and nutritionist who improve the eating and drinking habits, blood pressure levels, and exercise–relaxation rituals of their patients will ultimately have a greater impact on health than those involved in the necessary work of treating stroke, heart disease, and cancer. Health promotion is thus as central to health care as the treatment of existing disease.

An analogous issue exists concerning the second challenge to health care: interpersonal issues. There is increasing evidence that a significant improvement in health care can result from scientific attention to interpersonal relations among practitioners, patients, and families. Interpersonal issues are almost always present. For example, a major issue facing cancer patients is relations with others. Similarly, practitioner–patient rapport af-

3

fects patient cooperation with treatment, and cultural and family factors affect the perception and presentation of symptoms. There are many other related issues as well (see DiMatteo & Friedman, 1982, for an introduction to and overview of these issues). Yet like prevention and health promotion, interpersonal issues are sometimes seen as somehow less important to health care than a direct attack on existing disease and physical deterioration. The contributors to this book demonstrate that the contrary is true: Interpersonal issues are central to effective health care.

One reason for the insufficient attention given interpersonal issues in health care concerns the standard medical viewpoint of the patient's nature as a human being. Health care personnel, especially physicians, have amassed extraordinary power in almost all matters of health. Patients often yield even their most basic human rights, including the ability to make decisions regarding their own bodies. As is common in such instances of vast power differential, the patient is often treated as an *object*. The technical revolution in medicine has accelerated the trend toward impersonal treatment and has, as Wexler (1976) observed, "created an array of tools with which to do things *to* people, thus resulting in less and less time to do things *with* people [p. 276]." With technological advances, it becomes ever easier for the health care provider to place the patient in the role of object or "medical case." The disease tends to be separated from the human being who has been struck down by it.

The vision of health care as an assembly-line operation is in reality neither very efficient nor very beneficial. There are many psychological reasons for viewing patients as active, responsible, and thoughtful participants who have something important to contribute to their medical care. For example, patients who are treated as persons by their health care professionals are more likely to be satisfied with and cooperate with their treatment. And they are less likely to become helpless and depressed when hospitalized. In addition, there is a sense in which the perception of the patient as a person not an object is necessary to avoid some insidious attributions that could be detrimental to health care. People are very willing to blame victims for their fate (Lerner, 1970; Ryan, 1971) and to draw incorrect inferences relating behavior and disease, or personality and affliction. Patients undergoing an abortion, for example, may be seen as deserving the pain they experience. Most striking is the particular stigma associated with cancer, not fully accounted for by its association with death. Sontag (1978) has pointed out that a person with serious heart disease is probably at least as likely to die soon as is a person with cancer. In fact, there are various types of cancer for which the prognosis is far better than it is for heart disease. Yet health care personnel and family are not afraid to tell a patient that he or she has had a heart attack. Perhaps because cancer is poorly understood, it evokes a host of negative feelings ranging from disgust and fear to anger and blame directed at the patient. Such reactions often go hand in hand with the patient's loss of humanity.

Medical practitioners are not wholly to blame for overlooking interpersonal issues. There is another important reason why interpersonal issues have not received the attention they deserve. This reason involves the fact that social science matters are sometimes applied in excessively general terms to health problems. For example, a health practitioner may be interested in learning how to establish rapport with patients but may then be told about commonsensical "manners" that apply to all social interaction. Or, a hospital administrator may be advised to make hospitalized patients feel at home and in control, whereas in reality many patients, because of the demands of their medical care, can do neither. Such nonspecific advice is not sufficient and may reduce more than enhance practitioner concern with interpersonal issues.

At times it appears that just about every theory and concept in social science has some "important" applications in medicine. Such enthusiasm is admirable but may lead to a blurring of important conceptual distinctions. Most notably, applications of social science to medicine may be characterized by insufficient attention to discriminant validity. That is, it is easy to be too glib in applying social science to medicine. Should not practitioners be supportive and empathic like good clinicians? Should not practitioners understand the attributional processes that operate when people come to grips with their poor health or that of others? Should not practitioners understand psychosocial issues of power and attitude change, helplessness and reactance, stigma and self-presentation? Yes, but much more is needed.

For any construct to be useful, different measures of the construct must be positively related to one another. However, the measured construct must also be *different* from other constructs (Campbell & Fiske, 1959). This latter condition is known as discriminant validity. An example is the concept of "social intelligence." For this construct to be valuable, it must be shown to differ from the usual brand of "intelligence." Whereas construct validation usually involves a specific scale or measurement, the process also has implications for theories that underlie hypothesized relationships (Crano & Brewer, 1973). Discriminant validation is an important part of the process of validating social psychological constructs relevant to health care.

The key to a valid science of social psychology and medicine is to isolate those aspects of human behavior that are *unique* to medical issues. This effort involves observation and study of the relative importance of various interpersonal concerns in various situations. An example is the case of cancer. Should there be a "social psychology of cancer"? First of all, it is necessary to establish that interpersonal problems are sufficiently serious to warrant speaking of a "cancer patient" rather than of a patient who has cancer. Then, it must be demonstrated that certain social psychological matters are especially important for cancer patients. Finally, and most importantly, the ways in which such matters are unique to cancer must be analyzed. A good example of proper concern with discriminant validity comes from Rodin's (1978a) work on attribution. She begins by asking, ''While attributional processes are occurring all the time, they are especially likely to occur when a person feels sick. Why should this be true? [p. 531].'' This question directs attention to the special qualities of illness. It cannot be answered without some knowledge of medicine. Fortunately, the chapters in this book pay attention to the special demands of the health care situation.

This book has four main parts, each with a brief introduction. The first part presents a basic orientation to healing as an interpersonal process, built around the concept of *social influence.*

HEALING AS AN INTERPERSONAL PROCESS

Recently, a noted cardiologist was addressing first-year medical students at a major university medical center on the importance of the medical interview and medical history in the treatment of heart disease. In a lecture replete with medical terminology, the physician stressed the importance of inquiring about the patient's drinking and smoking history and present habits, of obtaining a complete description of the patient's daily activities and anxieties, and of forthrightly asking about the patient's sexual behavior. During the discussion period, a student asked, ''How can I tell if the patient is anxious, or is not answering the questions completely?'' Rather abruptly, the physician replied that such matters were common sense.

This incident serves to illustrate the attitude prevalent among health professionals that the interpersonal issues involved in practitioner–patient interactions are naturally and automatically understood and acted upon. Many practitioners believe that interpersonal issues do not require active concern and scientific study. In considering various aspects of practitioner–patient relationships, the three chapters that follow in this first part of this book detail the complexities involved in therapeutic communication. The transfer of information and the reception of feelings are actually quite difficult.

The complexities of the practitioner–patient relationship arise from three basic forces. First, the constraints of the medical care environment are often enormous. Second, the interactions are heavily influenced by the existing strong societal expectations about each role—the role of practitioner and of patient. Finally, there is the emotionally charged character of the relationship between practitioner and patient. As these chapters demonstrate, the understanding of interpersonal factors in the practitioner–patient relationship cannot be attained simply through intuition but requires a knowledge of social psychological issues. They show that these matters are anything but common sense.

In the first part of this book, the authors deal with the most central of interpersonal relationships in health care—that between the practitioner and the patient. This relationship is the focus of much thought and feeling on the part of patients, who typically recollect with vivid detail the emotional (affective) quality of their interchange with health practitioners, even though their recollection of the technical details (such as what they were told to do to follow the regimen) is often limited. A second important matter in this part involves the development of operational definitions of effective interpersonal relationships. DiMatteo and DiNicola trace the historical notion of the art of medicine as social science; Rodin and Janis emphasize referent power and the practitioner as normative referent in the patient's life; and Friedman analyzes nonverbal communication. In this way, this part specifies the exact meaning of rapport and effective communication between practitioners and patients. These chapters strongly support the notion that the means to achieve effective interpersonal relationships in medicine are decidedly *not* obvious.

The arguments presented in this book, pursued to their extreme, lead to a revolutionary model of medicine. In all of the contributions the emphasis is not on drugs, technology, or the physical environment; rather, it is on social, psychological, and emotional factors in the treatment of illness. Healing is seen as a process that is partially interpersonal. No one is advocating abandoning the technological and pharmaceutical efforts of modern medicine. But we do advocate the serious consideration of interpersonal factors. We are not saying merely that the physician should smile, as did the old family physician, when prescribing a particular treatment regimen. Nor are we saying merely that modern physicians should remember that the patient is a person with feelings and should be treated as such as a matter of civility. Rather, we are proposing that interpersonal relations are a *part* of the basic process of healing. From this perspective, it is inappropriate to think about the effects of drug regimens, medical procedures, or surgical interventions without at the same time considering the interpersonal aspects of these procedures. Ignoring these factors is not an error of ethics or courtesy; it is a scientific error. And the scientific evidence supporting this point of view is rapidly accumulating.

Fortunately, social science interventions are likely to be economically effective as well. Enlightened use of social science can reduce the cost of medical care by such processes as eliminating the waste resulting from patients' lack of cooperation with medical regimens, by reducing patients' tendencies to ''shop'' for physicians who satisfy them, by decreasing the incidence of malpractice suits as the vent for patient anger, and, most importantly, by improving the actual outcome of treatment.

2

M. Robin DiMatteo
D. Dante DiNicola

Social Science and the Art of Medicine: From Hippocrates to Holism

> *Medical science is intrinsically and essentially a social science, and as long as this is not recognized in practice we shall not be able to enjoy its benefits and shall have to be satisfied with an empty shell and a sham.*
>
> [Salomon Neumann, 1847, p. 64–65, cited in Rosen, 1972]

From the time of Hippocrates in the fourth century B.C. to the beginning of the twentieth century, physicians paid strict attention to the art of medicine. They took care to control their own interpersonal behavior toward patients, to develop their "bedside manner," and to cultivate their sensitivity to patients' emotional needs (Sigerist, 1951). This attention to the art of care was prompted at least in part by the more positive therapeutic results that accompanied it. The remedies of the early physicians (practicing prior to 1900) were by and large found, in later years, to be wholly ineffective when scrutinized from the perspectives of pathophysiology and clinical experimentation. Interestingly, these remedies were sometimes rather dangerous, as were, for example, the widely prescribed strychnine and arsenic tonics. Yet, many physicians saw their patients recover and return over and over again, and their incomes consequently increase, when they were sensitive to issues of interpersonal rapport. Hippocrates (1923 translation) noted that "the patient, though conscious that his condition is perilous, may recover his health simply through his contentment with the goodness of the physician." In fact, it has been suggested (Shapiro, 1960) that the entire history of medicine reflects little more than the positive

9

therapeutic effect of the physician's behavior. Thus, the physician was once, of himself, an extremely potent therapeutic agent.

After 1900, effective medical remedies were beginning to be developed. Antibiotics became available and their therapeutic effects understood. Successful surgical procedures came into practice, and their efficacy was demonstrated. Physicians began to apply the developments of many scientific disciplines to the care of patients. American medicine was indeed becoming a "science"—or more precisely, a composite of many scientific disciplines. A major catalyst for this development was the Flexner report to the Carnegie commission in 1910 (Flexner, 1910). This report argued for an end to the purely clinical teaching of the proprietary (privately owned, profit motivated) medical schools of the day. Mere clinical instruction in medicine was labeled by Flexner as inadequate to the task of preparing doctors. Instead, only university-based, basic-science-oriented medical schools were legitimized. New, stringent licensing laws led to the close of the proprietary schools, giving rise to a model of medical education firmly rooted in the basic sciences. Anatomy, physiology, microbiology, pharmacology, pathology, and neurology were then taught as separate and distinct disciplines. In this model, medicine itself was taught no longer in terms of the patient's particular signs and symptoms but instead in terms of negatively altered biology (Ebert, 1977). Particularly after World War II and during the early 1950s more and more of the discoveries from the basic sciences found important applications to medical practice. The sheer volume of relevant scientific material forced a significant rift between the technological aspects of medicine and the care of the patient. The new technology was experienced as both powerful and efficient. The interpersonal aspects of care, considered so very important in the earlier days of medicine, seemed by comparison superfluous and even a waste of time.

As medicine's scientific side grew in importance, physician–educators began to recognize a separation between the science of medicine and its actual practice. Frederick Shattuck (1907), for example, warned that the disease is one phenomenon but the diseased person quite another. He proposed that the gap between the science of medicine and its actual practice could be bridged by the *art* of medicine. Shattuck warned that the scientific aspects of medicine should never replace compassion, sympathy, cheerfulness, and gentleness. Shattuck argued that *the care of the patient,* not basic science research, should remain the primary goal of medicine. Similarly, in 1904 another prominent medical educator and physician, Sir William Osler, told medical students, "The practice of medicine is an art, not a trade; a calling, not a business; a calling in which your heart will be exercised equally with your head [p. 369]."

As scientific medicine developed, warnings like Shattuck's and Osler's continued to be heard. These warnings began to follow close upon empirical investigation of patients' growing dissatisfaction with medicine itself. Early surveys of patients' evaluation of their medical care suggested that it was the interpersonal aspects of care not the technical that were most important to them. Patients felt, for the most part, that they were not receiving the interpersonal care they desired (Caplan & Sussman, 1966; Freidson, 1961; Koos, 1955; Reader, Pratt & Mudd, 1957; Skipper, 1965). Eisenberg, an eminent physician, thus noted,

> It is . . . curious that dissatisfaction with medicine in America is at its most vociferous just at a time when doctors have at their disposal the most powerful medical technology the world has yet seen. The "old fashioned" general practitioner, with few drugs that really worked and not much surgery to recommend, is for some reason looking good to many people—in retrospect, at least [1977b, p. 235].

> Present-day disenchantment with physicians, at a time when they can do more than ever in history to halt and repair the ravages of serious illness, probably reflects the perception by people that they are not being cared for. . . . The patient wants time, sympathetic attention, and concern for himself as a person [1977b, p. 238].

What, then, is the art of medicine? Certainly it involves how a physician treats his or her patient. Is the art of medicine merely the sum total of positive interpersonal behaviors directed toward patients? Is it a reflection of the physician's whole personality, or a skill that might conceivably be developed and sustained? Does the art of medicine simply bring about the patient's pleasure and satisfaction at being treated respectfully and with compassion, or are there other effects as well? Is it a cure for the ills of high-technology medicine? Were the early physicians correct in stressing the importance of the art of medicine in effecting patient recovery? If medicine is the science of caring for patients, are the traditional medical–scientific disciplines sufficient to comprise it? The goal of this chapter is to attempt to answer these questions and to develop a more complete understanding of the art of medical care.

TIMELY DEFINITIONS OF THE ART OF MEDICINE

Today's classic textbook of medicine, *Harrison's Principles of Internal Medicine* (Isselbacher *et al.*, 1980) constitutes 3 in., 6½ lbs, and 2000 pages of small print covering the basics of medicine as a clinical science. On page 1 of this scholarly tome, the editors write,

> The crucial importance of understanding the scientific base of modern medicine is well known; the significance of the art of medicine is not as well appreciated. Thus, to extract from a mass of conflicting physical signs and laboratory data the ones that are of crucial significance, to know in a borderline case when to initiate and when to refrain from a line of investigation or treatment involves judgments

based on "assimilated" experience. Skill in accomplishing these necessities of
medical art is not usually the outcome of laboratory study alone.

Indeed, skill derives from both knowledge and experience, but is the art of
medicine something more than the skillful application of technical
knowledge?

Many modern physicians have developed a very narrow view of what is
"scientific" and have come to believe that medicine is a much more specific
science than it actually is. They often ignore both ancient and modern
evidence that patients' responses to their physicians are no less real than
their responses to drugs and other treatments, and that patients benefit (or
suffer) not only from the medications they are given but also from their
physicians' behavior toward them (Eisenberg, 1977b; Engel, 1977a,
1977b).

Samuel Bloom (1963) in his now classic book *The Doctor and His Patient: A
Sociological Interpretation* cited Richard Shryock, an eminent medical
historian, as saying, "Medicine, in the ordinary sense, represents a group
of biological sciences, but . . . medicine as an art is closely related to the
social sciences. This is true, at least, if one may employ the term 'art' in the
rather broad sense of including both medical practice and the social relations which this involves [pp. 33–34]."

This idea that the art of medicine involves both social and technical
science was, of course, not new. In fact, during the mid-nineteenth century,
when American medicine was dominated largely by traveling medicine
men and their shows, German and French physicians were developing
what has since come to be known as the "true" science of medicine—such
disciplines as microbiology, pathology, and cellular physiology (Brown,
1979). Interestingly, these founding scientific physicians felt quite strongly
that medicine rightly encompassed much more than the physician's
technical ministrations. They recognized the importance of the social side
of medicine. It was in this vein that Rudolph Virchow, a prominent German pathologist best known as the father of modern cell physiology, stated,
"Medicine is a social science in its very bone and marrow [Virchow, 1849,
cited in Robinson, 1978, p. 1]."

Some more recent attempts to understand and examine the social side of
medicine have suggested that it comprises the latter of two dimensions in
patient care (Bloom, 1963). The "instrumental dimension" was seen by
Bloom to involve the purely technical aspects of the physician's treatment of
the patient (his or her ordering of the appropriate laboratory tests, the collection, examination, and integration of relevant data toward a diagnosis,
and the implementation of an appropriate treatment). The "expressive
dimension," on the other hand, represented art. This was seen to include
the affective or "socio-emotional" components of the interaction—*how* the
physician did whatever he or she did to the patient. This dimension in-

volved primarily the physician's interpersonal behaviors toward the patient. Chafetz (1970), Kaufman (1970), and Headlee (1973) proposed that the art of medicine consisted merely of good manners, politeness, respect, and compassion. They argued that it is simply a matter of common sense and etiquette to reassure patients and to communicate to them that their welfare is indeed important. Similarly, McDermott (1977) referred to the art of medicine as the "samaritan" component of the actual practice of medicine—that collection of acts that provide reassurance and understanding to the patient.

Theories may be useful, but empirical research is crucial to understanding the art of medicine. In order to do so, we must first examine the empirical studies that relate various aspects of this "expressive dimension" of patient care to measurable effects and consequences. An overview of these studies will be used in outlining our empirical knowledge to date concerning the art of medicine. As such, this overview points to the influence of the art of medicine on patient satisfaction with medical care, on patient cooperation with treatment regimens, and on the actual outcome of medical treatment. This overview will aid in developing a more precise definition of the art of medicine.

CONCOMITANTS OF THE ART OF MEDICINE

Patient Satisfaction with Medical Treatment

Theoretical suggestions of the importance of the art of medicine to patient satisfaction are supported by research evidence. Doyle and Ware (1977), for example, found that a physician's conduct toward his or her patient was the strongest influence on the patient's satisfaction with medical care—stronger even than such important factors as access to the delivery of care and the quality of the treatment setting. In analyses of the verbal interaction in 800 tape-recorded clinic interviews between pediatricians and mothers and later follow-up visits with the mothers, Korsch, Gozzi, and Francis (1968) found that dissatisfaction occurred most often as a result of "communication barriers." These barriers involved the physician's lack of warmth and friendliness, the physician's failure to take account of the patient's concerns and expectations from the medical visit, lack of a clear-cut explanation concerning the diagnosis and causation of illness, and use of medical jargon. Methodological problems limited the wide generalizability of these findings, but they were indeed suggestive. These early studies stimulated some of the more recent findings on verbal and nonverbal communication in the physician–patient relationship. We consider these findings later. A review of the literature on the measurement and the meaning of patient satisfaction is available (Ware, Davies-Avery, & Stewart, 1978).

When the art of medicine is deficient, it is not surprising to see patients turn completely from the medical profession and seek nonmedical healers (often quacks and charlatans) in the hope of obtaining both a caring attitude and a cure. Cobb (1954), for example, found that cancer patients who rejected the medical establishment and sought help from nonmedical healers did so because of a lack of understanding and reassurance from their physicians and because of a lack of information about what would be done for them. These patients needed emotional support, sympathy, and most of all hope, however slim it might be. Their physicians, insisting upon labeling their cases as hopeless, also abandoned them emotionally since no more could be done medically to cure them.

Some economic issues in medical care seem to be related also to the art of medicine. It has been suggested, for example, that the medical malpractice suit serves as an important medium through which patients express their anger toward their physicians for ineffective interpersonal treatment. Blum (1957, 1960) provided some evidence that suit-prone physicians were indeed quite deficient in the art of medicine, although the direction of the causal effect remains unknown. Mechanic (1968) pointed out: "Much criticism of medicine in recent years and many medical malpractice suits against physicians reflect the impersonal nature of doctor–patient relationships and patients' doubts concerning the doctor's interest in their problems and the care and concern accorded to them [p. 169]." Vaccarino, a lawyer, argued to physicians that many malpractice suits could be avoided with clear communications of caring and concern to patients (1977). Sound prospective research, likely of course to be somewhat difficult, is needed in order to establish a direct causal link, and to specify the impact of the physician–patient relationship on malpractice litigation.

Finally, a patient's commitment to his or her provider tends to be highly influenced by interpersonal factors. Studies have shown that patients rarely change physicians because they believe the physician to be technically incompetent. Rather, they change because of inadequate interpersonal treatment and attention. Adults in the United Kingdom's National Health Service reported that they terminated the physician–patient relationship if the physician was too busy to talk with them or appeared to be uninterested in them as people (Gray & Cartwright, 1953). More recently, in a survey in the United States, Kasteler, Kane, Olsen and Thetford (1976) found that patients' dislike of their physician as a person, their dissatisfaction with the amount of time spent with them, and their perception of the physician's lack of interest in them were significant contributors to patients' doctor-shopping. Relatedly, DiMatteo, Prince and Taranta (1979) and DiMatteo and Hays (1980) found that patient satisfaction with the affective and communicative aspects of care from their physicians was significantly correlated with patient commitment to the therapeutic relationship. Data from a study by Roghmann, Hengst and Zastowny (1980) demonstrated that satisfaction with the physician's devotion was significantly *predictive* of patients' utilization of service (but not vice versa). This finding is important in establishing the direction of the relationship between satisfaction and health behavior, suggesting that satisfaction is a causal factor in patient commitment to care from the physician.

Patient Cooperation with Medical Regimens

Despite the time and trouble of seeking medical advice, and despite the dangers of avoiding treatment or of conducting unhealthy and self-destructive lifestyles, at least a third of all patients fail to cooperate with their physicians' recommendations for care (Davis, 1966; Haynes, Taylor, & Sackett, 1979). Rates of noncooperation vary with the characteristics of the regimen recommended, and with the measure of cooperation used. Research on this topic also suggests that the quality of the physician–patient relationship may be a significant factor in patient cooperation and motivation to overcome resistance and adhere to recommendations requiring behavior change (see DiNicola & DiMatteo, 1982).

A brief review of the literature supports the importance to cooperation of the physician–patient relationship. Francis, Korsch, and Morris (1969), for example, found that lack of cooperation was related to the pediatrician's insensitivity to and failure to meet the mother's expectations for her visit. Relatedly, Alpert (1964) found that patients who were most likely to fail to keep appointments in an out-patient referral clinic were those who felt they had no physician who cared about them and with whom they could talk. Davis (1968a, 1968b) analyzed the verbal communications from tape recordings of doctor–patient interactions and determined patient cooperation by content analyzing medical records and interviewing patients and physicians. He found that patients consistently failed to cooperate with treatment recommendations when physicians were verbally antagonistic. If the physician collected information from the patient and provided little or no information in return, or if tension was built up in the interaction and was not released through joking or humor, patient cooperation with treatment was unlikely to occur. Other studies have shown that a physician's anger or hostility toward a particular patient or toward patients having the same specific problem (such as alcoholism) could predict patients' missing follow-up appointments and refusing to enter long-term rehabilitative treatment programs (Milmoe, Rosenthal, Blane, Chafetz, & Wolf, 1967; Salzman, Shader, Scott, & Binstock, 1970). Thus, correlational research to date suggests that the quality of the physician–patient relationship may indeed influence the patient's willingness to accept and follow prescribed treatment regimens. Because these data are correlational, however, we cannot appropriately make a causal inference and argue that the physician's behavior is a cause of patient compliance. Indeed, it might be the other way around. Further research into the behavioral components such as physician sensitivity, communication, and rapport and the relationship of these to patient cooperation is critically important. Experimental research is desperately needed in this field (Becker & Maiman, 1980).

The Outcome of Treatment

The art of medicine—the physician's interpersonal treatment of patients—may significantly influence the outcome of medical treatments. This may be true even of those treatments that at first appear to depend solely upon the technical aspects of care. For example, Egbert, Battit, Welch, and Bartlett (1964) demonstrated that the interpersonal treatment of the patient before surgery and the provision of information and encouragement reduced patients' needs for pain-killing narcotics and helped patients attain a significantly quicker recovery. The explanation for this phenomenon involves patients' emotions—specifically, anxiety. Pain and illness are usually accompanied by a high level of anxiety on the part of the patient, and this anxiety quite often has health-related consequences (Janis, 1958; Langer, Janis, & Wolfer, 1975). Further, patient confidence in the physician's technical expertise can be brought about by the physician's effective interpersonal care of the patient (Ben-Sira, 1976). It has been argued that effective care of the patient's illness first demands a successful reduction in patient anxiety—especially likely to be achieved when the physician shows interest and devotion to the patient. Such interest and devotion were found by Ben-Sira (1980) to be particularly important when the patient was concerned about his or her health or had few resources with which to cope with problems. The greater their anxiety and concern and the fewer their resources, the more emotional support patients needed from their doctors (Ben-Sira, 1980).

There is some evidence that the physician's interpersonal behavior toward the patient can have a profound effect upon the observable physiological condition of the patient. Järvinen (1955) found a significant increase in the sudden deaths of coronary patients during or shortly after ward rounds conducted by the medical staff. These ward rounds were formal procedures carried out with little regard for patients as individuals. They focused instead on patients as medical cases, and they increased patients' fear and anxiety to dangerously high levels. This is not surprising, since human contact in frightening, upsetting, or negative emotional situations has been found to have major effects on the cardiac rhythms and electrical impulses of the hearts of cardiac patients (Lynch, Thomas, Mills, Malinow, & Katcher, 1974). This objective evidence supports the suggestions made long ago by Hippocrates that a patient's physical condition can be influenced significantly by the physician's behavior toward him or her.

THE EMPIRICAL SEARCH FOR THE ART OF MEDICINE

After examining some of the research on physicians' interpersonal behavior toward patients and the effect of this on patients' health and health behavior, we move closer to an understanding of the art of medicine. We have already mentioned a few specific definitions of the art of medicine, but as yet we have no systematic outline of the particular behaviors that constitute it. Delineation of each minute, specific behavior would of course be difficult and of doubtful utility. The broader categories into which these behaviors would fall can be specified, however. This specification is necessary if the art of medicine is to be evaluated and taught.

There is strong evidence that the art of medicine—the physician's ability to establish rapport with patients—is uncorrelated with medical-school admissions screening variables such as the Medical College Admission Test and the premedical grade point average (Flom, 1971; Gough, Hall, & Harris, 1963, 1964; Richards, Taylor, & Price, 1962). This suggests that scientific preparation is neither positively nor negatively predictive of the art of medicine. The art of medicine is also not clearly related to personality. A few personality measures have been found to correlate with a physician's ability to establish rapport with patients. These are sociability, self-confidence, and insight into people (Flom, 1971; Gough *et al.,* 1964; Howell, 1966). However, the results of these studies were often weak and equivocal, differing from study to study. No truly consistent patterns of personality traits have been found to relate to the art of medicine. (In these studies, it should be noted, the criterion measures consisted of ratings by other physicians of the target physicians' rapport with patients. The actual expressed views of patients regarding their physicians' treatment of them were not considered.)

The results of empirical investigations suggest that McDermott (1977) was correct in his theoretical assertion that the measurement of the physician's technical skill and skill in the art of medicine would be very difficult (if not impossible) to distinguish and to assess independently of one another. Ben-Sira (1976), for example, found empirical support for the hypothesis that the affective component of the physician's behavior toward the patient (also known as the interpersonal mode of behavior) would be a major factor in patients' assessments of the instrumental component of the physician's behavior (also known as the content of behavior). In another study, Ben-Sira (1980) found rather high correlations between patients' evaluations of the technical and interpersonal aspects of their care. This was particularly true when patients exhibited a high degree of concern about their health, or had a relatively low level of education. Ben-Sira (1980) suggested that the physician's mode of behavior (the art of medicine) reduces patient anxiety and consequently helps to relieve the patient's illness. Ben-Sira also suggested that this high correlation between patients' perceptions of the mode and the content of physicians' care may reflect simply their naiveté about health matters and their inability to judge technical performance separate from their reaction to interpersonal factors. Some recent findings suggest, however, that the raters' naiveté may not be an adequate explanation for these findings.

A recent study by DiMatteo and DiNicola (1981) examined performance evaluations of the technical and interpersonal skill of physicians in four different residency programs, involving three different disciplines (internal medicine, family practice, and general surgery). Physicians were rated by their attending (supervising) faculty physicians, by their peers on the house staff, by their patients, and by themselves. The reliabilities of the measures from all four sources were high. Within each source (physicians and patients), ratings of technical and interpersonal skill were found to be highly intercorrelated not only when these ratings were made by patients but *also when ratings were made by attending physicians.* That is, the supervising physicians and the patients saw the residents' interpersonal and technical skills as interrelated. The ratings made by the residents themselves and by their peers were not as highly intercorrelated as those made by attending physicians and patients but still reflected an interdependency among the two aspects of care. Thus, the findings of earlier research on patient satisfaction with medical care (reviewed by Ware *et al.,* 1978), which showed that patients usually do not distinguish between technical and interpersonal aspects of care, were replicated. These findings were further extended to physicians' ratings in which substantial correlations between these two dimensions were evidenced.

The argument (see Ben-Sira, 1980) that patients' naiveté prevents them from distinguishing between the technical and interpersonal aspects of care is thus weakened by these findings—that these two dimensions are *also* highly intercorrelated in ratings by supervising physicians (who are not technically naive). Furthermore, research evidence suggests that patients *can* make a distinction between these two aspects of care when the stimuli they are rating actually reflect a distinction. In a study using videotapes of physician behavior displaying high versus low interpersonal skill varied experimentally with high versus low technical skill (Ware *et al.,* 1980), patients were able to make accurate, independent assessments of these dimensions. The fact remains, however, that in naturally occurring physician–patient encounters, patients *do not make a distinction* between technical and interpersonal skill—between the content and the mode of care delivered.

As we have seen, then, patients and faculty physicians tend to make little distinction between the technical and interpersonal aspects of care. These distinctions *can* be made (by patients at least) when the distinctions actually exist. This pattern of empirical findings suggests the possibility that in the everyday practice of medicine, the divergence between the technical quality and the art of care does not actually occur, but rather the art and the science of medicine are substantially intercorrelated.

COMPONENTS OF THE ART OF MEDICINE

According to Engel (1977a), traditional medicine—the biomedical model—has been dominated by a dualism that has separated body and mind. Medicine throughout this century has stubbornly clung to the notion that the study of disease is a science and the care of the patient is an art (Engel, 1977b). The art of medicine has been thought to be more dependent upon the personal qualities of the care giver than upon principles that can be taught and examined. Such a viewpoint relegates the art of medicine to a semimystical realm while pointing to the disciplines of anatomy, physiology, and pathology as true science. It promotes the definition of disease in terms of altered biology instead of in terms of its effect on people.

Medicine's usual dichotomies—between mind and body and between art and science—form a basis for the frequently heard complaint that physicians have become too scientific and not sufficiently concerned with their patients as human beings. The latter complaint may be true enough. Consider, however, the possibility that just the opposite of the former complaint is valid—that medicine's neglect of a scientific approach to its human side may mean that in fact medicine is not yet scientific enough (Engel, 1977b).

> Attention to a scientific approach to feelings has special pertinence for clinical medicine, the practice of which so much depends on the ability of the physician to understand and to help thinking, feeling human beings. . . . The ultimate goal of a scientific approach to patient care is to render rational and accessible to conscious awareness and reporting the basis for the decisions and the means of their implementation. They must be predicated on reliable data correctly interpreted and on principles amenable to scientific study and validation. Such standards must apply as much to minute-to-minute microdecisions as to more major decisions, whether to linger a moment longer at the bedside as well as when and how to propose open heart surgery [pp. 222–223].

Patients' thoughts and feelings are inextricably intertwined with their physical condition. Thus, clinical medicine depends upon the ability of the physician to understand and to help thinking, feeling human beings. The care of patients requires a specificity of knowledge concerning the relationship of psychological and social phenomena to illness, a sensitivity to the existence and character of these phenomena in each individual patient, and an ability to deal successfully with them on many levels. Thus, the physician needs not only to work within the immediate physician–patient interaction but also to understand the meaning of the illness to the patient and the influence of the social, cultural, and family environment on the patient. We suggest that the art of medicine is, in fact, based upon the physician's awareness of, interest in, and skill in dealing with the many aspects of the psychosocial care of patients. The art of medicine may, in fact, involve a holistic approach to the patient—the treatment of him or her as a whole person whose physical, social, and emotional life affects and is affected by the illness (Pelletier, 1979). In the light of nearly 2 decades of empirical

research, Bloom's (1963) suggested definition of the art of medicine appears
to have a great deal of validity. He wrote that the art of medicine is not at all
nebulous. Rather, *it is precisely the body of knowledge that we refer to as social science*
applied to medicine and the care of the patient.

Psychosocial aspects of medical care are complex and multifaceted. In
their thoughts and feelings and interpersonal and social behavior human
beings are every bit as complex as they are in their anatomy, physiology,
and pathology. Theory and empirical research on the art of medicine
reviewed thus far suggests that respect, concern, and devotion to patients
can develop and be communicated only with skills based on complex,
multifaceted knowledge of psychosocial issues. Thus, many areas of social
psychology as they apply to medical practice contribute to a workable
definition of the art of medicine. This approach, of course, supports Engel's
(1977a, 1977b) contention that respect, compassion, and reassurance are
skills that are developed with a knowledge of many facets of human
behavior as they apply to illness. The "manner" in which the physician
treats the patient is dependent upon both knowledge attained regarding
psychosocial issues in medical care and interactional skills developed. This
all-important emphasis on "attainment" and "development" points to the
art of medicine as a dynamic changing process—a skill that can be
mastered.

In the following sections, we review a number of areas of social science
relevant to the practice of medicine and to the care of patients. We consider
social psychological factors in the immediate physician–patient interaction
as well as issues related to the context in which medical care is delivered. We
propose that these issues constitute the art of medicine. Research on them
suggests that ignorance of their relevance to the care of the patient is likely to
lead to errors in treatment and to the ineffective care of patients. Attention
to their relevance, on the other hand, is likely to lead to the development
and enhancement of the art of medicine.

Interpersonal Communication—The Verbal Dimension

Possibly from the very beginning of the practice of medicine, physicians
and observers of the physician–patient relationship have emphasized the
importance of effective verbal communication with patients. The word *doc-*
tor is originally from the Latin *docere,* which means "to teach". Indeed, the
physician as teacher is a potentially central figure in the life of the patient,
teaching and encouraging ways of prevention, explaining the meaning of
illness to the patient, and helping to guide appropriate and adaptive reactions to illness and toward recovery. Studies of the physician–patient relationship and patient satisfaction have emphasized the need for effective
physician communication to the patient. Explanations, education, and en-

couragement need to be offered—particularly in terms that avoid medical jargon and enhance patients' understanding (Korsch et al., 1968; Stone, 1979).

Some important research on verbal communication (Stiles, Putnam, Wolf, & James, 1979) has described three distinct parts of the typical physician–patient encounter: the initial phase, in which the physician takes a history and gathers information from the patient about the presenting problem; a second phase, in which a physical examination takes place; and a third phase, in which the physician provides recommendations for treatment to the patient. In this research it was found that patient satisfaction with care was most highly correlated with the physician's informativeness and verbal acquiescence in the third segment of the physician–patient visit. That is, patients were most satisfied with their doctor's communication and understanding when the doctor provided information about the illness condition and its treatment, and when the doctor shared with them control of the interaction. Interestingly, it was necessary for the physician to maintain his or her informativeness and acquiescence not throughout the whole visit, but only in the concluding phase. This suggests that the medical visit is experienced as a relatively dynamic process in which expectations for appropriate behavior continually change. It also points to the importance of the physician's sensitivity to the changing needs in communication with patients in an effort to establish rapport successfully (Bernstein & Bernstein, 1980).

A second aspect of physician–patient verbal communication is relevant to the art of medicine. This is the extent to which the physician *listens* to the patient. Research suggests that the traditional method of asking specific closed-ended questions and awaiting an often expected response is not very effective in patient care. Instead, the physician must allow the patient to tell his or her story in his or her own words, particularly in the initial phase of the medical visit. In their studies of verbal interaction in the medical visit, Stiles *et al.* (1979) found that patients' satisfaction with the affective dimension of care depended on their physicians' listening to them. According to Sir George Pickering, ''Hearing the patient's message is the *sine qua non* of a great physician. To hear that message requires first the physician's interest, second his understanding of the meaning of language, and third his sympathy toward and his knowledge and understanding of the circumstances of the patient's life; these again he hears best by listening to the patient [1978, pp. 554–555].'' Sir William Osler (1899) too emphasized that the physician should listen to the patient, for in doing so the physician will learn the diagnosis. Of course, in an examination of the social psychology of the practitioner–patient relationship, some possible explanations for the importance of listening to patients become apparent. First of all, the patient is usually attentive to all aspects of his or her own condition, including the detailed quality of the symptoms and the times and the circumstances under which they occur. The patient may have even gathered some clues to the condition and may know enough about the workings of his or her own body to provide the physician with valuable information. Second, the family of the patient usually observes aspects of the patient's condition and may remind the patient to tell the doctor about these. Third, listening fully to all the patient has to say and only then consolidating the information into a diagnosis can help to prevent the all-too-common problem among physicians of formulating a theory about the patient's problem too quickly and then fitting all the subsequent data to that theory (Elstein, 1976). The formulation of a theory only after collecting all the empirical evidence could help to prevent a premature, inaccurate diagnosis. Fourth, the patient may have the best knowledge of his or her own history, and in many cases accurate history may be the best predictor of the present problem. Fifth, a physician may miss a key to differential diagnosis if he or she fails to listen to and explore the patient's specific description of his or her own problem. Finally, listening to the patient's story told in his or her own words suggests that the physician respects the patient as a person and is willing to share control of the interview. Listening to the patient suggests that the physician–patient relationship is a joint problem-solving venture on the part of both physician and patient—a mutual transaction—which is likely to result in the patient's continued cooperation with treatment regimens (Stone, 1979).

Relatedly, the art of medicine involves a knowledge of and comfort with basic counseling skills such as reflecting patients' communications in order to check on the accuracy of interpretations. The importance of these skills for physicians has been demonstrated by Kagan (1974). The art of medicine also involves the persuasiveness of the physician—his or her capacity to mold patients' attitudes and motivate changes in their behavior (Balint, 1964). This persuasiveness and capacity to motivate are based partly upon the physician's (a) capacity to communicate to the patient in language he or she can understand; and (b) formulation and presentation of convincing arguments for the desired behavior, and against opposing behavior (Zimbardo, Ebbesen, & Maslach, 1977).

Interpersonal Communication — The Nonverbal Dimension

Related to issues of effective instrumental and affective communication, counseling, and attitude change are issues of nonverbal communication skill—the ability of the physician to detect and understand, as well as to express, nonverbal cues of emotion.

The art of medicine depends partly upon the physician's ability to interpret the emotional or affective information that is conveyed by a patient's nonverbal communications (facial expressions, body movements, and voice tone). The ability to "decode" or interpret the nonverbal cues of another is called "nonverbal sensitivity." It has been linked significantly to patient satisfaction with care from the physician (DiMatteo, Friedman, & Taranta, 1979; see also review by Friedman, 1982). The art of medicine involves the physician's sensitivity to indications of distress and other negative affect in the nonverbal cues (particularly body language) of the patient. Only with this recognition can the physician begin to deal with problems before the patient becomes dissatisfied with the physician, or uncooperative with the treatment regimen. By understanding the patient's nonverbal cues alone or as they accompany verbal cues, the physician may be better able to identify signs of confusion and discontent in patients (Friedman, 1979a).

The art of medicine also involves the physician's ability to communicate caring and concern to patients through his or her own nonverbal behaviors. In the fourth century B.C., Hippocrates suggested the importance of this when he remarked that the physician must "bear in mind [his] manner of sitting, reserve, arrangement of dress, decisive utterance, brevity of speech, composure, bedside manners, care, replies to objections, calm self-control . . . his manner must be serious and humane; without stooping to be jocular or failing to be just, he must avoid excessive austerity; he must always be in control of himself [1923 translation]." Ben-Sira (1976, 1980) showed that the communication of positive affect from physician to patient is essential to the development of patient confidence in the physician. Research in the field of counseling has demonstrated the importance of nonverbal cues in the communication of empathy, warmth, and caring and has suggested that nonverbal cues may be even more important than verbal cues in some cases (Haase & Tepper, 1972). Effective counseling and psychotherapy require warmth, genuineness, and empathy on the part of the therapist. All of these have been operationalized successfully in nonverbal terms (Friedman, 1979b; LaCrosse, 1975; Smith-Hanen, 1977). Finally, the physician's nonverbal behavior provides the patient with social comparison information and social validation and engages the patient in a process of social influence (Friedman, 1979a). DiMatteo, Taranta, Friedman, and Prince (1980) reported two studies that measured the nonverbal expressiveness of physicians directly and documented a significant relationship between their communication ability and the satisfaction with care expressed by their patients.

The Patient in a Context

The effective care of the *whole patient* is part and parcel of the art of medicine. Therefore, in addition to studying the therapeutic interaction itself, we must also focus on understanding the patient as he or she functions within a context. This context includes factors that influence the patient's feelings and experiences such as the patient's family and culture, as well as the setting of medical care. The patient's context provides certain blueprints and expectations for patient behavior, and the art of medicine involves the physician's understanding of the facets of this context and his or her ability to work within it while caring for the patient.

The Family

The family comprises the primary reference group for the patient. As such, it has a tremendous influence on three facets of health and illness (Pratt, 1976). Family history, values, and interactional patterns play an important role in the development of illness. The family can provide a rich history of the patient, as well as a context for the illness. Family values influence the patient's definition of symptoms as illness, and they influence the patient's dependence on the medical profession.

Psychosomatic illnesses, or those exacerbated by stress, may be made worse by unpleasant, strained, or dysfunctional family interactions (Minuchin, 1974). Patients' continuing self-destructive behaviors, such as excessive drinking, may be the result of family dysfunction as well. These behaviors may be used as attempted solutions to the psychosocial problems within the family, and unless this is understood by the physician, efforts at behavior change are unlikely to be successful. The patient's reactions to illness and the meaning that the illness holds for the patient (in terms of social roles lost, for example) are also partly determined by the family context. Finally, the course and even the quality of patient recovery may be influenced by the family. As a support system, the family may provide the ill patient with physical and psychological support. The family may help to reduce the patient's stress and anxiety and to provide encouragement for the patient's compliance with medical regimens (Caplan, Robinson, French, Caldwell, & Shinn, 1976). On the other hand, the family may provide "secondary gains" (e.g., sympathy, attention) that may encourage the patient to remain ill (Mechanic, 1968).

Thus the physician's knowledge of the influence of family on the patient's illness is likely to enhance the effectiveness of the treatment he or she delivers. Although the physician may not have enough time to deal fully with these issues, he or she should be able to recognize family problems and their potential effects on health and illness, as well as be prepared to make the appropriate referrals to psychologists, social workers, and related clinicians. (For more information about family issues, see Goldenberg and Goldenberg, 1980; and Medalie, 1978.)

The Cultural Context

Another contextual issue involves the patient's ethnic group, culture, subculture, and social class and the influence of each of these on health. The art of medicine demands some understanding on the part of the physician regarding these issues. Culture and social class influence the meaning attributed to illness. Thus, it is critical for the physician to recognize the ways in which illness is different from disease. Although the latter is specifiable in technical terms—in terms of a specific pathogen or tissue damage—the former includes the *meaning* of the problem to the patient. The cultural and social context influence the patient's beliefs about the cause of disease (for example, improper diet or sinful thoughts) as well as the symptoms to which the patient attends (Koos, 1954). The social context strongly influences the patient's reactions to medical care and his or her belief in its efficacy. The social acceptability of the patient's symptoms, strongly influenced by the cultural context, will affect the patient's willingness to seek care as well as his or her presentation of symptoms once care is sought (Zborowski, 1952; Zola, 1966). (Further examination of this issue can be found in Mechanic, 1968.)

The Role of the Patient

A final issue of context in the art of medicine involves understanding the role of the patient in the medical world (Parsons, 1958). The art of medicine involves recognizing when the expectations of the patient (for example, for total passivity) are detrimental to his or her recovery. To help patients fully, the physician must understand the frustrations patients face and must have some feeling for the difficulties inherent in the patient's attempt to make sense of an often confusing medical care system. Studies have found that providing patients with information regarding the sensations they are likely to experience and with aid in maintaining cognitive control has helped them to control their reactions to medical treatment and hospitalization (see Kaplan, 1982, for review). The art of medicine involves recognizing patients' needs for such information and aid and providing them effectively or referring when necessary.

In the previous sections, we have examined factors that comprise the art of medicine. We have, however, been able to provide only a brief overview within a broad structure. Nevertheless, we have provided some appropriate references from which considerably more can be learned. We recognize the difficulties of integrating these factors into medical practice, since in fact there are significant time and training limitations placed upon physicians. For example, we by no means suggest that physicians become accomplished family therapists and carry out intensive therapy with their patients. Although some physicians might be inclined toward this activity, most would do well to make skillful diagnoses of particular problems, make knowledgeable referrals, and offer reliable follow-up. The art of medicine need not involve the ability to deal directly with every psychosocial problem of the patient, but it must involve recognizing psychosocial issues and acting upon them in some capacity, often indirectly.

UNDERSTANDING THE PHYSICIAN IN A CONTEXT

It is important to recognize that a physician's behavior—his or her capacity to develop the art of medicine—will be influenced and shaped by the role expectations of the medical profession. These include a high degree of technical expertise, an orientation toward the collective good, and a position of emotional neutrality (Parsons, 1951). Successful development of the art of medicine demands the physician's understanding of his or her own values, status vis-à-vis other doctors, and standards of professional behavior and conduct. The physician needs to be keenly aware of how these factors influence the treatment of the patient. It is important to understand the extent to which a physician's behavior toward patients is constrained by preference (attitudes) and the extent to which it is constrained by role expectations (the situation).

The Role of Attitudes

As we have seen, the art of medicine demands knowledge and skill. The psychological and social aspects of medical care must be fully understood and managed by the physician. The patient's emotional needs must be considered, along with the impact of the social environment on both the course of illness and reactions to care. The physician's verbal and nonverbal interactional skills are central to this care and must be developed and maintained. But knowledge, skill, and practice are not sufficient conditions for the maintenance of the art of medicine. Something more is needed.

Judging from research findings on human communication, it is unlikely that a physician will be able to establish rapport with patients, comfort them, show caring, concern, and devotion, and exert a profound interpersonal influence on them in the absence of feelings of goodwill, or while harboring negative attitudes toward patients. Although there is no evidence that positive attitudes toward patients guarantee positive interpersonal behavior toward them, some evidence does suggest that negative interpersonal attitudes may show through in the physician's nonverbal behavior. Research by Ekman and Friesen (1969, 1974) demonstrates that although negative feelings may be hidden in verbal communications and in facial expressions, true feelings may "leak" through body movements, postures, and gestural cues. Milmoe et al. (1967), for example, found that the hostility detected in the voice tone of physicians when they were talking about alcoholics was negatively correlated with their ability to persuade alcoholics to enter a detoxification program. The greater the hostility in their voice tone, the less likely they were to be able to persuade alcoholics. The hostility felt by the physicians may have been evident to the alcoholics, who were sensitive to interpersonal rejection. Further, if a physician communicates a positive verbal message to a patient while "leaking" a negative nonverbal communication of affect, the overall communication is likely to be experienced as very distressing (Friedman, 1979b). Finally, the literature on counseling and psychotherapy points not only to warmth and empathy but also to genuineness as critical conditions for the therapist–patient relationship and the initiation of therapeutic change (Rogers, 1957). Genuineness is thus central to the physician–patient relationship. The evidence considered so far then suggests the possibility that selection procedures for physicians should include measures of physicians' attitudes, at least as they relate to the potential for learning the art of medicine. Of course, attitudes can be changed, and the situational factors that influence them can be altered.

Situational Constraints on the Physician

A full understanding of the art of medicine demands an appreciation of the factors that interfere with it. Medical training and practice are physically, intellectually, and emotionally taxing for the practitioner. Requirements that the physician develop interpersonal skills as well as technical ones, hold positive attitudes toward patients, and be aware of the psychosocial influences in patients' lives seem to add to the burden. In the medical care setting, the physician's daily routine is often determined by immediate demands, with rare opportunity to decide on a precise course of action. Under such circumstances, it is easy for the physician to lose awareness of the art of medicine in his or her behavior toward patients. Several factors in the medical care setting, in the training of physicians, and in the conduct of medical practice are likely to influence strongly whether the physician will fulfill these demands effectively, with sensitivity and perceptiveness to all aspects of the care of patients.

The first of these factors involves the character of the medical school and residency environment to which the physician is exposed during training, and its effects on the development of the physician's ability to relate to patients as human beings. Cartwright (1979) reviewed research on medical education (e.g., Rosenberg, 1971) that suggested that the usual character of medical education in the United States is cold and hostile in its approach to the medical student, undermining his or her self-confidence and idealism and placing more value on traditional scientific disciplines and research than on the care of the patient. Students receive little if any reinforcement of their concern for human-service issues. Further, students are encouraged to be obsessive and compulsive in their attempts to cope with the demands placed on them. Of course, the exacting nature of medical work demands a degree of compulsivity. But the consistent use of this, and of the defense mechanisms of intellectualization and emotional isolation (actually encouraged in medical training), causes many students to compartmentalize their feelings and deny normal human emotions in the care of patients (Cartwright, 1979). Moreover, the values taught to physicians in their clinical training (in internship and residency) strongly influence how they treat their patients. Mumford (1970), for example, found that a scientific–technical approach was emphasized by residents in a university-based hospital program, but a person-oriented holistic approach was emphasized by residents in a community hospital. Seeman and Evans (1961a, 1961b) found that interns who trained on wards in which status differences between them and their senior staff were minimized (low stratification) tended to minimize status differences between themselves and their patients. They tended to offer their patients more information and psychological support than did interns who had trained on wards with a high status differential between themselves and staff physicians (high stratification).

A second related issue involves the stresses on physicians in the care of patients. Medicine is a profession that offers high income, prestige, and numerous opportunities for exposure to a wide range of intellectual and emotional challenges. These challenges carry with them many hazards, however (a fact suggested by the significantly higher probability of suicide, heart disease, alcoholism, and drug abuse among physicians compared with the general population) (Cartwright, 1979). There is evidence that stressed health professionals suffer measurable impairment in their thinking and their technical performance. Their relationships with patients also suffer as a result of overwork, fatigue, demands on their emotional and decision-making capabilities, and limitations of opportunities for humanizing activities such as their family, relaxation, and physical fitness pursuits (Cartwright, 1979). Furthermore, in order to deal with the sometimes overwhelmingly distressing aspects of caring for patients—the everyday occurrences of enormous human suffering and death—physicians may learn to deny their emotional reactions completely. In the short run, this coping mechanism might be effective, but in the long run, physicians, like all human-service workers, are likely to develop emotional exhaustion, cynicism, and a dehumanizing attitude toward patients. This phenomenon is known in the literature as "burn-out" (Maslach, 1976). Studies of the prevention and treatment of burn-out have suggested that physicians, as well as other health professionals, need to receive support in order to deal with their emotions. They need help to cope with the stresses they experience, for as the evidence considered earlier suggests, the treatment that physicians receive is likely to influence the treatment they give to their patients.

Finally, a physician's attention to the psychosocial aspects of patient care is unlikely to continue if it receives no reinforcement. Genuine organizational support is needed if physicians (as well as nurses, pharmacists, and other health professionals) are to provide effective psychological support for their patients and attend to issues of the art of medicine (Caplan, 1979). Beginning with medical school and residency training, specific behavioral goals in the realm of the art of medicine must be set, and some methods for assessing them must be specified (for example, with periodic measurements of patients' perceptions of care or the analysis of audiotaped or videotaped patient visits). The health care organization or training institution should provide esteem and recognition for attention to the art of medicine.

IMPLICATIONS

In this chapter we have attempted to provide a better understanding of the art of medicine. We have proposed and examined various components of the art of medicine and have considered how this art might be developed and maintained. Our examination of the art of medicine has important implications for the theoretical development of this issue and for research. It also has important implications for the practice of patient care. This chapter argues that understanding the nature of the physician–patient relationship requires an interpersonal science. Bloom (1963) noted this long ago when he argued that the art of medicine comprises both knowledge of and skill in applying social science.

It is important to recognize, of course, that the physician has by no means complete control over the practitioner–patient relationship. The art of medicine and the physician–patient relationship depend partly upon the social, economic, and political context in which the relationship occurs. For example, patients' expectations about their physicians and the care they receive may differ as a function of their demographic characteristics, education, social class, and culture (DiMatteo & Hays, 1980; DiMatteo, Prince, & Taranta, 1979). The physician–patient relationship is influenced by the reference groups of both physician and patient, and by their value orientations based on class, race, religion, and ethnic origin. Such factors may affect the conduct of health care quite profoundly in many cases (Adler & Stone, 1979). In addition, the public's trust of science, determined in part by the prevailing political climate, may strongly affect the degree of influence that physicians can have over their patients and the patients' willingness to trust the physician with the burden of uncertainty that is bound to exist in the medical treatment setting. Related to this, the physician's treatment of patients is likely to be affected by issues regarding the philosophy, ethics, and legality of medical care. The treatment of disease brought on by "self-destructive behavior" (Knowles, 1977) is one such arena in which these issues are becoming prominent. Current societal and economic forces are tending to influence patients' acceptance of personal responsibility for their health and hence may profoundly influence the physician–patient relationship. Finally, economic issues such as the shortage and/or maldistribution of physicians and cost containment (particularly in health maintenance organizations) may strongly influence practitioners' relationships with patients. Thus, we recognize that many factors beyond the physician's immediate control are likely to dictate some aspects of the relationship he or she has with patients and hence affect the art of medicine.

A more complete understanding of the art of medicine is a potential solution to a significant problem facing medicine today (DiMatteo & Friedman, 1982). As we noted earlier, many people believe that the present quality of medical care is deficient and that more can be done by physicians to care effectively for their patients. Patients, as a result, may reject many life-saving remedies (such as chemotherapy) and search for quacks and proponents of "natural" remedies. Some suggest (e.g., Pelletier, 1979) that the answer to this dilemma is alternative medicine—a holistic approach. The holistic concept advocates attention to the patient as a whole being, substituting many homeopathic (or natural) remedies in the place of invasive ones (Pelletier, 1979). In its basic concept, the holistic approach is sound and is not incompatible with traditional medical practice. Unfortunately, however, the holistic approach has been associated in modern times with an adversarial position toward medicine. Many proponents of the various holistic approaches question the very efficacy of science in modern medicine. They advocate, instead, remedies based more upon folklore and fancy than upon research and experimentation. The holistic movement has, in effect, become a battleground for physicians and patients to vent their frustrations over the limitations of medical science.

A solution to this stalemate demands that patients and physicians work together toward an integration of mind and body (interestingly, the basic principle of holistic medicine). It is clear, of course, that the care of patients without attention to the technical, scientific side of medicine is quackery. It must also become clear that the application of purely technical principles of medicine without regard to psychological and social issues is also ineffective. In part because of the medicine-versus-holism controversy, we are tempted to stray too far in one direction—to ignore the psychosocial side of medicine, on the one hand, or to brand drugs and surgery ineffective or harmful and devalue technical medicine, on the other. Any dramatic distinction between the two should be avoided, since both these aspects of medical care must coexist. In fact, as we have seen, the art and the science of medicine may be so interdependent as to be indistinguishable. Thus, as the sage has pointed out, "Problems that remain persistently insoluble should always be suspected as questions asked in the wrong way, like the problem of cause and effect. Make a spurious division of one process into two, forget that you have done it, then puzzle for centuries as to how the two get together [Watts, 1966, p. 54]." The merging again of medical art and science, like the merging of body and mind, may be the solution for developing a modern scientific medicine that is both effective and accepted. Investments in the development of all aspects of the art of medicine might well produce gains in modern health care, but this is likely only if the art of medicine remains firmly grounded in a rigorous science of human behavior.

3

Judith Rodin
Irving L. Janis

The Social Influence of Physicians and Other Health Care Practitioners as Agents of Change

THE PROBLEM OF INDUCING ADHERENCE

It is probably safe to say that patients' failure to adhere to prescribed medical regimens is one of the most serious problems in health care today. Although it is difficult to estimate how effectively health care professionals induce patients to adopt their recommendations, the evidence clearly indicates that there is enormous room for improvement.

Numerous studies suggest that physicians' communications often are ineffective in influencing patients to accept their recommendations for diminishing or preventing health hazards. (See reviews of the literature on adherence by Kasl, 1975; Kirscht & Rosenstock, 1977; Sackett, 1976; Stone, 1979.) For example, in a study of 47 men and women treated at an outpatient clinic in Liverpool, England, more than half of the medical recommendations given by the physicians could not be recalled accurately by the patients immediately after they left the consulting room (Ley & Spelman, 1965). Investigations of American women with acutely ill children suffering from rheumatic fever, streptococcal pharyngitis, and otitis media revealed that from 34% to 82% were seriously endangering the health of their children because they were not giving them the proper doses

33

of penicillin that had been explicitly prescribed by their physicians (Bergman & Werner, 1963; Charney, Bynum, Eldredge *et al.*, 1967). A study of 154 new adult patients in the general medical clinic of a large teaching hospital in a northeastern city of the United States showed that 37% failed to comply substantially with the physicians' recommendations and only 14% fully complied (Davis, 1971). Reviews of the large number of studies on patients' failure to comply with physicians' recommendations report wide variation in different circumstances, with noncompliance rates ranging from 15% to 93% (Davis, 1966; Sackett & Haynes, 1976).

These and many other such findings indicate that physicians' recommendations frequently go unheeded. As these examples show, the rate of adherence varies, but it is nearly always less than 100%. Defective communication has been linked to a variety of indicators of nonadherence (Mohler, Wallin, & Dreyfus, 1955; Stimson, 1974; Wilson, 1973). But we have no clear indications as to how often lack of success is primarily attributable to defective communication on the part of the physician, to predispositions of the patients, or to a combination of these or other factors. Although there are undoubtedly many reasons for failure to act in accordance with medical recommendations, it is striking that from the patients' perspective nonadherence is often related to difficulties in relationships with health care professionals. Patients frequently assert that their physicians fail to explain the purpose of the treatment and do not find out the patients' reasons for wanting to be examined. Patient satisfaction with a particular visit has been found to relate positively to compliance with the prescribed medical regimen and to keeping the next appointment (Becker, Drachman, & Kirscht, 1972; Francis, Korsch, & Morris, 1969).

Undoubtedly, there are many social, motivational, and structural barriers in the relationship between patients and health care providers that prevent a freer exchange about the disease, the treatment, and the relationship itself (Cartwright, 1964; Ley & Spelman, 1965; Merton, 1976). After reviewing the pertinent studies, Kasl (1975) has suggested that the crucial element in the typical relationship between a patient and a health care professional is probably not the exchange of information, but the nature of the expectations the two persons have about their roles, the congruence and mutuality of their role expectations, and their potential for exploring and revising those expectations.

It is probably essential in some cases to deal explicitly with these expectations during the course of treatment since social psychological research has shown that not only adherence but also the actual course of illness and recovery can be greatly affected by the patient's cognitive appraisals and expectations (see Abrams & Finesinger, 1953; Johnson, 1975; Jones, 1982; Rodin & Langer, 1980). Patients' attributions regarding the cause of their illness and of changes in their symptoms may be critical determinants of a variety of health-relevant outcomes (Rodin, 1978a).

Health care providers are inclined to neglect the patient's expectations in their communications with patients when they view the relationship as involving the onesided delivery of information. Often, professionals see themselves as experts who have special knowledge to be imparted to patients, which will lead to improvement or cure. Their implicit assumption is that because they possess and know how to use this special knowledge, they can influence patients to undergo medical treatments or to do anything else they prescribe. The expert's ability to exert this type of influence, of course, is based on genuine skill and experience, but it is fully retained only so long as the practitioner is able to keep the patient from acquiring comparable expertise (Thibaut & Kelley, 1959). There may actually be built-in negative incentives that keep professionals from sharing the mysteries of their craft and from explaining the reasons for their recommendations in less mysterious ways. In the sections that follow, we shall consider how expertise and other sources of social influence naturally develop and affect the relationship between the patient and the health care professional. Further, we shall consider the utility for health care of understanding the nature of social influence processes in the patient–practitioner dyad.

SOURCES OF SOCIAL INFLUENCE IN THE HEALTH CARE SITUATION

Social psychologists use the term *social power* to designate a person's capability to shape another's behavior, which is equivalent to his or her potential influence (see Tedeschi, 1976). There are several sources of social power that allow physicians and other authority figures to influence their patients. French and Raven (1959) and Raven (1965) have identified six sources of power: (*a*) expert power; (*b*) informational power; (*c*) legitimate power; (*d*) coercive power; (*e*) reward power; and (*f*) referent power.

Expert, Informational, and Legitimate Power

The availability of expert, informational, and legitimate power in the patient–practitioner relationship is the most obvious. These powers are based, respectively, on the professional's genuine skill and superior knowledge, and on the legitimacy of the professional's role, which carries with it the right to tell others what to do in order to improve or preserve their health. These bases of power are dependent upon the influencing agent's credentials and what he or she says but do not rely on direct surveillance for their effectiveness.

Health care often begins when the patient has a problem that is brought to the expert. According to Stone (1979), this is generally reformulated by the expert after he or she examines the symptoms and the results of medical tests. Throughout the diagnosis period, the physician is "in charge" of the problem-solving process by virtue of expertise and legitimacy, and the patient is usually expected to comply without questioning ("You're the doctor"). But physicians who rely exclusively on expert and legitimate power tend to concentrate entirely on the purely medical aspects of the patients' problems, excluding from consideration other aspects of the patients' life situations, such as work commitments or child care, which may be critical determinants of their ability to carry out medical recommendations (see Innes, 1977). As Stone (1979) points out, the expert often does not know and fails to inquire about patients' resistances arising from anticipated consequences such as pain, impairment of sexual function, or embarrassment from public (or even private) display of therapeutic devices.

Physicians also have at their disposal considerable informational power, which involves drawing upon their knowledge to induce cognitive changes by presenting impressive facts that are inherently persuasive. Once these changes have taken place, they may continue relatively independently of the continued contact with the influencing agent (Raven, 1965).

Not surprisingly, investigators have found that patients who were able to recall the medical information given to them by their physicians had lower error rates in following recommendations (Hulka, Cassel, Kupper, & Burdette, 1976). Kristeller and Rodin (1980) suggest that patients' failures to grasp what the physician is recommending is sometimes attributable to· disturbances in attention that lead to poor comprehension. For example, early in treatment, when the patient must understand the diagnosis and the recommended courses of action, a great deal of vigilance is required. At such times, the patient's anxiety regarding the illness is a common source of interference with attention. A busy, complex environment may also distract the new patient. Important information probably should not be presented during a stressful physical examination. Subsequently, it may have to be given in small doses to keep the messages simple and to prevent informational overload. Otherwise, adherence is likely to drop off sharply as the complexity of the treatment regimen increases (Blackwell, 1973; Hulka, Cassel, & Kupper, 1976; Latiolais & Berry, 1969).

Presenting certain types of information may reduce rather than increase the effectiveness of a physician's communication (see Stone, 1979). Although specifics about what to do and the main reasons for the regimen are essential, details about the nature of the illness and alternative treatments can prove to be far from helpful (Haynes, 1976; Kasl, 1975; Matthews & Hingson, 1977). Nevertheless, giving patients appropriate information about available alternatives may have the advantage of inducing efficacious changes without requiring continued surveillance. It could help to build up the patients' sense of self-efficacy by enabling them to exercise some degree of choice.

Among the central tasks of ongoing research is to specify the types of information that tend to have favorable rather than unfavorable effects and to determine the conditions under which each type of information is most likely to have the intended effect.

Reward and Coercive Power

The interpersonal context of the patient–practitioner interaction provides considerable opportunity for the professional also to use coercive and reward power. Coercive power stems from the ability of the influencing agent to mediate punishment for failures to comply; reward power, from his or her ability to mediate rewards for desirable behavior. Coercive and reward power generally require surveillance to be effective. Praise, warmth, time, and availability are but a few of the tokens of the practitioner's esteem that he or she can convey or withhold, contingent on patients' performance. Some physicians give their favorite patients free drug samples or even reduced rates, so economic incentives also contribute to the bases of their reward power. Patients seeking tangible or intangible rewards may consciously engage in ''good patient behavior,'' sometimes at great personal cost to their health and well-being (Taylor, 1979, 1982).

Referent Power

Of all the sources of power, referent power is probably the least used in health care at the present time. Referent power is the source of social influence based on the target's identification or desire for identification with the influencing agent. Persons have referent power for those who perceive them as likable, benevolent, admirable, and accepting. Their motivating power derives from the social–emotional aspect of the patient–practitioner relationship.

Health care providers can foster in several different ways the type of relationship that results in their becoming significant reference persons for their patients or clients (Berscheid & Walster, 1969; Byrne, 1971; Janis, in press; Levinger & Breedlove, 1966; Tedeschi, 1974). One way is to make salient the similarities between themselves and their patients, particularly with regard to beliefs, attitudes, and values. A second way is to talk and act in a manner that conveys a benevolent attitude toward each client, an unselfish willingness to provide help out of a genuine sense of caring about the client's welfare. Still another technique, which may overlap somewhat with the second way, is to be seen as accepting, which conveys to the client that he or she is held in high regard as a worthwhile person despite whatever weaknesses and shortcomings might be apparent.

Quite clearly, some physicians cannot spend enough time with their patients to become referent individuals. But others, such as oncologists, do see their patients for a longer period of time and might therefore make effective use of referent power. In clinical settings or hospitals, where physicians and nurses may be too busy to do this, paramedics, acting as members of the team and thus representatives of the staff, are often used to make sure that health regimens are clearly understood and followed. Their effectiveness might be greatly enhanced by developing referent power.

It is likely that contact with an authority figure who is exercising referent power can be anxiety reducing. By giving reassurance and satisfying the patients' stress-induced desire for interpersonal contact, practitioners can alleviate fear and related emotional states, which is likely to augment their referent power (Janis, 1971; Schachter, 1959). This, in turn, may better enable patients to attend to and learn the information being given (Kristeller & Rodin, 1980). Further, since health care warnings themselves may have fear-provoking components, and since high levels of fear can motivate patients to ignore, minimize, or even deny the importance of the threat, a reassuring health care provider can have a major impact on whether the recommended protective actions in such warnings are attended to and carried out (Janis, 1967; Rogers & Mewborn, 1976; Rogers & Thistlethwaite, 1970).

There are marked individual differences among physicians and other practitioners in the degree to which they use one or another means of building up their referent power, and also in the extent to which they rely upon the other sources of social power (see Janis, in press). Years ago, many family physicians developed their referent power to such a high degree that their patients would strive to get well partly because they did not want to disappoint their lovable "old doc." This component is often missing in present-day treatment by specialists. Some health professionals fail to do anything to build up their power as reference persons. These are to be found among physicians and nurses who conscientiously concentrate on their professional tasks and tell their patients exactly what they ought to do without paying much attention to patients' psychological resistances. Some are so businesslike that they do not express any concern about the patients' current plight or future welfare. These practitioners, in effect, appear to rely heavily on their coercive, reward, legitimate, informational, and expert powers but neglect the potential increase in their ability to influence patients that could come from acquiring referent power as well.

Even if a businesslike physician, nurse, or counselor is using the other five sources of power to the very limit, his or her effectiveness would be expected to increase by adopting one or another of the means for augmenting social influence as a significant reference person in the life of each client. Of course, to do so may be seen as too time-consuming and as diverting the practitioner's attention from the strictly medical problems at hand. But by adding referent power to the other bases of social power, according to the foregoing analysis, a practitioner would become an even more highly esteemed helper with whom the patients are more likely to identify. Then his or her health-promoting recommendations not only would meet with less initial psychological resistance but would also be more conscientiously adhered to long after the consultations have come to an end. This is clearly a testable hypothesis. An explicit assessment of the hypothesis will require investigators to develop cost–benefit analyses and comparative outcome studies on each of these different sources of power alone and in sequential combination with one another.

The effects of the different sources of a physician's influence on a patient's perceptions of control are crucial to understand because perceptions of control mediate significant health-relevant outcomes (Rodin, 1980; Rodin & Langer, 1977; Seligman, 1975). On the basis of social psychological research bearing on the differential effects of the various sources of influence, we expect that when patients comply because of the expert, legitimate, coercive, or reward powers of the health care professional, they will attribute their compliance to the external incentives and will be less likely to perceive themselves as having personal responsibility or control over their own health-relevant actions (see Deci, 1975; Kelman, 1958). We hypothesize that this will usually prove disadvantageous to their long-term health care when they are no longer under direct supervision. Systematic studies are needed to investigate this hypothesis to determine the long-term versus the short-term effects of using extremely salient external incentives on behavior change and adherence to prescribed regimens.

On the other hand, it is likely that referent and informational power are likely to promote internalization of recommendations under conditions where salient external inducements for decision making are absent. Internalization is the propensity to perform a recommended behavior even when one is removed in time and place from the source of influence. We expect that the same circumstances that promote internalization also serve to increase patients' feelings of choice and control because they perceive themselves to be acting on the basis of internal, self-motivated norms and goals. It has already been shown that the use of informational power does indeed determine the extent to which causality is attributed to the individual being influenced (Raven & Kruglanski, 1970). Research in other contexts has shown that greater feelings of causality increase behavioral commitment and play an important role in facilitating adherence (Collins & Hoyt, 1972; Klemp & Rodin, 1976; Lazarus, 1966; Pranulis, Dabbs, & Johnson, 1975; Seligman, 1975). These are indeed reasons why referent and informational power may be especially important for the practitioner to develop.

So far, we have focused primarily on times when patients are suffering from acute or chronic symptoms. People may also be more likely to take *preventive* health measures if they believe that they are actively involved in making choices and in implementing their own decisions. Consider, for example, adherence to a long-term program for subclinical hypertension, which might include keeping referral appointments, coming back for recommended medical checkups, taking prescribed medication, and changing lifestyle factors such as smokng, diet, and daily exercise. Feelings of personal responsibility deriving from internalization of prescribed behaviors should be extremely important in such instances because adherence to the medical regimen cannot be monitored continuously. Dieting is an especially good example, since patients do most of their eating under unsupervised conditions. Those who engage in self-monitoring and self-reinforcement appear most successful (Mahoney, 1977).

Under some circumstances, the use of expert, legitimate, and coercive power may actually diminish feelings of personal control if patients feel that the doctor's or nurse's admonitions limit their freedom. According to Brehm (1966), under these conditions people feel reactance, a psychological state that motivates them to restore their lost freedom and regain a sense of control. This type of reaction may help to explain why patients sometimes act against what appears to be their own best interests by quitting treatments before they are completed. These patients may be attempting to restore freedoms that they perceive as having taken away from them by health care professionals who use expert or coercive power, especially when they are told to eliminate pleasurable activities, food, or drugs that they feel are an important part of their lives. As a young convalescent cardiac patient put it, "No smokes, no booze, low salt, low fat, low energy, low sex or no sex—I feel like a cardiological capon!" (quoted in Hackett & Cassem, 1975, p. 36).

Lack of adherence may sometimes be an active coping strategy on the part of the patient to restore a lost sense of control. The conditions under which such reactions are most likely to occur in health care have yet to be investigated and merit further research.

STUDIES OF REFERENT POWER

In our own research, we have each separately been studying different ways in which referent power can be established and used in a dyadic relationship between a professional and a patient seeking help for weight control and, less often, for smoking. The goal is to motivate patients to adopt and stick to the recommended low-calorie diet, or to stop smoking even though they may at first be deterred by the threat of deprivation or other short-term losses. When referent power is used effectively, the relationship presumably will be one in which patients feel a gain in their socioemotional goals (such as esteem), anticipate improved physical and psychological well-being as a result of carrying out the actions recommended by the practitioner, and internalize those recommendations. Prior research on the effectiveness of counselors in clinics that offer professional help to heavy smokers and to overweight men and women has documented a high incidence of failures. In the United States, many of these clinics are part of a profitable industry. Each year hundreds of thousands of new consumers and recidivists pay for their services. But most of their successes appear to be short-lived. A high percentage of the men and women who come to the clinics do cut down on cigarette smoking or lose weight for a few weeks, but most of them fail to adhere to the prescribed regimen after supportive contact terminates (see Atthowe, 1973; Lichtenstein & Danaher, 1976; Sackett & Haynes, 1976; Shewchuk, 1976). In a review of the literature on the effectiveness of clinics for heroin addicts and heavy drinkers, Hunt and Matarazzo (1973) found that, just as with heavy smokers, many people begin to abstain in response to whatever counseling treatment they receive, but a very high percentage relapse within a month or two.

One of the assumptions underlying our research is that the incidence of long-term failure can be reduced if health care practitioners take the time and trouble to build up their referent power. There is no doubt that the various sources of power can interact with one another. Building up referent power, for example, may also increase informational or reward power. One of the conceptual tasks for future research will be to partial out, where possible, the separate and interactive effects of the various bases of power on relevant health outcomes. For the present, we have chosen to focus specifically on referent power because we believe it is often neglected in modern medicine and because of its hypothesized effects on patient internalization of the recommended courses of action, which may serve to increase rather than decrease the patient's sense of control.

Observations in a variety of clinical settings suggest that there are three critical phases in establishing and using referent power to help patients to change their behavior and to be motivated to adhere to a prescribed regimen (Janis, in press). In the first phase, the practitioner attempts to build up motivating power. In the second phase, the practitioner uses his or her motivating power to encourage the patient to embark on the needed course of action and provides help through strategies such as stress inoculation. In the third and final phase, the practitioner handles termination of contact in a way that retains his or her motivating power as a change agent to promote further internalization of the recommended behavior changes.

Phase One: Establishing Referent Power

In the first phase, the health professional has to encourage the person to disclose his or her personal feelings, troubles, or weaknesses. In certain circumstances some level of reciprocal self-disclosure might also be effective in the initial stages of such relationships (Jourard, 1971). Referent power is

acquired as the professional responds to the self-disclosures with unconditional positive regard (Bennis, Berlew, Schein, & Steele, 1973; Rogers,
1951). This type of acceptance leads patients to view the practitioner as a
warm, understanding person who will enhance their self-esteem, someone
who can be counted on to accept personal weaknesses and defects. For example, during initial interviews in a weight-reduction clinic, the clients'
self-defeating statements often fall in three categories. These are self-critical
statements about: (a) their appearance, such as "Look how fat and ugly I
am"; (b) overeating in general, such as "I'm a pig about desserts"; and (c)
uncontrollable cravings for specific foods, such as "I just keep thinking
about how good that piece of pie looks [Rodin, 1978b]." In addition to encouraging overweight patients to talk freely about their past dieting failures
and their concerns about being able to control their eating in the future, the
health counselor can build up referent power by providing consistent
understanding and encouragement, regardless of how "awful" the patients
characterize themselves.

Another aspect of encouraging a moderate degree of self-disclosure about
personal problems, such as craving rich desserts, is that the professional can
use those disclosures to help the patient reappraise specific difficulties and
to develop a more facilitating set of cognitions that are incompatible with
self-defeating thoughts (Rodin, 1978b). For example, the belief that "I'm a
pig about desserts" can interfere with successful dieting because eating any
dessert confirms the belief, leads to self-blame, and contributes to
demoralization. Patients can be shown how to identify the situational context where desserts are most troublesome (e.g., certain restaurants or parties) and change the cognition to one that is not as demoralizing (e.g.,
"French restaurants have irresistible-looking pastries that turn me on").
Although the individual must learn to take personal responsiblity for his or
her actions, it requires some elementary insights, which a practitioner can
provide, about when, where, and how to do so. Self-blame per se is not bad,
but it is likely to have more positive behavioral outcomes when the causes
are seen by the patient as situational and not dispositional (Janoff-Bulman,
1979; Rodin, 1978b).

In addition, the health care practitioner must also encourage patients to
disclose expectations regarding their health and treatment. These include
attributions for the locus of their troubles and beliefs about treatment and
recovery, as well as expectations about the therapist's role, the hoped for
level of concern, and the like. Patients' expectations about the initial visit to
the doctor, including what the doctor will say and how they will be treated,
have been shown to influence whether patients are satisfied, the degree to
which they commit themselves to follow the physician's recommendations,
and the level of anxiety they experience (Francis *et al.*, 1969; Korsch, Gozzi,
& Francis, 1968). There is also evidence that unfulfilled expectations at the
initial contact may threaten continuation of the therapeutic relationship.

Zola (1973) observed that patients are more likely to break off treatment when doctors do not adequately attend to the specific problems that brought the patient in. Even when the patient has presumably come for a routine checkup, there is often a hidden agenda—something that the patient is worried about but is a bit hesitant to disclose. If the physician fails to explore this possibility, the patient may not keep the appointment for the next checkup (Zola, 1972). Since initial expectations and concerns have been shown to influence adherence and treatment outcomes, the health care professional can develop motivating power by assessing patients' views and responding to them with interest and concern.

In a study designed to test the effects of positive versus neutral feedback in response to self-disclosures, Dowds, Janis, and Conolley (in press) carried out a controlled field experiment in a weight-reduction clinic. Overweight women were given a standard initial interview that was designed to elicit a moderate amount of self-disclosure of personal failures, negative feelings about the self, and other personal information that is normally withheld in everyday conversations. Subjects were assigned on a random basis to two experimental conditions. One condition consistently provided positive feedback; that is, the interviewer made explicit comments of approval for cooperating and ''acceptance'' comments reflecting the key content of the subject's answers, as is done in the Rogerian client-centered style of counseling. The contrasting condition provided only *neutral* feedback, that is, the interview made neutral comments or gave no response at all following the subject's answers. After the self-disclosing interview, in both experimental conditions the interviewer became a norm-sending communicator by presenting explicit recommendations concerning adherence to a 1200-calorie diet.

The results of this initial study indicate that noncontingent positive feedback from a counselor, as compared with neutral feedback, when given during an interview that encourages self-disclosure of personal weaknesses, has the effect of fostering not only more positive ratings of the counselor but also more adherence to the recommended low-calorie diet, as measured by weight loss 2 months later. Other studies have replicated these findings (Chang, 1977; Conolley, Janis, & Dowds, in press; Greene, in press). Greene's study further suggested that for positive feedback to be effective, the counselor must use it *consistently* throughout the initial interview, abstaining from saying or doing anything that could be construed by the clients as withdrawing from them or criticizing them.

In a number of further studies in the weight-reduction clinic and of a Red Cross blood-donation campaign, Janis and his coworkers have investigated the effects of different levels of self-disclosure by varying the content of the counselor's questions, while holding constant the personality of the counselor, the length of the interview, the recommendations being made, and a variety of other variables that might affect the outcome. One group of studies supports the hypothesis that counselors or health care practitioners will be more effective in inducing adherence to their recommendations if they first elicit a moderate degree—rather than a very low degree—of self-disclosure in the initial session with each of their clients, provided that they generally give positive feedback in the form of acceptance responses and never display any signs of rejection or unfriendliness (Colten & Janis, in press; Mulligan, in press; Quinlan, Janis, & Bales, in press). However, a second group of experiments shows that eliciting a relatively high degree of self-disclosure—as compared to a moderate degree—results in less behavioral adherence (Quinlan & Janis, in press; Riskind & Janis, in press). The high-disclosure interviews used in these studies elicited a great deal of confidential material about the client's weaknesses and shortcomings.

Thus, one set of experiments shows that moderate disclosure is more effective than low disclosure, and another set shows that high disclosure is less effective than moderate disclosure. This implies that the relationship between amount of induced disclosure and adherence to the counselor's recommendations is nonlinear, perhaps an inverted U-shaped function, similar to that postulated for other types of independent variables that have both facilitating and inhibiting effects. This implication will have to be tested systematically in parametric experiments, in which self-disclosure is varied from very low through intermediate levels to very high, within a single study, before we can hold it with confidence.

What accounts for the relatively detrimental effects of high disclosure? From intensive interviews of some clients immediately after the high- and moderate-disclosure interviews, two main types of detrimental effects are suggested (Janis & Quinlan, in press). First, there are numerous signs that participating in a very high disclosure interview makes the clients somewhat demoralized, despite all the positive comments and acceptance statements made by the counselor. After having revealed all sorts of personal weaknesses, some clients feel dissatisfied with themselves, as well as with the counseling session; their self-confidence is shaken. When this occurs, the clients feel less certain than ever that they can succeed in carrying out a difficult task, such as adhering to a low-calorie diet. The second type of detrimental effect, suggested by more indirect and subtle indicators, involves feelings of vulnerability from having revealed so much. Some clients seem to manifest overinvolvement in the emerging relationship by indicating that they really want the counselor to give them more time and more directive advice, not just about the problem at hand (such as being overweight) but also about other problems that were discussed in the high-disclosure interview (such as what to do about marital difficulties). Since this kind of advice is not part of the short-term counseling being offered for the overweight problem, these clients feel frustrated by the counselor.

The clients given a moderate-disclosure interview seem less likely to regard the counselor as someone who could become an affectionate parental figure or a savior who will solve their problems by telling them exactly what to do. At the end of the initial session they appear to accept an open but businesslike relationship with the professional person they are consulting and do not feel deprived because of the limited amount of help that he or she is offering. They regard the counselor as friendly, genuinely helpful, and doing a good job.

All the various research studies we have just reviewed, including the controlled field experiments and the qualitative analyses of individual case studies, converge on the following conclusion: When a practitioner expresses consistently positive regard, referent power is fostered by eliciting a *moderate* degree of self-disclosure (rather than a very high or a very low degree of self-disclosure), which results in *enhancement of the client's self-esteem* and makes for *increased adherence* to the practitioner's recommendations.

Phase Two: Using Referent Power

Once referent power is established, the relationship is characterized by cohesiveness and trust. In the second phase, the practitioner can then use his or her power to encourage the patient to become motivated to embark on the needed course of action, such as going on a diet, self-monitoring, and changing eating behavior and lifestyle. The professional is now functioning as a norm-setting communicator. He or she should be able to surmount the problems arising from recommending a difficult course of action by making it clear that the demands are as limited in scope as possible and by encouraging the patient to set realistic, flexible goals—with specific behavioral recommendations—in order to achieve the desired outcome. Some effective weight-control programs, for example, include joint patient–practitioner goal setting (Mahoney & Mahoney, 1976) and drawing up a contract (Foreyt, 1977), which lead to increased commitment to the goals.

Professionals can also use their motivating power to encourage vigilant decision making, based on the information that they are providing. When referent power is used, clients who come to a weight-reduction clinic, for example, may feel in a more colleague-like relationship with the counselor, who is seen as teaching them skills and sharing knowledge with them so that they can actively make fully informed choices regarding their diet and weight-control program (Rodin, 1978b). Correct information about what to expect in terms of reactions to treatment provides a normative standard against which patients can make appropriate judgments on their own about their actions and may have a reassuring effect since patients can assume that they are feeling and doing what most people do in a similar situation (Rodin, 1976). Providing the information necessary for informed behavior change and adherence to medical regimens is most likely to be effective after referent power has been established. There are many studies showing that simply being given correct information about a disease or a medical regimen by itself is, at best, weakly related to a patient's adherence (Blackwell, 1972; Charney, 1972; Finnerty, Mattie, & Finnerty, 1973; Wilson, 1973).

During phase two the health care professional can also use the trust built up in the relationship to prepare the patient realistically for the potential discomforts, difficulties, and problems that lie ahead. This procedure is called stress inoculation (Janis, 1958; Meichenbaum, 1977). Without a trusting relationship based on referent power, such procedures could be viewed as threats or high fear-provoking statements, which may prove under certain conditions to be ineffective or to have effects on behavior opposite to those intended (Janis & Terwilliger, 1962; Rogers & Thistlethwaite, 1970).

The principle underlying stress inoculation is that accurate preparatory information about an impending crisis gives people the opportunity to anticipate the loss, to start working through their anxiety or grief, and to make plans that might enable them to cope more adequately (see Janis, 1971). We would expect stress inoculation to be effective for any decision that entails severe short-term losses before substantial long-term gains are attained. Most decisions concerning personal health problems belong in this category because they usually require painful treatments or deprivations before physical well-being improves. Much of the evidence on the effectiveness of stress inoculation comes from studies of such decisions—voluntarily undergoing abdominal surgery, painful medical treatments, and the like (Egbert, Battit, Welch, & Bartlett, 1964; Janis, 1958; Johnson, 1966; Schmitt & Wooldridge, 1973; Turk, 1978; Vernon & Bigelow, 1974).

We expect that stress inoculation will prove to be most effective when the health care provider is exercising referent power because the patients need to be highly motivated to accept the unpleasant information about difficulties they are likely to encounter and to carry out the recommended courses of action for coping with the difficulties. In the treatment of obesity, Rodin (1978b) has used stress inoculation to deal mainly with those environmental problems that cannot be eliminated through stimulus control or cognitive reappraisal. Behavioral rehearsal is used in conjunction with providing preparatory information by a professional who has gained referent power. Patients are taught that they often fail to cope adequately with certain recurrent problem situations simply because they do not have readily accessible alternatives. Role playing, imagery, and preplanning are used to make them aware of new possibilities in line with their goals, by providing them with a repertoire of desired behaviors and cognitions in advance of the problem situation. For example, patients are encouraged to plan what they will eat before going to a restaurant where they will be bombarded with cues from the menu and the sight and smell of food. Similarly, they are encouraged to shop for food from a shopping list, prepared before they leave home. Since Rodin (1977) and her colleagues have found that many overweight people are aroused and become physiologically more responsive when salient food cues abound, these techniques can serve as effective forms of stress inoculation.

Phase Three: Maintaining Referent Power

In the third and final phase, the practitioner must retain his or her motivating power as a change agent to promote further internalization of the recommended behavior changes in anticipation of the termination of contact. During this period the influence of the supportive, norm-sending practitioner can be threatened by the patient's disappointment and resentment about termination. Patients whose chronic diabetes has been stabilized, for example, may stop following the prescribed medical regimen after a period of several months when they no longer have any appointments to see their physician (Kasl, 1975). Adverse reactions to separation may be minimized by giving assurances of continual positive regard and arranging for gradual, rather than abrupt, termination of contact (Janis, in press). The likelihood of maintenance of weight loss (Brownell, Heckerman, Westlake, Hayes & Monte, 1977) and smoking cessation (Shewchuk, 1976) can be increased if periodic contact with the relevant practitioner, even by telephone, is maintained.

The health care professional must attempt, during this third phase, to give communications that continue to build up the patient's self-esteem. Feelings of self-efficacy will serve to increase a sense of personal responsibility and are crucial mediators of behavior change. This may have begun in phase two, but patients must now feel fully confident that they are able to go forward on their own. In diet programs, the health counselor can emphasize that the clients' initial weight loss and changes in eating habits demonstrate their capabilities for successful self-control; these dispositional attributions for success increase the likelihood of long-term maintenance (Rodin, 1978b). On the one hand, when patients try to attribute their success to the therapist, it is important to point out that it was they themselves who were able to give up eating their favorite high-calorie foods and make the necessary behavioral commitment that led to successful changes. On the other hand, if a client initially does not lose weight, the failure should be attributed to plausible situational factors, such as overexposure to temptations during the holiday season, or to other changeable events in the environment, rather than to the client's lack of willpower or other dispositions.

Studies by other investigators also provide some evidence that appears to be consistent with hypotheses about the effects of the variables specified in the foregoing theoretical analysis (see DiMatteo, 1979; Elling, Whittemore, & Greene, 1960; Freeman, 1971; Korsch *et al.*, 1968; Stone, 1979).

Part of the art of effective health care may require dealing with each of the three phases in a way that minimizes adverse reactions. Perhaps only a small proportion of practitioners have the interpersonal skills that enable them to function with great artistry when treating the majority of their patients. Nevertheless, practitioners with modest amounts of talent and skill in dealing with people in trouble may be able to improve their percentage of successful cases by taking account of the main prescriptive hypotheses that follow from the foregoing analysis.

CONCLUDING COMMENTS: DEFINING THE CIRCUMSTANCES FOR THE BEST USE OF REFERENT POWER VERSUS THE OTHER SOURCES OF POWER

First, it is clear that research needs to be directed to the conditions under which referent power is and is not an effective source of motivation in the relationship between health care professionals and their patients. Thus far, there has been little systematic investigation of the bases of social power that are best suited for different types of patients, for different settings, and for different types of changes in behavior. It is possible, for example, that referent power is most effective when behavioral options are seen as available and controllable by the patient and when long-term adherence to medical regimens is desirable. Referent power may also be effective when patients are somewhat upset and need to have their anxiety reduced by an open and reassuring person before they can attend to and follow health-relevant measures. On the other hand, when patients are extremely anxious or depressed, their dependency needs are so great that expert or legitimate power may become more effective.

Attempts to build up referent power clearly have their limitations, as the studies of very high disclosure indicate. Further, Janis and Rodin (1979) have pointed out that a major deterrent to expressing understanding and acceptance is that it is necessary for the practitioner to take account of the patients' point of view, or to empathize with their feelings, in order for his or her positive comments to be impressive and believable. But this is difficult for anyone, no matter how well trained, when a patient is weak, miserable, and lacking in self-control, as many patients appear to be.

Aside from the problem of empathy, considerable skill is needed to avoid the pitfalls of giving unconditional acceptance. Clients are just as aware of the norms of social equity as are practitioners, and they are likely to be suspicious when given overzealous unearned praise or compliments. Practitioners' attempts to use acceptance can have boomerang effects if they give so much praise that they are presumed to be either habitually insincere or attempting to be ingratiating with a hidden manipulative intent (see Jones, 1964). The conditions under which acceptance by health care practitioners will and will not be perceived as ingratiation by their patients need to be systematically investigated.

There is evidence from other short-term counseling studies that authorities who have expert and reward powers also can be effective, even though they do not enhance self-esteem (Janis, in press). This can occur especially under conditions where the health care professional continually monitors the patient's behavior. Where constant monitoring is not possible or practical, the use of referent power to promote internalization of recommended actions may prove to be most successful.

Expert, coercive, or reward power may be more effective than referent power in situations in which feelings of control are stress inducing, especially when the individual believes that there are actions that he or she ought to be taking but is not able to initiate (Averill, 1973). Expert power may be especially advantageous in those instances where the patient would suffer from making futile attempts to control symptoms, such as high blood pressure, or accepting responsibility for health-relevant outcomes that are uncontrollable. But these possible generalizations are speculations that require systematic investigation.

Many of the ideas presented in this chapter are offered in the form of testable hypotheses, only a few of which have already been fairly well confirmed. Whatever the actual data on the effects of specific variables may eventually show, it is undoubtedly true that the relationship between health care provider and patient may be the most significant component in the entire health maintenance and treatment process. Viewing it as a dyad in which there are significant issues regarding the sources of social influence and opportunities for control may help to further our understanding of health seeking and illness behavior, including stress reduction, effective coping, adherence to treatments, and recovery.

4

Howard S. Friedman

Nonverbal Communication in Medical Interaction

Face-to-face interaction is a crucial aspect of medical care. Since ancient times, physicians and other healers have relied upon careful observation to diagnose illness and have developed bedside manners to promote recovery. Medical education emphasizes the need for careful attention to the patient's subtle clues of pain, anxiety, emotion, and disease (O'Brien, 1974). Medical lore offers numerous suggestions for proper comforting of patients, for correct demeanor, and for appropriate reactions to patient behavior (see DiMatteo, 1979). In practice, many experienced practitioners rely heavily on the subtleties of face-to-face interaction. However, although scientific procedures have replaced art in much of medical practice, the dynamics of interpersonal interaction in medicine remain mostly unattended by systematic research and training (Bennett, 1976). Even in the face of the past decade's advances in behavioral science and communication, words such as *intuition, faith, empathy, sensitivity, caring, will to live,* and similar pregnant but imprecise terms are still the bywords of direct patient care.

In recent years, the medical establishment has become increasingly cognizant of the importance of modern social science to health care. For example, the American Board of Internal Medicine has explicitly included "Interpersonal Skills" as one of the four categories of competencies required of an internist (American Board of Internal Medicine, 1979). They see interpersonal skills as having eight components, four of which are of direct relevance to this chapter. They are the skills to (a) develop a strong relationship that inspires confidence in patients and conveys a feeling of interest and concern; (b) interact in a nonjudgmental manner; (c) recognize and be attentive to the patient's emotional needs and recognize their potential influence on the symptoms and course of the illness; and (d) be alert to and interpret nonverbal cues from the patient (American Board, 1979, p. 404). Unfortunately, in medical schools and residency programs, it is not uncommon for physicians to tell their students that such communication issues involve "intuition" or "common sense." Actually, there is a quantity of available scientific information on the use and meaning of nonverbal communication that is of direct relevance to medical interactions. As we will see, nonverbal communication is especially crucial in accurate diagnosis and the communication of expectations.

Nonverbal communication involves those subtle cues that complement and illustrate aspects of the verbal interaction and often provide messages and express feelings that are not subject to direct conscious analysis by the interactants. A patient's grimace, smile, or expression of fear, as well as a nurse's comforting touch or facial expression of disgust, are communicative acts that may be even more important than the matter under verbal discussion.

HEALTH CARE TRANSACTIONS

Analysis of what actually occurs in health transactions can be usefully divided into those nonverbal cues that the patient receives, those that the patient expresses or sends, those that the practitioner receives, and those that the practitioner expresses or sends.

Patient Sensitivity

A number of factors combine to make it likely that most patients will be especially observant of and sensitive to the nonverbal communication of health practitioners. First of all, illness generally provokes fear, anxiety, and emotional uncertainty not only because of the possibility of disability or death but also because of encounters with unfamiliar scientific terminology and medical jargon, reactions to drugs, the presence of imposing medical equipment, and separation from loved ones and familiar surroundings. Under these conditions, many patients will have a strong need for others to help them define their situation and understand their feelings. That is, they will have a need for "social comparison" and will look to those around them—health care personnel—for reassurance and subtle clues as to what they are or ought to be feeling (cf., Ellsworth, Friedman, Perlick, & Hoyt, 1978; Schachter, 1959). Second, most patients are likely to be searching for factual information about the nature of their disease, its severity, its course, and their prognosis. Of course, some of this information is provided in the form of a verbal diagnosis, lab reports, and statements of current condition. However, this information may not be fully understood by patients. More importantly, it may not be fully believed. Practitioners may withhold or distort the whole truth for a variety of legitimate and not-so-legitimate reasons, and patients know that this may be happening in their cases. Since people commonly believe that clues about possible deception are expressed and "leaked" through nonverbal channels (Knapp, Hart, & Dennis, 1974), such cues are likely to be afforded special consideration by patients. Third, patients playing the role of the "good" (compliant) patient (Taylor, 1979) may be hesitant to question or confront a busy, high-status professional; they may prefer to rely on messages left "unsaid" for clues about their medical condition. Fourth, patients are especially likely to attend to nonverbal cues because of their position of relative powerlessness. There is evidence that subordinates may closely monitor the nonverbal cues of their bosses to ascertain which actions are having a positive and which a negative effect (Exline, 1972; Henley, 1977). Hospitalized patients are in a "total institution" where the rules are made by the medical establishment. Patients thus are often completely at the mercy of the practitioner and are probably especially motivated to see how their actions are being viewed (cf. Taylor, 1979, 1982). Finally, certain medical matters that interfere with normal verbal communication, such as speech or throat impairments, orders to hold still, attachment to a respirator, need for the practitioner to concentrate, and even a thermometer in the mouth, all limit the patient's ability to question the practitioner and increase the importance of nonverbal cues.

Patient Expressiveness

Some of these same factors and other additional ones make it likely that patients will be especially nonverbally expressive and that important information will be emitted through nonverbal channels. First of all, patients are likely to experience a number of emotions, and we have noted that competent practitioners must recognize patients' emotional needs. Emotions are more often clearly revealed nonverbally rather than verbally, especially through facial expressions (Argyle, 1975; Ekman, Friesen, & Ellsworth, 1972). Relatedly, some of these emotional states, such as pain, fear, depression, and various bodily disturbances, may be states that the patient rarely experiences otherwise and thus are not readily described in words. They can be detected, however, by a trained observer of nonverbal cues. Second, patients are unlikely to have had much experience hiding or controlling these emotions, especially in medical settings. For example, people may learn to control anger at an interpersonal slight in a supermarket, but fear, surprise, or pain at a doctor's probing may be directly revealed. Third, patients may be hesitant to communicate their feelings about certain difficult matters—concerning death, embarrassing disabilities, desires for additional services, and so on—and thus communicate them only through channels that are not deliberate, that is, through nonverbal communication. Fourth, many illnesses affect a patient's movements, odors, facial expressions, and other nonverbal signals in ways not fully recognized by the patient. Such cues cannot be described or controlled by the patient but could be important clues for practitioners. Finally, various medical conditions resulting from disease, drugs, or other treatment may disrupt verbal communication and leave the patient communicating only by nonverbal means. For example, weakness of the seriously ill may make verbal conversation too difficult but leave nonverbal messages, such as a glance or gesture, still available (Blondis & Jackson, 1977).

Thus it is probable that patients will (a) be especially observant of and sensitive to the nonverbal cues emitted by health practitioners; and (b) communicate a significant amount of important information through their own nonverbal cues. The relations of specific nonverbal cues to diagnosis and health maintenance are presented later in this chapter.

Practitioner Sensitivity

Since so much important information is revealed by the patient through nonverbal communication, the importance of practitioner sensitivity to these matters in diagnosis and treatment should be obvious. However, typical is a recent study of medical house officers which found that among 10 identified interpersonal skills such as "explains the nature of prescribed medication and therapy," the house officers were least skilled at "ascertaining the patient's emotional response to illness" (Duffy, Hamerman, & Cohen, 1980). The physicians were more comfortable concentrating on "medical" (i.e., organic) problems. Physicians may feel poorly trained in psychosocial issues and may rationalize their deficiencies by viewing such matters as outside the realm of medicine. Unfortunately, valuable patient nonverbal communication will be lost on an insensitive physician.

Practitioners, like other people, vary in their sensitivity to nonverbal cues. More specifically, people vary in how well they understand communication in different nonverbal channels such as facial expression, voice tone, and body movements. The channel of communication is especially important in embarrassing situations often faced by patients since there is increasing evidence that people may control their facial expressions of emotions in such situations but may "leak" their true feelings through body movements (Ekman & Friesen, 1969). One research project measured patients' satisfaction with medical treatment as a function of physicians' nonverbal sensitivities. Physicians were measured with the PONS test (Rosenthal, Hall, DiMatteo, Rogers, & Archer, 1979), a film test of abilities to decode facial expressions, voice tones, and body movements. In two studies, patients' satisfaction with their physicians was found to be positively related to physicians' abilities to decode the meaning of body movements (as measured by the PONS) (DiMatteo, Friedman, & Taranta, 1979). Physicians who are sensitive to subtle nonverbal cues may be better able to detect and then satisfy the social and emotional needs of their patients.

Yet attention to and interpretation of nonverbal cues is not sufficient. As we have mentioned, practitioners must also communicate in a manner that transmits concern and creates respect and trust. The effects of practitioner communication are an important but often overlooked aspect of medical care.

Practitioner Communication and the Placebo Effect

In most medical research involving patients, the methodological safeguard known as the "double-blind" procedure is essential. In this procedure, neither the patient nor the physician (or clinician) knows whether the patient has received the experimental treatment or is in the control group. For example, in a pharmacological study of pain reduction, neither the patient nor the physician is told whether the patient is receiving a traditional analgesic such as aspirin or a new experimental narcotic. This procedure is necessary to protect the validity of the experimental design from the well-known but misunderstood *placebo effect*—the psychological or psychophysiological effect of a therapy that does not have specific activity for the condition being treated (Shapiro, 1971). Often, improvement results from the expectation of improvement. However, this research "problem" points up two processes essential to many aspects of healing: the patient's expectations and the practitioner's role in creating these expectations.

The placebo effect remains overlooked and underresearched, although it is central to the healing process. Much of the history of medicine before modern times was the history of the placebo effect, and it is understandable that medical practitioners would want to disavow any association between modern medicine and such therapies as bleeding, leeching, purging, shocking, and such drugs as crocodile dung, eunuch fat, and swine's teeth. Yet throughout history, physicians have retained relatively high status because such treatments often worked (Shapiro, 1960, 1971). They worked, in part, because of the importance of psychological and emotional factors to "physical" health. Rather than being a threat to the science of medicine, placebo effects are intimately related to the well-being of many patients.

Placebos may produce definite, strong physiological effects (Shapiro, 1971), and placebo effects may disrupt the usual action of a standard treatment.

One prime element of a placebo effect is expectation (Frank, 1978; Jones, 1977; Rosenthal, 1976; Shapiro, 1971). If the practitioner can transmit positive expectations to the patient, real benefits may ensue; negative expectations may produce negative effects. It is important to keep in mind that placebo effects involve a therapy with nonspecific activity for the condition being treated; drugs or pills may function as placebos, but so may various other therapies, including psychotherapy (Shapiro, 1971). In fact, it seems likely that placebo effects more often result from procedures described and prescribed by the practitioner—exercise regimens, diets, rest patterns, and other medical rituals—than from pills. Certainly in such areas as pain reduction, which have relatively strong psychological components (Johnson, 1973), expectations can significantly influence outcomes (cf. Jones, 1977). Yet, positive expectations do not arise miraculously. Patients' expectations arise from interactions with health practitioners. Expectations are social psychological in nature. And, for the various reasons described earlier, patients are especially likely to obtain information on which these expectations are based through nonverbal cues. Patients will observe the nonverbal actions of the health providers and decide whether they are liked, cared for, and expected to improve, or are repugnant, worthless, and untreatable.

One indication that a physician's interpersonal effectiveness is related to his or her nonverbal expressive skills comes from a study of "charisma" and physician popularity (Friedman, Prince, Riggio, & DiMatteo, 1980). In this research, a valid, self-report measure of individual differences in nonverbal expressiveness was developed and was administered to 25 family practice residents (physicians). Each physician's patient load was measured over a period of 6 months. This research found a strong relationship between the nonverbal emotional expressiveness of the physician and the number of patients seen by that physician. Of course, patient load may merely be a measure of efficiency, but in this family practice clinic setting, the number of patients seen can probably be considered a measure of the physician's popularity; in many medical settings, there is consensus that certain primary-care physicians are always in demand. Such physicians deal effectively with patients on an interpersonal level.

ELEMENTS OF NONVERBAL COMMUNICATION

A number of recent writers in medical psychology recognize the importance of the face-to-face practitioner–patient interaction itself, discussing such matters as tone, warmth, rapport, empathy, and support. Unfortunately, relatively little use has been made of the specific advances of the last decade in the field of nonverbal communication. This field has identified key nonverbal cues and has begun to examine how they combine with other cues and with the social situation to produce unique meanings. A number of ideas, hypotheses, and findings concerning facial expressions, touch, smells, gestures, and related cues are directly relevant to medical settings.

Touch

For hundreds of years during the Middle Ages, Europeans sought relief from the disease of scrofula (a tubercular lymphatic disease) through the "King's touch" or the "royal touch" (Bloch, 1973). People traveled long distances to sessions in which they thought they would receive the transfer of the divine spirit. The persistence of the belief in the curative powers of the royal touch, despite a very low "cure" rate, attests to the tremendous symbolic value of touch in healing as well as to the important role of expectation in health care. The healing power of the royal touch tended to wane with the disappearing divinity of kings, but it may in fact have been transferred to physicians. Patients may feel better after a routine physical exam in which the doctor uses his or her special expertise to examine rather than merely question them. Certainly the desire to be touched by high-status political leaders, entertainers, sports figures, and the like has not disappeared in this modern age; touch has retained its symbolic value as a kind of blessing involving the transfer of special powers.

Faith healers have long used the technique of the "laying on of hands," and this "therapy" is still popular in American society. Since its efficacy is supposedly derived from the transfer of a healing spirit, just as the king transferred the divine spirit, this technique is generally viewed as quackery by modern medicine. However, the practitioner's touch may indeed promote healing if it is imbued with a special symbolic value for the patient. In the last two decades, the concept of touching as basic to the process of healing has been enthusiastically adopted by the so-called human potential movement. In fact, even the "most timid and conservative T-groups are assailing cultural taboos against touching. It is rare to find a group whose members do not at some point take turns being lifted up in the air from below by the hands of others [Howard, 1970, p. 146]."

At the very least, touching may have a significant psychological effect on many patients. Although therapeutic touching has been left as a relatively unresearched "art," medical practitioners are well trained to palpate, poke, feel, and otherwise touch their patients for purposes of diagnosis. Furthermore, diagnostic procedures such as temperature taking, blood testing, ear, nose, and throat examinations, and reflex testing all necessitate invading the patient's bodily integrity with a scientific instrument. Often, as in routine examination of the breasts, vagina, rectum, prostate, and testes, the touch is in intimate areas not usually invaded by relative strangers. This touching will produce reactions on two levels: emotional and interpersonal.

On the emotional level, there is little doubt that being touched is sometimes comforting and sometimes emotionally (or sexually) arousing. However, whether a certain type of touch at a certain part of the body can be shown to have a general, predictable effect is doubtful. There are tremendous individual differences in response to different types of touches, ranging from the type of pat that is reassuring to the type of stroke that is sexually arousing.

Many other differences arise from interpersonal matters: the meaning of the touch for the specific matter at hand. Two likely interpersonal meanings of touch involve *intimacy* and *power*. In usual interaction, the part of the body touched is clearly related to the intimacy of the relationship (Jourard, 1966); for example, the genitals are generally only touched by a close friend of the opposite sex. Violations of such norms in the medical setting may produce confusion. Nurses often report incidents in which patients begin disclosing very personal information or become flirtatious during or after a backrub, a bath, or other usually "intimate" forms of touching, even though such behavior violates role constraints (Johnson, 1965). Touching also often communicates power (Henley, 1977). In normal social interaction, high-status persons are much more likely to touch low-status persons than vice versa. In the medical setting, practitioners touch patients routinely, but there is usually very little occasion for the patient to touch the practitioner. Of course, most of this onesided touching is for instrumental purposes in the technical side of medical care. But the possible implication of a power difference remains. In one study of touching in a hospital setting, female nurses touched patients on the hand and arm during a presurgical explanation session (Whitcher & Fisher, 1979). A series of measures assessed the patients' responses to the session. It was found that female patients who were touched reacted more positively than control patients who were not touched, but male patients who were touched reacted more negatively. Although it is not clear from this study what interpretations by the patients mediated their reactions, it is interesting that such a seemingly minor change in practitioner behavior—the touch—could have definite measurable effects.

Not all benefits of touching are due to expectations and other psychosocial factors. Since Harlow's classic studies of monkeys raised with wire and cloth surrogate mothers (Harlow & Zimmerman, 1959), the importance of touch to healthy social development has been widely accepted. Research continues to support the idea that tactile stimulation in infancy is crucial to normal development of the organism (Denenberg, 1967; Russell, 1971).

The comfort of contact is physiologically based; indeed, lack of touch has been implicated in skin disease (Montague, 1978). Certainly back scratching, patting, gentle massaging, and other touches can be tension reducing. In fact, nursing instructors will now acknowledge that "in nursing, touch may be the most important of all nonverbal behaviors [Blondis & Jackson, 1977, p. 6]." An ill, anxious patient, surrounded by cold equipment, may be especially reassured by a warm touch. A similar conclusion was reached by Ashley Montague (1978), who wrote that "in every branch of the practice of medicine touching should be considered an indispensable part of the doctor's art. . . . Touch always enhances the doctor's therapeutic abilities [p. 223]."

In sum, touch has various significant functions and meanings in medical settings. Touch may have symbolic value in healing, may create positive expectations, may have important physiological effects, and, even when used for strictly diagnostic purposes, may affect the interpersonal nature of the practitioner–patient interaction. Certainly this topic is deserving of much additional research that reflects the multidimensional meaning of touching.

Gaze

One of the most influential nonverbal cues is gaze. Looking at someone may open or intensify a social interaction. People generally know and respond when they are stared at (Ellsworth, 1975) and know when someone is avoiding eye contact. Eye behavior is like touching in that its meaning depends heavily upon other factors in the situation: A stare may be comforting if it intensifies a pleasant situation or opens communication in an uncertain situation, but a stare may be arousing or threatening if the context is negative (Ellsworth, 1975; Ellsworth et al., 1978). Glances from a sympathetic nurse or an unhurried doctor may encourage a patient who is having a difficult time or help a patient bring up a sensitive subject. Failure to look a patient in the eye, on the other hand, may be part of the process of dehumanization, common in medical settings, in which the patient is seen as (and comes to feel like) a body not a person.

Excessive staring at a patient, with no apparent cause, will likely have a negative effect, perhaps making the patient feel like a freak or like a bad person. Presumably, health providers will generally not stare at a patient's physical deformity, but constant eye contact to avoid so doing is also likely to be noticed by a patient. Although studies have not found systematic effects of stigmata on eye-contact behavior, interaction with a handicapped person (including eye contact) does tend to be less variable, that is, more rigid and unchanging (Kleck, 1968). Refusal to look at or constant staring at the chest of a mastectomy patient, or avoidance of or excessive eye contact with a dying patient, may have similar effects: a signal to the patient that something is awry in the interaction and an intensification of the emotions being communicated through other channels.

The gaze of the patient may indicate something about the patient's mood. For example, one physician wrote the following about patients who are facing death: "A downcast look, a seemingly undetected tear, a sigh, an expression, or an inappropriate laugh can reveal a great deal about one's patients and their anxieties in dealing with the death dilemma [Flexner, 1977, p. 179]." In fact, research tends to support the conclusion that depressed people have downcast looks and generally engage in less eye contact (Harper, Wiens, & Matarazzo, 1978).

The Face and Facial Expression

The most specific and detailed information about states and emotions is communicated through facial expressions (Izard, 1977). First of all, the face is a key area for diagnosis because it has many muscles, detailed innervation, several sense organs, and high visibility. Long ago, Hippocrates urged the physician to study the patient's face first. A face with "the nose sharp, the eyes sunken, the temples fallen in, the ears cold and drawn in and their lobes distorted, the skin of the face hard, stretched and dry, and the colour of the face pale or dusky" usually portends death [1950 ed., p. 113]." In modern times, facial features have proved very useful in diagnosing genetic disorders (Goodman & Gorlin, 1970).

Facial *expression* (as opposed to facial features and states just mentioned) is an important element in the communication of pain and other feelings. Although pain is not one of the basic facial expressions of emotion in current categorizations, it is closely related to them (Ekman & Friesen, 1975; Izard, 1977). There is little doubt that valuable information about the intensity and stage of pain and related negative feelings (fear, distress, sadness) is communicated to the health practitioner through the face, even when the patient is not fully conscious. For example, facial expression has been used to assess amount of distress of women in labor (Leventhal & Sharp, 1965). In fact, the concept of pain itself has a communicative component in that its expression generally brings help from others (Szasz, 1957); pain is, in part, a request for comfort. Facial expression of pain may thus be expected to vary in part as a function of the nature of interpersonal relationships. If the expression of pain brings rewards other than pain relief, the patient may show more and more pain. On the other hand, if the expression of pain is ignored or punished, it may decrease, though sometimes at the cost of the possibility of relief through treatment.

This communicative function of pain expression is especially important because theory and research suggest a role for facial expression in the perception and management of pain. At the very least, facial expression plays an important mediational role in the subjective experience of emotion (Izard, 1977). Controlling the facial expression of pain (hiding pain) may help to reduce the pain (Lanzetta, Cartwright-Smith, & Kleck, 1976). For example, one study found that hiding pain led to lower pain than did a facial expression that showed exaggerated pain, especially so long as the expression was not inconsistent with one's thoughts about the pain (Blackman, 1980). Thus it may advantageous for health providers to reinforce patients' suppression of facial expressions of pain. However, since such suppression will, in turn, affect other responses of the health care providers and family members, the issue is a complex one, which should continue to be researched.

The practitioner's expectations and judgments are often clearly and forcefully communicated to the patient through facial expression. The human face is fantastically expressive and is most often the object of our attention (Vine, 1970). People can easily and quickly recognize distinct emotional states from facial expression (Ekman *et al.,* 1972; Ekman & Friesen, 1975), and thus such expression can effectively communicate a nurse's disgust at a wound or deformity, a physician's anger at a patient's failure to follow treatment regimens, or a technician's fear of a patient's deterioration. On the other hand, facial expressions can be effectively controlled by most people (Ekman & Friesen, 1975). With proper training and motivation, practitioners' expressions might just as effectively communicate a nurse's sympathy or a physician's positive outlook. This psychological power of facial expression was not lost on tribal medicine men, who wore elaborate masks during healing. In fact, in Ceylon, different masks were worn for each disease (Liggett, 1974). Patients, paying special attention to nonverbal cues and being especially influenced by the affective nature of the interaction (Ben-Sira, 1976) may be heavily affected by the provider's facial expression.

Olfaction

Although communication through odors is very important throughout much of the animal world, it appears to be relatively insignificant among humans, especially in American society (e.g., Knapp, 1978). However, the medical field may be an important exception. Most obviously, strong smells of alcohol and tobacco may be important diagnostic cues. Various illnesses and treatments also act directly to produce distinctive or unpleasant odors in the patient. Cyanide poisoning may be diagnosed by the characteristic "bitter almond" odor on the breath of the victim, halitosis may indicate respiratory tract infection, and malodorous stool may be indicative of gastrointestinal disease (Isselbacher, Adams, Braunwald, Petersdorf, &

Wilson, 1980). There is even some promise of a breathalyzer device for diagnosis ("Breath and body odors," 1978). On the other hand, practitioners too may be associated with particular odors. The use of disinfectants, chemical treatments, anesthesia, and so on, as well as the lingering odors of other patients, may all transmit olfactory messages to the patient. And there is no doubt that many of these patient and practitioner odors arouse strong negative feelings.

In the area of "person perception," it has been noted that negative personal attributes are often associated with malodor. A bad person may be labeled a "stinker" or "stinkpot." In fact, perceiving the outgroup as smelly is a prime characteristic of prejudice (Allport, 1954; Largey & Watson, 1972). The diseased person suffering from malodor may be reacted to with negative feelings. Some health care personnel may come to see foulsmelling patients as less good or moral, especially if the patient has at least some control over the odor. Such reactions of distaste are then likely to be transmitted to patients through facial expressions of disgust and the distances used in face-to-face interaction (cf. Hall, 1966).

The particular, uncommon smells of medical settings may also affect the health care process in another way. For unknown reasons, odors often have tremendous power to evoke memories of forgotten times and places (Allport, 1954; Meerloo, 1964). Hence, a doctor's office, a hospital, or a sickroom may evoke vivid memories of the previous negative experiences of an ill relative or a childhood trauma and thus may create significant negative expectations. The many implications of olfactory communication in medical settings remain to be systematically investigated. The first step probably should be the collection of impressions and observations regarding odor in medical settings to serve as a basis for more systematic research.

Voice

As with facial expressions, the specific emotional and motivational states of patients and practitioners may be revealed through their tone of voice (cf. Davitz, 1964). The tone of voice refers to those sounds, primarily pitch variations, that accompany the spoken word but are independent of the verbal content. Feelings like fear, anger, sadness, joy, and pain are readily transmitted through vocal cues.

Although tone of voice is probably an important element of the overall "tone" the practitioner sets for an interaction, surprisingly little research has been conducted in this area. One research project found a relationship between a physician's ability to express emotions through voice tone or through face and voice and the way in which the physician was evaluated by his or her patients (Friedman, DiMatteo, & Taranta, 1980). Physicians who could on demand accurately express emotions through tone of voice were more likely to have patients who were satisfied with the interpersonal manner of their physicians. Another study found that doctors who had anger in their voice while talking about alcoholics to an experimenter were less successful in getting alcoholic patients to continue treatment in an alcoholic clinic (Milmoe, Rosenthal, Blane, Chafetz, & Wolf, 1967). Presumably, these physicians were not acting in a "nonjudgmental manner" around alcoholic patients. Other studies have implicated voice in the transmission of experimenter expectancies (e.g., Duncan & Rosenthal, 1968). Voice tone is thus likely to be of importance to placebo effects. However, the effects of voice tone are not necessarily direct ones. Since voice cues are so closely tied to the verbal message actually being spoken, voice tone may combine with the verbal message to create unique new meanings. This point is discussed later in this chapter. Nevertheless, voice tone can clearly express emotion and is relatively easy for patients to detect. Thus, additional research should continue to address such questions as the effects of the voice tones of health care providers on the expectations and emotional reactions of various types of patients.

A final important aspect of the health practitioner's voice tone involves the use of "baby talk" in discussions with patients. Baby talk—the special speech adults use in talking to toddlers (Snow & Ferguson, 1977)—involves simplified words and language patterns, presumably to facilitate comprehension. However, baby talk also uses tone of voice to communicate messages of dominance and/or intimacy. In addition to interactions between parents and children, it may appear between lovers and between caretakers and patients. In a study of baby talk at a nursing home, Caporael (1981) found that baby talk—characterized by high pitch and wide pitch variability—was a significant aspect of the speech directed toward the institutionalized elderly. Although generally positive in affect, the practitioner's baby talk may communicate that the patient is dependent and in need of sympathy. Such communications may encourage patient passivity and thereby affect health. There is a need for additional research that identifies other such aspects of vocal communication that are especially likely to occur in medical settings.

Other Nonverbal Cues

There are many other nonverbal cues that are important to face-to-face interaction and take on a special meaning in medical settings. Although relatively little is known about these cues (with a few exceptions), the basic scientific approach of the field of nonverbal communication can do much to inform the untrained observer of medical interactions.

A major category of nonverbal communication involves body positions and gestures. Posture, hand movements, gait, lean, foot tapping, and so on, are included in this category. These cues generally receive little attention from the interactants; furthermore, not too much is known about the meaning of such individual actions in isolation. However, such behaviors do have important effects on the "immediacy" or mutual stimulation of an interaction (Mehrabian, 1972). That is, direct orientation and forward lean increase the mutual sensory stimulation of an interaction, thus conveying concern. One especially active area of related research involves the nonverbal detection of deception. As we have mentioned, there is theoretical and empirical reason to suspect that cues of deception are often emitted through body behavior rather than through facial expression, presumably because the body is under less conscious control (Ekman & Friesen, 1969; Riggio & Friedman, 1981). For example, nurses learn to recognize a patient's squirming, gesturing, pacing, and similar body signs of general restlessness (Blondis & Jackson, 1977); practitioners should also learn to watch these cues when questioning a patient.

The complementary issue of whether many patients, with their heightened vigilance, can generally detect practitioner lying and thus develop negative expectations about treatment has not been investigated in controlled studies but is certainly deserving of immediate attention. Practitioners often speculate that certain patients who have been denied the whole truth really "know" it anyway, and if so, it is possible that deception actually hurts rather than helps treatment.

There are also a number of sounds that may affect the nature of face-to-face interaction and are more likely to appear among patients than in the general population. For example, stomach rumbles, belches, flatulence, sneezes, coughs, and so on, may be especially common. Although these signs may be valuable for diagnostic purposes, they also may violate some subcultural norms of polite society. The effects of such disturbances on practitioner–patient interactions have not generally been investigated but could be fruitfully addressed. For example, one study monitored coughing in a number of natural situations and found that coughing is influenced by social psychological factors (Pennebaker, 1980). It was found that people were more likely to cough in large rather than in small groups and when in boring rather than in interesting situations. Hence it is possible that nonverbal cues like coughs may appear in medical interactions as conscious or unconscious messages from patients to practitioners about their health expectations.

Finally, many other factors in the health care environment, ranging from the clothing worn by practitioners and patients to the color and design of hospital rooms, will likely have a significant effect on the health care process. For example, doctors wear white coats and hospital patients wear gowns even when such clothing is not required by the technical demands of care. However, the present chapter focuses mainly on the dynamic aspects of face-to-face practitioner–patient interaction, since these elements are likely to be psychologically most salient. Nevertheless, environmental factors are also deserving of increased attention (Moos, 1979).

VERBAL AND NONVERBAL COMMUNICATION

One of the most critical aspects of effective treatment involves neither just what is said nor just how it is said. Rather, what is often more important is the degree of consistency between verbal and nonverbal cues. Stigmatized people in general are quite vigilant in watching for clues as to how they will "really" be treated (cf. Goffman, 1963). As noted earlier, such vigilance is probably even greater in the ill who are also seeking factual information about the nature and severity of their illness and social comparison information as to what they should be feeling in a time of emotional uncertainty. So even the slightest inconsistency is unlikely to go unnoticed.

A positive verbal communication, such as "You're looking better today," accompanied by a negative facial expression may be perceived as insincere or sarcastic (Argyle, 1975; Friedman, 1979b). However, negative nonverbal cues may be useful if they do not explicitly contradict the verbal message; for example, a negative voice tone may indicate that the practitioner is being serious and concerned. On the other hand, a relatively submissive, negative verbal message, such as "I hope you won't mind if I tell you that you need some additional tests," will probably be perceived as sincere and sympathetic, despite the negative content, if accompanied by a sad face but might be seen as patronizing if accompanied by a happy face. The degree and type of consistency between verbal and nonverbal cues create the "innuendo" that can be either very distressing or comforting to an ill person. One study examined the verbal and nonverbal (voice tone) communications between patients and two female physicians in an outpatient clinic (Hall, Roter, & Rand, 1981). Verbal communications were assessed by having observers (judges) rate written transcripts of conversations on scales of emotion; nonverbal voice tone was rated using content-filtered audiotapes (in which the words were made unintelligible). Patients' self-reported contentment with the health care transaction was found to be related to physicians' communications in an interesting way. When physicians uttered words that were less anxious and more sympathetic, patients were more content; however, when the physicians' voice tones sounded more anxious and angry, the patients were again more content. In other words, on the average it was a combination of positive words and negative tone that pleased patients most. It may be that this cue combination produces a serious, controlled, but explicitly (verbally) positive atmosphere that is admired by certain patients. Additional research is needed before we can fully understand such subtleties of cue combinations, but the illustrations given here show that we need not remain tied to vague notions of "empathy" and "sincerity" but can instead define specific behaviors.

CONCLUSION

For a number of reasons, nonverbal communication takes on a special importance in the medical setting. Attention to patients' nonverbal cues deserves a key place in diagnosis and monitoring, alongside the newest computerized, mechanized techniques. And appropriate expectations and encouragement, communicated both verbally and nonverbally, must be an important part of medical regimens. Although this importance is increasingly recognized, the topic is generally not approached with the scientific rigor applied to most other medical matters. Fortunately, it is no longer necessary for medical practitioners to rely solely on vague concepts such as intuition, sincerity, and empathy in dealing with the subtle interpersonal aspects of health care. Further, it is an oversimplification for behavioral scientists studying medical care to discuss in vague terms the "tone," the "atmosphere," or the "rapport" of practitioner–patient interactions. There is a scientific literature on the meaning and impact of touch, facial expression, voice tone, and related elements of nonverbal communication. Our knowledge now provides the concepts, tools, and strategies necessary to understand the crucial face-to-face aspects of health care.

II

RELATIONS WITH OTHERS, SOCIAL SUPPORT, AND THE HEALTH CARE SYSTEM

To provide for closer family ties, we have changed our policy regarding maternity visiting hours. Fathers, grandparents, and siblings of the newborn may visit at any hour, although only two visitors are allowed at a time. All visitors are requested to wash their hands before handling the newborn.

The above recent statement of visiting hours in a New England hospital reflects a dramatic shift in care during childbirth. Such policies are a far cry from the days of not too long ago when childbirth had many of the trappings of major surgery for a deadly disease and family members were excluded. In contrast, there is evidence that during the last two-thirds of the nineteenth century, many American men attended the births of their children (Suitor, 1981). These husbands in fact were often valuable sources of psychological, emotional, and even physical support in the "lying-in" room. In addition, they were able to check up on the practices of the attending physician. However, questions about the morality of the husband's participation in this intimate female event were raised, and many physicians objected to the interference with their authority. By the twentieth century, with hospital childbirth becoming increasingly common, husbands' participation began to wane.

By delegating to fathers the task of isolated pacing while clutching a box of cigars, banishing siblings from the hospital, and removing healthy newborns to a glass-enclosed nursery, modern physicians believed they were acting in the "best interests" of the mother and child. Unfortunately, their belief was incorrect. This case illustrates the dangers of viewing the doctor–patient relationship as separate from the larger context of family and culture. At the extreme, this separation from the larger society has led to what some critics refer to as the excessive use of power by the medical establishment.

Patients do not exist in a vacuum. In the first part of this book, we presented frameworks for understanding the importance of interpersonal relations to health care. In this part, we focus directly on the specific issues faced by patients in social interaction outside the hospital. In general, patients' needs involve desires to understand and deal with their new life situations created by the uncertainties of illness. To do so, they look to others—medical personnel, family, friends, and community. It is becoming increasingly apparent that most patients have a great need for social support. This is a need to which health professionals must attend, as evidence is mounting that social support may be directly and indirectly relevant to physical health.

Social support involves a host of related concepts. The term itself is used in a number of different ways. In one sense, social support involves love and caring, respect and admiration, and sense of community. In other uses, social support involves the provision of information and even physical resources. Social support also sometimes refers to the provision of psychological resources for coping with illness. In general, the term is used to refer to some assistance that comes directly from relations with others. The following three chapters expand on these meanings. In any study of social support, of course, it is important to try to isolate conceptually the precise type of social support involved and its consequences, even though the various types of social support often occur together in practice.

In this context, the terms *psychosocial* and *psychosomatic* are sometimes confused or erroneously interchanged. *Psychosocial* properly refers to the influence of the social situation. Psychosocial factors in the workplace or family environment may induce stress or interfere with a treatment regimen, but they may also induce calm, provide support, or facilitate cooperation with treatment. *Psychosomatic* properly refers to illness in which physical symptoms have been caused by psychological, especially emotional, influences. Most commonly, psychosomatic illness results from changes in the autonomic nervous system or through the action of hormones. Thus, psychosocial factors such as divorce, loneliness, and employer demands may for some people produce psychosomatic illnesses such as skin rashes, ulcers, migraines, or colitis. However, it should be remembered that psychosocial factors are relevant to almost all illnesses, and therefore the provision of social support is a key ingredient of effective medical care.

5

Christine Dunkel-Schetter
Camille B. Wortman

The Interpersonal Dynamics of Cancer: Problems in Social Relationships and Their Impact on the Patient[1]

One in four Americans develops cancer and two out of three families are touched by it (American Cancer Society, 1978). Even more alarming, the incidence of cancer has been rising for many years, yet little progress has been made in discovering its primary causes. In a substantial proportion of cases cancer is fatal. In fact, next to heart disease it is the most frequent cause of death in the United States (American Cancer Society, 1978). However, cancer is no longer synonymous with death; for many it is an acute or chronic disease that can be treated.

A notable feature of cancer as compared to other life crises is that it is usually not a single event, but a series of events that may last over several years. At the beginning there is the initial diagnosis and surgical, radiation or chemotherapeutic treatments. Later on, periodic checkups are necessary, and recurrence, extended treatment, remissions, metastases (disease spread), or a terminal phase may follow. Indeed, the ultimate outcome is typically unclear for long periods of time. Thus, considerable ambiguity

[1] The preparation of this chapter was supported by N.I.H. Contract No. IT 32MH15786 in the form of an N.I.M.H. predoctoral training fellowship to the first author, and by N.S.F. Research Grant BNS 78-04743 to the second author.

Interpersonal Issues in Health Care

usually accompanies the other physical and psychological stresses of the disease.

These factors—the prevalence of cancer, its rank as a major cause of death, its potential to be treated over long periods of time, and the ambiguity surrounding the outcome—suggest that its psychological aspects merit attention. How do individuals live and cope with the disease on a day-to-day basis? What difficulties are typically encountered by the person with cancer? What factors influence the patient's psychological distress and quality of life? A person's psychological reactions to the disease are not only important in their own right but also may influence the patient's physical condition and ultimate prognosis (Derogatis, Abeloff, & Melisaratos, 1979; Rogentine, van Kammen, Fox, Docherty, Rosenblatt, Boyd, & Bunney, 1979; Weisman & Worden, 1975). For this reason as well as for those just mentioned, greater knowledge of the psychological aspects of cancer is greatly needed.

This chapter focuses on one psychological aspect of living with cancer: the effect of the disease on the patient's interpersonal relationships, and the ultimate impact of these relationships on the patient's emotional adjustment to the illness. One factor that has influenced our approach to this problem is our former work, as social psychologists, on the question of how victims of uncontrollable life events are treated by others. As we have detailed elsewhere (Coates & Wortman, 1980; Dunkel-Schetter & Wortman, 1981), people undergoing life crises often experience a strong desire for social support. Furthermore, there is evidence that support from others can be highly beneficial in ameliorating the effects of negative life events. Yet others are often threatened and made uncomfortable by the victim's status and are therefore unable or unwilling to provide effective support. In fact, the more unfortunate the victim's plight or the more distress the person shows, the more threatened, uncomfortable, and rejecting others may become (see Coates, Wortman, & Abbey, 1979, for empirical evidence on this point). Thus, individuals in greatest need of social support may be least likely to get it.

To our knowledge, this social psychological "victimization" perspective has not been applied to the social environment of the cancer patient. Yet, because of the intense fears and the stigma associated with the disease (Public attitudes toward cancer, 1980), those who have cancer may be especially likely to experience problems in their interpersonal relationships. Few investigations have carefully probed the interpersonal problems experienced by cancer patients, but numerous authors describe them (e.g., Cobb & Erbe, 1978). For example, Vachon, Lyall, Rogers, Formo, Freedman, Cochrane, & Freeman (1979), Parkes (1974), and Abrams (1966) have each discussed problems between cancer patients and physicians, and Cobb (1956) discusses difficulties with nurses. Investigations on the impact of cancer document varying degrees of family and marital problems

(Greenleigh & associates, 1979; Lee & Maguire, 1975; Meyerowitz, Sparks, & Spears, 1979; O'Malley, Koocher, Foster, & Slavin, 1979) resulting from cancer. The existence of problems in at least some proportion of families when a member has cancer is further substantiated in anecdotal and data-based descriptive accounts (Dyk & Sutherland, 1956; Kaplan, Grobstein, & Smith, 1976, Parkes, 1972b). In addition to difficulties in relationships with family and physicians, problems with friends, acquaintances, and social life seem to occur in some cases (Greenleigh & Associates, 1979; O'Malley *et al.*, 1979; Silberfarb, Maurer, & Crouthamel, 1980; Sutherland, Orbach, Dyk, & Bard, 1952). Particularly high rates of interpersonal difficulties have been demonstrated to occur among adolescents with cancer, probably because of the added problems of this life stage (Boeck & Leventhal, 1979; Moore, Holton, & Marten, 1969; Tebbi, Tull, & Koren, 1980).

Especially notable in the literature is the frequent mention of communication problems (Cobb & Erbe, 1978; Harker, 1972; Klagsbrun, 1971; Krant, Beiser, Adler, & Johnston, 1976; Kubler-Ross, 1969; Spiegel, 1979; Wellisch, Mosher, & Van Scoy, 1978; Winder, 1978). For example, Gordon, Freidenbergs, Diller, Rothman, Wolf, Ruckdeschel-Hibbard, Ezrachi, & Gerstman (1977) asked 136 patients with breast, lung, and sarcoma cancers whether or not they had experienced any of 100 problems. Of the 20 problems most frequently noted by all patients, seven were of an interpersonal nature (e.g., "people acting differently after the cancer"), and three of the seven were explicitly concerned with communication issues (e.g. "communication about the cancer with friends difficult," "discussing future with family difficult"). In another study of 33 outpatients, Bean, Cooper, Alpert, & Kipnis (1980) found that over half of the comments made by subjects dealt with the communicative aspects of their relationships. We know of no studies that have compared cancer patients with other populations, so it is not clear whether they experience greater interpersonal distress than do other ill populations or well individuals. However, the evidence noted earlier suggests that such problems are reported frequently enough to merit attention.

A second factor shaping our approach in this chapter is our personal experience with cancer patients. For the past 5 years the authors have been serving as facilitators in peer support groups for cancer patients and their family members. These groups are part of a national organization called Make Today Count (see Make Today Count, 1977; Peebler, 1975; Pellman, 1976), the purpose of which is to provide a setting where patients and family members can engage in open communication about problems encountered in attempting to live with cancer.

Although it is not clear how representative the group members are of the total population of cancer patients, we have been struck by the high frequency of interpersonal problems reported at group meetings. People frequently report being upset and bewildered by the responses of family members and friends. For example, group participants often indicate that spouses show an unwillingness to acknowledge the disease and its ramifications and to discuss these with them. Perceived avoidance by friends, and awkwardness and tension while in the patient's presence are also common themes. In addition, group members report that others are generally intolerant of their negative affect, close off discussion of issues the patients would like to pursue, and minimize the importance of these issues.

AN ANALYSIS OF THE INTERPERSONAL DYNAMICS OF CANCER

A Brief Overview

A person diagnosed with cancer is likely to be highly fearful and uncertain. The intensity of these feelings may lead patients to worry that they are coping poorly or losing their grip on reality. Many patients experience a need to clarify the meaning of their responses to the illness in order to learn whether their reactions are reasonable and normal. People with cancer also experience intense needs for emotional support from others. However, communication barriers make it especially difficult for cancer patients to obtain the clarification and support they need.

The reactions of others who are prominent in the life of the patient (family, friends, health care personnel) are likely to be determined by two factors: by their feelings about the patient and the illness, and by their beliefs about appropriate behaviors to display when in the patient's company. Although their feelings about the patient's illness are largely negative, they believe that they should remain positive, optimistic, and cheerful in their interactions with the patient. This contradiction may result in behaviors that are unintentionally harmful to the patient, including (a) physical avoidance of the patient; (b) avoidance of open communication, especially about the disease and its effects; and (c) contradictory or inconsistent behaviors.

The person with cancer often interprets these ambiguous and negative actions as rejection at the very time when communication with and support from others is especially important. He or she may try subsequently to increase the support and attention received from others by one of two opposite strategies: exaggerating and stressing difficulties, or hiding problems from others, thus conveying the impression that he or she is coping well. Unfortunately, these solutions only serve to make it more difficult for others to know how to react to the patient and may therefore exacerbate their interpersonal problems rather than solve them. This analysis of the cancer patient's situation is described in more detail with reference to relevant evidence in the following subsections.

The Cancer Patient's Situation

Fears and Uncertainties

The individual who has just been diagnosed with cancer is likely to be profoundly fearful and uncertain about many things. An environment that was previously at least tolerable has now become increasingly unpredictable and threatening. Former assumptions and beliefs about the world and one's self are brought into question. The person is confronted with a web of fears, including fear of pain, of recurrence, of progressive deterioration, of dependency on others, and of death (Davies, Quinlan, McKegney, & Kimball, 1973; Hackett & Weisman, 1969; Katz, Weiner, Gallagher, & Hellman, 1970; Lewis & Bloom; 1978–1979; Meyerowitz, 1980). Patients worry, for example, about whether the doctors have been honest with them, whether they are receiving the best care, and how their illness will affect their families. They are also forced to contend with a variety of physical changes and problems, which may include pain, energy loss, disfigurement, nausea, hair loss, and unpleasant odors. Clearly such things can be unsettling and can have a profound effect on the patient's self-concept. Countless descriptive sources and some empirical work corroborate the contention that the diagnosis of cancer elicits terror and uncertainty about the future (e.g., Greenberg, 1961; Milton, 1973; Orbach & Tallent, 1965; Quint, 1965; Rollin, 1976; Sutherland *et al.*, 1952).

Within the context of this fear and uncertainty, the person with cancer is often called upon to function more competently than ever before in making a multitude of decisions. These may range from questions about what hospital to enter, which physician to contact, and what treatment to have to questions about if and what to tell their children, friends, and coworkers. Many patients are overwhelmed by the number and complexity of decisions to be made. Although these decisions are similar to those that people make in everyday life, they are linked to graver consequences for the cancer patient. Furthermore, the person is usually emotionally and physically less able to tackle them. In addition, a large number of these decisions concern matters with which the patient has no expertise or prior experience. Because of the considerable ambiguity within the field of medicine about how to treat certain types of cancer, there are often no clear-cut answers to some of the problems facing the patient. Thus, it will frequently be impossible for the patient to feel confident that the chosen alternatives are the best ones. Evidence that cancer patients experience anxiety and emotional distress is consistent with the above description of patients' fears and uncertainty. (Achte & Vauhkonen, 1971; Chesser & Anderson, 1975; Craig & Abeloff, 1974; Forester, Kornfeld, & Fleiss, 1978; Hinton, 1963; Lee & McGuire, 1975; Lewis, Gottesman, & Gutstein, 1979; McGuire, 1978; Meyerowitz, *et al.,* 1979; Morris, Greer, & White, 1977; Parkes, 1972b; Peck, 1972; Silberfarb, *et al.* 1980).

A Need for Clarification and Support

Because of the uncertainties they face and because their sense of self is threatened, many people with cancer experience intense needs both to clarify what is happening to them and to be supported and reassured by others. Concerning clarification, the intensity of their fears and uncomfortable feelings may lead many cancer patients to worry that they are coping poorly or are losing their grip on reality. They experience a need to understand the meaning of their responses. Are their reactions to the crisis reasonable or "normal"? How *should* they be responding? How long will their fears and anxieties last? There are at least three distinct ways that patients may gain clarification: by receiving comparison information, by being encouraged to discuss feelings openly with others, and by interacting with others whose experience enables them to provide feedback to the patient about the meaning of his or her responses to cancer. Each of these is elaborated upon in the following discussion.

One way to learn more about the meaning and appropriateness of various behaviors is through gaining relevant comparison information. As Festinger (1954) and Schachter (1959) have pointed out, confusion and ambiguity can often be resolved through social comparison. For example, a patient can learn from exposure to others that it is normal to become angry or depressed after diagnosis, to fear recurrence, and to be avoided by some of one's former friends. Comparison information can be obtained from educational materials (articles, books, or specially prepared pamphlets about cancer, films or television programs, lectures, symposia or public meetings), or from face-to-face encounters with other patients. Some of these sources may provide general information about how most cancer patients react to certain treatments or problems; other sources include individual accounts or "case studies" in which a patient describes his or her personal reactions to the disease. All of these can help the patient clarify his or her feelings by providing information about problems typically encountered, common or normal reactions, and strategies which might be employed to cope with them. However, personal accounts may be the most effective in influencing patients' beliefs because they are more vivid and thus more involving (Kahneman & Tversky, 1973; Nisbett & Borgida, 1975, Ross, 1977; and Sanders & Kardinal, 1977 on cancer specifically).

Few studies have probed patients' needs to clarify their responses. However, there are indications that under many circumstances, patients and family members would like to receive more information about treatments, side effects, and other reactions to the disease than they are normally given (Bloom, Ross, & Burnell, 1978; Cassileth, Zupkis, Sutton-Smith, & March, 1980; Greenleigh & Associates, 1979; Henriques, Stadil, & Baden, 1980; Messerli, Garamendi, & Romano, 1980; Krant & Johnson, 1977–1978; Morris *et al.*, 1977; Sheffer & Greifenstein, 1969). For example, Messerli *et al.* (1980) report that when breast cancer patients were asked if there were unanswered questions concerning their treatment, 86.2% answered in the affirmative. A survey of 15 hospitals by these same investigators revealed that information on stages of breast cancer, choices of surgery, postoperative therapy, prosthesis information, reconstructive surgery, and personal counseling was conspicuously absent. Similarly, in a survey of information preferences among cancer patients, Cassileth *et al.* (1980) found that a large majority of patients desired information on such issues as the possible side effects of treatment (98.0%), whether all parts of the body are involved (94.9%), and exactly what the treatment would do inside the patient's body (96.3%). There is also empirical evidence to suggest that such information is beneficial to the patient. In one study, women who were provided with information about breast cancer surgery were subsequently more satisfied than those who were not (Blum, 1980). Similarly, Gerle, Lundin, and Sandblom (1960) report that a group of cancer patients who received all the facts regarding their illness showed considerably less anxiety and depression and a resultant decrease in the use of psychotropic drugs, compared with a group told little or nothing regarding the nature of their disease.

A second way that patients can help to clarify the meaning of their feelings is to discuss them frankly and openly with a sympathetic listener. Articulating one's fears and feelings may be the first step in understanding them and in working out strategies for coping with them. By allowing the patient to express his or her concerns, by acknowledging these concerns, and by acting as a "sounding board," relatives, friends, or health care personnel can help the patient to interpret and manage his or her experiences.

Some evidence suggests that patients would like additional opportunities to discuss their problems (Cobliner, 1977; Greenleigh & Associates, 1979; Kleiman, Mantell, & Alexander, 1977). For example, Mitchell and Glicksman (1977) conducted an interview study of 50 cancer patients undergoing radiation therapy. Only 22 patients were able to identify a person with whom they could discuss their emotional problems, and 86% of the patients wished to be able "to discuss the situation more fully" with someone. Despite apparent interest in discussion with others, the value of it is not well documented. As we discuss later, however, the available evidence suggests that it is advantageous (Binger, Ablin, Feuerstein, Kushner, Zoger, & Mikkelson, 1969; Cobliner, 1977; Cohen, Dizenhuz, & Winget, 1977; Derogatis *et al.*, 1979; Kaplan, *et al.*, 1976; Kellerman, Rigler, Siegel, &

Katz, 1980; Spinetta, Swarner, & Sheposh, 1981; Vachon, Freedman, Formo, Rogers, Lyall, & Freeman, 1977; see also Silver & Wortman, 1980, for a review).

A third, and perhaps best, way for patients to clarify their feelings is to have the opportunity to discuss these feelings and personal reactions with others who can provide feedback about their meaning and appropriateness (e.g., other cancer patients who have shared many of the same experiences as the patient, or health care professionals who have had considerable experience with the patient's disease). Because this approach includes both exposure to comparison information and opportunity to express one's feelings, it would seem to have an advantage over either of these alone.

Although the evidence is not entirely consistent (see Mitchell & Glicksman, 1972),[2] it suggests that patients generally wish to talk with others with the same disease or problems (Binger *et al.*, 1969; Bozeman, Orbach, Sutherland, 1955; Messerli *et al.*, 1980; Sanders & Kardinal, 1977). In one study, meetings with other cancer patients were among the most frequently mentioned services that cancer patients felt should be provided. Of those who had been personally offered the opportunity to meet with other cancer patients for support, 52% had taken advantage of it. In fact, more than one-third of the men and women surveyed indicated an interest in volunteering to help others through a peer support program for cancer patients (Greenleigh & Associates, 1979).

There is also some research to suggest that discussions with similar others are beneficial (Binger *et al.*, 1969; Bozeman *et al.*, 1955). For example, Bozeman *et al.* (1955) reported that other parents with leukemic children "were regarded by most mothers as the most important source of emotional support [p. 15]." In one study, Parkes (1979a) found that individuals dying from cancer in hospitals or a hospice frequently reported becoming acquainted with other patients. Such interactions were seen by the majority of those who had them as helpful and by very few as upsetting.

The uncertainties and fears of the person with cancer are likely to result in an enhanced need for social support as well as an increased need for clarification (Lieber, Plumb, Gerstenzang, & Holland, 1976; Schwartz, 1977; Thomas & Weiner, 1974; Vachon, *et al.* 1979). As the patient contends with the prospect of a shortened life, unpleasant and possibly mutilating treatments, and physical deterioration, the need for support may grow stronger. In fact, one of the many fears patients have during the early stages of cancer is that they will be rejected and abandoned by loved ones (Sutherland & Orbach, 1953).

Several studies have provided evidence that perceived support is

---

[2] The majority of the patients in Mitchell and Glicksman's (1977) study felt that it would be undesirable to spend additional time with other patients, but almost all of the patients who felt that way had not engaged in open discussions with other patients in the waiting room. Most of the patients who had discussed their problems openly in the waiting room expressed a desire to spend additional time with other patients to discuss common problems.

associated with positive outcomes such as improved emotional adjustment among cancer patients (see, e.g., Jamison, Wellisch, & Pasnau, 1978; Lewis & Bloom, 1978–1979; Weisman & Worden, 1976; see Meyerowitz, 1980, for a review). A positive relationship between social support and numerous outcome measures (e.g., physical health, emotional well-being) has also been found among individuals undergoing other life stresses (see Cobb, 1976; DiMatteo & Hays, 1980; or Silver & Wortman, 1980, for reviews). In most cases, these studies are correlational, so that it is unclear whether social support actually causes better physical and psychological adjustment. One alternative explanation for these findings is that stressed or victimized individuals who are poorly adjusted might alienate members of the support network to a greater degree than those who are doing poorly (and consequently receive less support). Alternatively, those who are doing well may be less critical in the judgments they make about the adequacy of their social support network. These and other ambiguities could be resolved by longitudinal research that assesses social support at one point in time as a predictor of subsequent distress or physical deterioration. In one such study (Vachon, 1979a), social support was associated with better long-term adjustment among both cancer patients and the bereaved. A causal relationship between support and effective long-term adjustment could also be established by intervention studies in which participants are assigned to treatments that mobilize their support system or supplement the support available to them (e.g., Bloom, et al. 1978). (For a more detailed discussion of the social support construct, including various types and components of social support, possible mediating mechanisms through which social support may influence outcomes, and possible deleterious effects of behaviors intended to be supportive, see Antonovsky, 1979; Caplan, 1979; Cobb, 1976; Cohen & McKay, in press; DiMatteo & Hays, 1980; Heller, 1979; House, 1981; Kahn & Antonucci, 1980; Silver & Wortman, 1980.)

Barriers to Social Validation and Support

Although persons diagnosed as having cancer may have many needs that could be satisfied through social interaction, they are likely to have difficulty in meeting these needs. In most cases, cancer patients have limited access to others suffering from comparable problems. They may be exposed to newspapers and other media coverage of cancer; however, such presentations may be biased toward patients who have a positive attitude and who are coping well. Other patients may be encountered by chance in a hospital waiting room or doctor's office, but these settings are ones in which only superficial exchanges are likely to take place.

In fact, three investigations confirm that cancer patients and mothers of children with leukemia interact very little with one another in hospital waiting rooms (Hoffman & Futterman, 1971; Mitchell & Glicksman, 1977; Peck & Boland, 1977). The majority of these patients spent no time talking to other patients during waiting periods before treatments or spoke only of "trivial subjects" during this time. This type of exposure to others with cancer could actually be detrimental, since it could lead patients to the erroneous conclusion that most people have few problems in coping with cancer and that their own confusion, doubts, and fears are deviant and abnormal. This research suggests that intimate discussions between cancer patients are unlikely to occur spontaneously. Moreover, because cancer is such a stigmatizing disease, many patients may feel inhibited about seeking out other cancer patients or publicly identifying themselves as such. For these reasons, patients are usually forced to rely on dissimilar others such as health care professionals, family members, and friends for validation and support. This is unfortunate, since other cancer patients are in a better position to provide consensus information that the patient's reactions are normal and understandable.

Although family, friends and health care professionals are more likely to be available to the patient than are other people with cancer, two particular factors may inhibit the patient from approaching these people and discussing their feelings. First, cancer patients may fear that open discussion of their feelings about the illness will upset or hurt others. This strategy of protecting others may be especially strong toward family members, because they are perceived by the patient as being already overburdened by their illness (Bean et al., 1980; Harker, 1972; Schwartz, 1977). Second, patients may believe that it is inappropriate to express their feelings or concerns to others, particularly their doctors. These beliefs may occur both because patients feel that doctors are too busy for such conversation (Mitchell & Glicksman, 1977) and because they believe that bringing up one's concerns will elicit a negative reaction from the doctor. In fact, being silent, passive, and accepting is the perceived role of a "good patient" (Greenberg, 1961; Tagliacozzo & Mauksch, 1972; Taylor, 1979).

Although the specific reasons have not been explored, there is evidence that the needs of cancer patients for social interaction are frequently not met by dissimilar others (Bard, 1952; Bean et al., 1980; Cohen et al., 1977; Gordon et al., 1977; Jamison et al., 1978; Krant & Johnson, 1977–1978; Mitchell & Glicksman, 1977; Sanders & Kardinal, 1977; Vachon et al., 1977; Wellisch, Mosher, & Van Scoy, 1978). The following analysis of the reactions of others to the cancer patient offers some additional perspectives on why this occurs.

Reactions of Others to the Person with Cancer

What types of behavior do cancer patients generally elicit from others? A person's behavior toward the patient is likely to be influenced by two factors: by a complicated set of feelings and attitudes toward the cancer patient, and by prior assumptions and beliefs about how one should behave when interacting with the person. Each of these factors is described in more detail in the following discussion. We then argue that the behaviors people see as desirable are often discrepant with their private feelings. For this reason, people are often uncomfortable about the prospect of interacting with the patient and may therefore behave in ways that are detrimental to him or her.

Feelings and Attitudes

For a variety of reasons, others' feelings about cancer patients are likely to be negative. Some of these feelings are specific to cancer; others may occur whenever individuals are exposed to victims of undesirable life events. In analyzing these feelings and attitudes, we draw both from research in the cancer area and from theory and research in social psychology.

Cancer appears to be somewhat unique in its ability to arouse fear and feelings of vulnerability. For example, medical students and residents have been found to hold significantly more negative attitudes toward cancer than toward heart disease (Kaye, Appel, & Joseph, 1980). In health surveys the general public has expressed considerable fear of developing cancer and has many misconceptions about the chances of contracting and dying from the disease (Knopf, 1976; "Public Attitudes toward Cancer," 1980). For example, individuals markedly underestimate the incidence of cancer in the population. People believe that only one out of seven persons will develop cancer, whereas medical statistics indicate that the true incidence is one out of four. However, the public is unduly pessimistic about cancer mortality rates. People believe that only one in five cancer patients survives, yet medical statistics suggest that the survival rate (i.e., living 5 plus years from diagnosis) is about one in three ("Public Attitudes toward Cancer," 1980).

The disease also seems to evoke physical aversion and disgust in others, particularly when it is associated with mutilating surgery or physical deterioration. These feelings may be increased when one encounters striking and visible changes in a previously healthy person. Even family members report being taken aback by changes in the appearance of the patient. Aversion may also stem from individuals' fears that they will catch the disease. Indeed, patients in our support groups have described instances where they have been the only one at a party to receive paper eating utensils, or where they have been asked not to use public rest rooms or swimming pools (see, e.g., Kelly, 1975; "Cancer, More than a Disease," 1977). In one case a neighbor would not allow her child to play with a boy who had cancer (Cooper, 1980). In another, a woman's husband forbade her to touch her two young children for 2 years after she was diagnosed with cancer because he was fearful that the entire family would contract cancer

(Vachon & Lyall, 1976). The fact that the causes of cancer are not fully understood has contributed to this belief. Indeed, Kleiman *et al.* (1977) suggest that this myth about contagion is pervasive even among health care providers and is a major cause of avoidance and rejection of the patient.

In addition to fear, dread, and aversion, cancer in another person is likely to arouse feelings of anger, sadness, and depression on their behalf. Sympathy and concern for the patient are also common. The closer the relationship between a patient and another person, and the more dismal the prognosis, the more intense these empathic and sympathetic reactions may be.

Still other motives may lead individuals to derogate and blame cancer patients. In principle, these points apply in any situation where contact with someone who is suffering occurs. Lerner and his associates (1970, 1971; Lerner, Miller, & Holmes, 1976) argue that individuals are motivated to believe in a "just world" in which people "get what they deserve and deserve what they get." If we can believe that people do not suffer unless something is wrong with them or their behavior, we will feel protected from undeserved suffering ourselves (Lerner, 1970, 1971; Lerner & Simmons, 1966; Simons & Piliavin, 1972; Walster, 1966). Since having cancer is regarded as an extremely undesirable fate, individuals may be strongly motivated to protect themselves by attributing the disease to others' undesirable personal characteristics or their past behavior. Such reactions toward cancer patients are probably most prevalent among strangers and acquaintances.

Another factor that may contribute to a person's motivation to derogate an individual who is suffering is that such an attitude more or less absolves the derogator from any guilt for not helping the suffering person. As many health care providers can attest, dealing with a cancer patient who is depressed, fearful, and in pain can be a very stressful experience. Those in close proximity to the patient may become frustrated if they notice little improvement in the patient's morale after providing reassurance and help. Attributing the patient's negative feelings and fears to his or her own inadequacy in coping with the disease can relieve the sense of personal responsibility for being unable, or even unwilling to help. Derogation of this type may be especially likely to come from family members and health care professionals, who have frequent and continuing contact with the patient (Kalish, 1977, for descriptive corroboration of this point).

In addition to these motivational factors, there may be cognitive biases that lead observers to derogate and blame cancer patients. One such bias has been identified by Jones and Nisbett (1971) in their influential paper on actor–observer differences in the attribution process. Jones and Nisbett (1971) have argued that actors tend to attribute the causes of their behavior to aspects of the situation, whereas observers attribute the actor's behavior to stable dispositions or personality characteristics of the actor. For example, an observer may reason that the cancer patient is complaining because he or she is ''weakwilled, selfish and cowardly,'' while the patient attributes his or her complaints to the difficult or stressful circumstances. Theoretically, this difference occurs because the actor has more information than does the observer about the situational factors that are impinging on him or her. In contrast, the observer focuses on the behavior itself.

Since cancer patients are confronted with a genuinely stressful and aversive experience, many of the behaviors they manifest are likely to be negative (e.g., fear, depression; see Harker, 1972). Thus, observer biases toward dispositional attributions will often lead to negative inferences about the patient. This bias may be especially prevalent among family members and health care professionals who are more likely to witness unbecoming behaviors than are casual acquaintances or friends. Over time, this attributional tendency may result in the accumulation of tensions between the patient and others that are difficult to correct or counteract.

Several different kinds of negative feelings toward a person with cancer may be experienced simultaneously or in succession. The spouse of a colostomate, for example, may feel physical aversion regarding the condition, sadness that the spouse is suffering, and anger and resentment that he or she must spend so much time caring for the patient (Dyk & Sutherland, 1956; Sutherland et al., 1952). In describing these negative feelings, we do not mean to paint others as intentionally cruel, unsympathetic, or unfeeling toward cancer patients. We do believe, however, that certain affective, motivational, and cognitive factors may unwittingly create negative reactions among them. These may occur even among individuals who have strong feelings of love, concern, and sympathy for the person with cancer.

Beliefs about Appropriate Behavior

Although most people have not had extensive experience in interacting with cancer patients, they often hold prior assumptions about how they should behave when with them. Some of these notions come from the acceptance of social norms and dictates for behavior toward the sick or dying. Others come from their conceptions about what types of comments and interactions are likely to be most helpful to the patient. Regarding the former, people are socialized to show concern for others who are seriously ill, and they learn ritualized behaviors of politeness such as visiting, calling, or sending cards. Consequently, they may feel strong obligations to behave in these ways toward a cancer patient. For example, if one's coworkers go to visit a fellow worker who is hospitalized with cancer, one may feel obligated to do the same.

Regarding their conceptions about what is beneficial for the patient, many people seem to feel that it is desirable for the patient to remain as cheerful as possible. It is often considered inappropriate for cancer patients to discuss problems they are having in coping with their illness, or to focus on a negative prognosis. These discussions are thought to be depressing to the patient, to encourage self-pity, or to undermine the patient's motivation to keep fighting the disease. The assumptions that patients should avoid thinking or talking about negative aspects of their situation and try to be as cheerful and optimistic as possible appear to be quite prevalent. According to Kastenbaum and Aisenberg (1972), a majority of nurses and attendants on a geriatric ward reported changing the subject when patients tried to discuss their feelings about death. The most frequent reason they gave for doing this was that they wanted to ''cheer up'' the patient, and they felt that the best way to do so was to focus the patient's attention on something else (see also Quint, 1965). Similarly, Harker (1972) and Garfield (1977) have suggested that most people believe open discussion of a cancer patient's difficulties would upset the person's emotional equilibrium. Kalish (1977) has argued that family members believe discussions about the disease and death will make the patient uncomfortable. Research also suggests that victims of other undesirable life events who discuss their problems are seen as coping poorly. For example, Coates, Wortman, and Abbey (1979) found that rape victims who made a brief negative comment about the incident 6 months after its occurrence were rated as less attractive and were regarded as more maladjusted than those victims who did not.

In fact, there are sound reasons to question the assumption that expression of negative affect is always maladaptive for the person with cancer. As discussed previously, many cancer patients are highly motivated to share their feelings rather than to conceal them so that they can clarify what is happening. Moreover, there is at least some evidence, indicated earlier, to suggest that the opportunity to express one's feelings is beneficial (Binger et al., 1969; Cobliner, 1977; Cohen et al., 1977; Derogatis et al., 1979; Kaplan et al., 1976; Kellerman et al., 1980; Spinetta et al., 1981; Spinetta & Maloney, 1978; Vachon et al., 1977; see also Silver & Wortman, 1980, for a review). For example, children whose families maintained an open level of communication during the course of the illness demonstrated higher levels of self-esteem and reported feeling closer to their families members than did children whose families did not maintain open communication (Spinetta, et al., 1981).

Although there are few studies in which the opportunity for ventilation has been experimentally manipulated, one experiment with widows has provided impressive support for the importance of ventilation. Raphael (1977) randomly assigned widows at risk for postbereavement morbidity to a treatment involving ''support for the expression of grieving affects such as sadness, anger, anxiety, hopelessness, helplessness and despair [p. 1451]'' or to a no-treatment control group. This treatment occurred for a maximum of 3 months and included an average of just four sessions. However, when assessed 13 months after their spouses' deaths, women in the intervention group reported significantly better psychological and physical health than those randomly assigned to the no-treatment control group.

Conflicts about How to Behave

As elaborated earlier, people harbor negative feelings about cancer and cancer patients but believe these feelings should not be expressed to the patient. Instead, they assume that they must act cheerful and encouraging in their dealings with a person who has cancer. This state of affairs interferes with the frequency and quality of time that others spend with cancer patients. The prospect of coming into contact with someone who is seriously ill is likely to produce a great deal of ambivalence and conflict: Should one obey his or her desire to deny or avoid the unpleasantness associated with the cancer patient? Or should one try to hide his or her negative feelings and attempt to reach out to the patient, to be positive and cheerful? These discrepant feelings may be immobilizing, and patients may interpret such conflict and indecisiveness as active avoidance of them. Some people may resolve this ambivalence by voluntarily deciding to contact the patient. Still others may be required to spend time with the patient (as is generally the case with family and medical personnel) or may "force themselves" to visit because they believe it is the right thing to do.

In all of these cases, the interaction is likely to evoke a certain amount of anxiety for nonpatients. Evidence consistent with this was found in a study by Krant and Johnston (1977–1978) in which 55% of the family members of terminal cancer patients reported feeling uncomfortable or ambivalent about visiting the patient. The reasons stated included being upset by the patient's pain, feeling helpless, not knowing what to talk about, and fear of being near cancer. The prospect of contact with the patient forces people to confront their negative feelings; indeed, it often heightens these feelings since the patient's suffering and deterioration are usually more evident in face-to-face interaction. At the same time, people assume that every effort must be made to control their feelings and conceal their anxiety and distress. Parkes (1972b) has noted that family members worry constantly that they will "break down" and "betray their feelings" to the patient. Direct exposure to another who is suffering, coupled with an ever-present concern that one will reveal his or her feelings, or "say the wrong thing," makes many encounters with the patient awkward, uncomfortable, and tense. Furthermore, many people have had few encounters with others who are seriously ill and thus have little experience to guide them in this difficult situation.

Behaviors of Others toward the Person with Cancer

These reactions of others often lead to behaving in ways that are unintentionally damaging to the person with cancer. There is considerable evidence that people avoid cancer patients, that they discourage open communication with the patient, and that they give off conflicting behavioral cues when in the patient's presence. Each of these is discussed below.

Physical Avoidance

According to several investigators, health care professionals often avoid cancer patients or express strong desires to do so (see Schulz, 1978, for a review). For example, Pinkerton and McAleer (1976) report data that suggest that counselors are likely to provide less counseling to cancer patients than to patients with other equally serious disease-related disabilities. Physical avoidance is probably most likely to occur when a cancer patient's condition is deteriorating. The results of one study revealed that nurses took longer to answer the calls of dying patients than those of other individuals who were hospitalized (LeShan, 1964, reported by Kastenbaum & Aisenberg, 1972). Similarly, Artiss and Levine (1973) reported that doctors were uneasy about encounters with dying patients and often dreaded and avoided them. In another report, 77% of interns and 48% of residents surveyed perceived that physicians in their hospitals withdrew from terminal cancer patients (Fosson, 1980). Investigations have also reported some avoidance of cancer patients by friends (Greenleigh & Associates, 1979; O'Malley *et al.*, 1979; Silberfarb *et al.*, 1980).

A cancer patient at any stage of the illness may also experience avoidance and reduced physical contact with his or her family. For example, Dyk and Sutherland (1956) found low levels of physical assistance from spouses of colostomates even though, in most cases, the patients desired more help from their spouses than they were receiving. A survey of 142 family members of cancer patients in California found that 18% reported physical contact with the patient had become "cooled or withdrawn" since the illness (Greenleigh & Associates, 1979). Many other studies report a reduction or change in sexual activity as a consequence of the disease (Jamison, *et al.*, 1978; Meyerowitz, *et al.*, 1979; Morris, *et al.*, 1977; Silberfarb, *et al.*, 1980). Ironically, this change may be occurring at a time when cancer patients especially need physical contact as a sign of reassurance (cf. Lieber *et al.*, 1976).

Avoidance of Open Communication about the Disease

A number of empirical studies suggest that open communication with cancer patients is infrequent (Jamison *et al.*, 1978; Krant & Johnston, 1978; Sanders & Kardinal, 1977; Vachon *et al.*, 1977). For example, Jamison *et al.,* (1978) found that 89% of the mastectomees in their sample reported having had little or no discussion with spouse or significant other prior to surgery, 87% reported little or no discussion while hospitalized, and 50% reported little or no discussion after returning home. Similarly, a study of families of terminal cancer patients by Krant and Johnson (1978) found that discussions with the patient about dying were rare. Sixty-nine percent of the family members in the sample indicated that they had thought about the possibility of the patient dying, but of these, a large majority (78%) indicated that this topic had not been discussed with the person. Furthermore, when asked if issues such as life insurance, a will, or intentions for belongings had been discussed, 76% of the sample stated no. The results of this study also suggest that there are discrepancies between patients' and family members' perceptions of the others' perspective. For example, only 46% of the patients felt that their families knew they had a malignancy whereas 87% of the family members reported that they did. Even more dramatic, only 26% of the family members gave an affirmative answer when asked whether the patient was getting better, yet 46% thought that the patient *believed* he or she was getting better (Krant & Johnson, 1978).

It is not clear from these investigations whether the lack of open communication is brought about by others or by the patient. However, other studies (some of which were cited earlier) suggest that it is common for family members, friends, and medical staff to react unfavorably to open communication and that patients see this as a problem (Bard, 1952; Gordon *et al.,* 1977; Kastenbaum & Aisenberg, 1972; Mitchell & Glicksman, 1977; Pearlman, Stotsky, & Dominick, 1969). For example, Vachon (1979a) has found that breast cancer patients feel that others will react negatively if they display any emotional distress once the treatment has been completed. Dyk and Sutherland (1956) quote one cancer patient who felt that his family members "would never have the patience to listen to the whole story of my illness. . . . Their desire was always to hear from me that I was all right [p. 74]."

Family, friends, and medical personnel not only refrain from initiating discussions of patients' feelings but they may also try to influence patients to conceal their feelings (Dyk & Sutherland, 1956; Quint, 1965; Vachon, 1979a). For example, Quint (1965) interviewed 21 mastectomy patients at five intervals postsurgery and collected observations on patient–staff interactions. She found that physicians and nurses made it difficult for patients to express concern or ask questions by directing the conversation into "safe channels." Both patients and nurses reported that nurses did not permit open communication. Patients also reported that family and friends blocked them from discussing their illness. Barriers to verbal communication were greater the more extensive the cancer was. Other evidence suggests that family members are as likely as medical care givers to attempt to control the level of discussion with the patient (e.g., Bard, 1952; Binger *et al.,* 1969; Dyk & Sutherland, 1956; Glaser & Strauss, 1965; Klein, 1971;

Quint, 1965). Studies with other populations of victimized individuals provide further documentation that blocking them from ventilating their feelings is common (cf. Andreason & Norris, 1972; Glick, Weiss, & Parkes, 1974; Helmrath & Steinetz, 1978; Maddison & Walker, 1967; see also Silver & Wortman, 1980, for a review).

There are a number of reasons stemming from the feelings and beliefs of others, discussed earlier, why those in the cancer patient's social network may discourage expression of feelings. Open communication may be avoided because it is not consistent with most people's beliefs regarding what is good for the patient (Garfield, 1977; Kalish, 1977; Kastenbaum & Aisenberg, 1972). In addition, individuals may wish to avoid listening to the patient's feelings simply because they are unpleasant (Buehler, 1975; Kastenbaum & Aisenberg, 1972). Open discussion may even serve to intensify negative feelings that are already present. Thus, if a family member is upset about a patient who is dying, it may add to his or her distress to learn that the patient is afraid to die. Finally, others may wish to avoid listening to the patient's difficulties because it is even more difficult to control one's own feelings in these situations (Parkes, 1972b).

In addition to those mentioned, there are also some obvious and more altruistic motives for physical avoidance and for the avoidance of open communication. Friends may be fearful of intruding on the family's privacy by visiting the patient, and on the patient's privacy by bringing up sensitive aspects of the disease. During particularly difficult phases, friends or family may wonder if the patient wants attention, or whether he or she prefers to be left alone. Even family members may be afraid of harming, angering, or offending the person by mentioning certain touchy issues such as the costs of medical care or the possibility of death. Thus, genuine ambivalence about what to do, and real dilemmas over what the patient wants and needs may contribute to these tendencies of others to physically or emotionally withdraw.

Discrepancies in Behavior

Because of the underlying conflict between one's negative feelings about the cancer patient and one's beliefs about how to respond to him or her, individuals are likely to behave in contradictory ways when they do interact with a cancer patient. Especially likely are discrepancies between verbal and nonverbal behaviors directed toward the patient. When with the cancer patient, individuals may make a gallant effort to appear agreeable, optimistic, and cheerful. Yet, despite the fact that most people can voluntarily make optimistic statements, the nonverbal behaviors that accompany these statements may be more difficult to control. And, since nonverbal behavior is often a clue to one's true feelings (see, e.g., Argyle, 1975), the negative affect underlying interactions with cancer patients may well be manifested in their nonverbal behavior.

To our knowledge, no one has systematically investigated the nonverbal behaviors that occur when well persons interact with cancer patients. However, experiments dealing with confrontations between ablebodied and handicapped individuals seem directly relevant. These studies have shown that the ablebodied often express their discomfort in such situations by more rigid and controlled motor activity, fewer smiles, greater interpersonal distance, and earlier exits than they demonstrate when interacting with other ablebodied individuals (see, e.g., Farina, Holland, & Ring, 1966; Kleck, 1969; Kleck, Buch, Goller, London, Pfeifer, & Vukcevic, 1968; Kleck, Ono, & Hastorf, 1966). If these results are generalizable to persons with other kinds of stigmata, there may be a considerable discrepancy between others' verbal statements and their nonverbal behaviors toward cancer patients. For example, an individual may offer reassurance while maintaining an awkward interpersonal distance or while talking in a sad or nervous voice.

There is evidence that patients are aware of negative nonverbal behaviors and find them disturbing. For example, in an interview study of 50 patients hospitalized with chronic illnesses including cancer, Cobb (1956) found that patients easily picked up signals of nurses' attitudes from their tone and manner and wished nurses would transmit more concern and compassion nonverbally. Perhaps for this reason, the importance of nonverbal communication modes in medical settings is being increasingly stressed (see, e.g., Bennett, 1977; DiMatteo, 1979; Friedman, 1979a; Parkes, 1972b; Verwoerdt, 1966).

The conflict between individuals' negative feelings and their desire to respond positively to the patient may also be evident in discrepancies between verbal behaviors in a given context. For example, a person may be supportive to a cancer patient one moment and rejecting the next. One of the women in the authors' support group reported that her daughter once said to her, ''Does your arm hurt, Mother? Well, don't tell me if it does.'' Discrepancies may also occur between behaviors in different situations and at different times. For example, a friend who has lavished attention on a cancer patient after the initial diagnosis may subsequently not visit or call at all when the prognosis worsens. There may also be discrepancies between a person's expressed intentions and his or her subsequent behaviors. People may promise to call or visit but then fail to fulfill these promises, perhaps because of their underlying ambivalent or negative feelings.

Discrepancies in behavior may be especially likely to come from family members, since it is the family members who generally have the most sustained contact with the patient (Aitken-Swan, 1959; Binger et al., 1969; Dyk & Sutherland, 1956; Klein, Dean, & Bogdonoff, 1967). No matter how much they love the patient, most family members are bound to resent the enormous responsibility thrust upon them and the changes the ill person has brought about in their lives. They frequently become emotionally drained from trying to keep pace with rapid fluctuations in physical condition, mood, and reactions of the patient. Frustration results from efforts to help the patient that have little impact on the course of a progressive disease. Physical exhaustion is common among close care givers, and the strain of financial difficulties often accompanies it. Family members' own needs, interests, and problems are neglected as they struggle to stay on top of a complicated and demanding situation.

Because of all the pressures upon them, even the most patient and understanding family members are likely to direct occasional negative outbursts toward the patient. As the stress of interacting and caring for a suffering and ill person continues with no improvement in sight, these outbursts may become more frequent. Yet, they conflict with the family member's feelings about how the patient should be treated, and thus, they are likely to be followed by strong feelings of guilt and remorse and by displays of love and concern for the patient. It may add to the patient's frustration and confusion to be treated harshly one moment and lavished with kindness the next.

Impact of Other's Behavior on the Person with Cancer

In summary, when a person learns he or she has cancer, that knowledge produces a need for clarification and social support. As the disease progresses and the patient attempts to cope with all of the events ensuing from the illness and its treatment, the need for satisfying social interaction becomes more intense. But most cancer patients find themselves in a situation where their needs for information and social support are thwarted.

The changes in their social relationships are likely to be profound. Casual friends and acquaintances may begin to avoid the patient completely. When people do visit, any attempts to provide reassurance and support are unlikely to be convincing. Despite others' best intentions, their interactions with the patient are often characterized by awkwardness, hesitancy, uncertainty, and tension. Many of those who interact with the patient may attempt to keep the conversation superficial and thus, avoid the topics that are really on the patient's mind. While this evasion may often be motivated by a concern for the patient's welfare, the patient may infer that others are not really interested in his or her feelings. Friends, family members, and health care professionals are likely to voice reassurance on the surface, but manifest negative nonverbal behaviors as well as inconsistencies in behavior over time. Moreover, their efforts to be reassuring and agreeable may often backfire into an oversolicitous and patronizing attitude toward the patient. Even from family members, patients may receive mixed messages and occasional negative outbursts as the stress of caring for an ill person takes its toll. Positive messages that are laced with subtle and sometimes overt negative signs can leave the patient feeling hurt, rejected, and certainly confused. As this cycle continues, the patient's need for social validation and support may reach overwhelming proportions.

Since they elicit signs of rejection from virtually everyone, and since the negative messages are fairly consistent across situations and over time, patients may draw the conclusion that they are worthless and unlovable. The impact of consistently negative or ambiguous feedback on the patient's self-esteem can be devastating (Dyk & Sutherland, 1956). Over time, patients may come to internalize the views they perceive others to hold (Kleiman *et al.*, 1977). What Goffman (1963) has stated about the stigmatized in general may hold for the cancer patient: he or she may incorporate the views of others into his or her identity and begin to feel shame and guilt, self-blame, self-derogation, and self-hatred. Mastrovito (1972), for example, has speculated that more than half of the cancer patients treated in his clinic over the past 3 years expressed self-revulsion and negative self-concepts. Ultimately, the self-doubt and isolation that result from disruption of one's social relationships can contribute greatly to the cancer patient's distress.

Attempts by the Person with Cancer to Solve the Interpersonal Dilemma

Because the disease and its associated problems may leave the patient physically and emotionally drained, most patients do not have a great deal of energy to divert to improving their social relationships. Yet, as the need for information, clarification, and support becomes more desperate, the individual with cancer may try any of several strategies to break out of the crippling interactional patterns that we have been describing. For example, he or she may exaggerate the negative aspects of the situation so that others will respond. However, the more a patient dwells on his or her problems, the more alienated and rejecting others are likely to become (Lerner, 1970, 1971).

At some point, it may occur to the patient that attaining useful information about one's own responses is probably incompatible with getting acceptance and approval from others. Although the best way to validate one's feelings may be to discuss them with others, the best way to get support may be to indicate that everything is fine and that one is coping well. Thus, the patient may try to stave off the rejection and avoidance of friends by adopting a more positive self-presentational strategy. Hackett and Weisman (1969), in a paper on reactions to imminent death, argue that the patient "learns that to pursue his doubts by asking questions seldom yields more than uneasiness between himself and those upon whom he depends for companionship. Therefore he stops asking and becomes a player in the death-bed drama in which optimism is the theme [p. 304]." And from the cancer patient's point of view, Rollin (1976) recalls, "I got many congratulations for being so brave and cheerful. I liked that, so I got more brave and cheerful. And the more brave and cheerful I was, the more everyone seemed to love me, so I kept it up. I became positively euphoric [p. 70]."

There are two problems with this approach to the patient's dilemma. First, this may stop avoidance responses from some people (e.g., those who cannot deal with the patient's pain and suffering), but not from others (e.g., those who fear the illness is contagious). Second, since the patient is aware that he or she is using false pretenses to gain approval from others, any support received may provide little information to the patient about his or her true worth (Jones & Wortman, 1973). Positive feedback may have little impact on the patient, since it is likely to be attributed to the patient's obvious need for it or the self-presentational strategy employed to obtain it. In fact, a general problem for the patient who wishes to correct their communication problems is that there is often little contingency at all between his or her behavior and the responses of others. Ambiguous and negative feedback from others stems as much from their own anxiety or distress as from the patient's actual behavior. Thus, the patient's attempts to alter the situation may be met with a seemingly random pattern of responses. As a consequence, the patient may learn over time to expect negative or ambiguous messages from others.

So most cancer patients find themselves in an uncomfortable situation, a "Catch-22": Either they can express their feelings and be themselves, thereby incurring others' avoidance and rejection, or they can enact a charade, pretending that everything is fine, and obtain at least some support from others. Because neither of these alternatives is satisfactory, the patient may vacillate between them, sometimes putting on a good face, and sometimes confronting others with his or her pain and anxiety. This vacillation, of course, pollutes the social environment still further and makes it even more difficult for friends and relatives to know how to respond. Most patients are not in a position to test the hypothesis that *all* cancer patients are treated in this manner by friends and loved ones, so they stay trapped within this dilemma indefinitely. If it continues unchecked long enough, this process may lead to complete withdrawal from the social environment and to severe and chronic depression.

IMPLICATIONS FOR TREATMENT INTERVENTIONS AND FOR SUBSEQUENT RESEARCH

Many authors have talked about the social isolation of the cancer patient (e.g., Forester, *et al.*, 1978; Giacquinta, 1977; Klagsbrun, 1971; Lewis & Bloom, 1978–1979). In principle, this process of social isolation may be stopped or reversed at any point by natural circumstances or by therapeutic intervention. Some patients may not experience this social breakdown as acutely as others because of exceptionally sensitive relatives or friends with whom they can openly communicate without rejection or avoidance. Occasionally patients' cancers may be effectively treated before interpersonal networks are disrupted. Yet for many cancer patients, especially those who are debilitated by their illness for a long period of time, none of these naturally occurring preventions may apply. These patients may benefit from psychological interventions that prevent or correct problems in their social relations and from health care providers' awareness and understanding of these problems. The following sections discuss the implications of what has been presented here for intervention with patients and their family members and offer some preliminary guidelines for the health care professional and for the general public.

Potential Treatment Interventions for Patients and Family Members

Family Counseling

One treatment suggested by our analysis is a family counseling program that makes cancer patients and their families aware of the complicated social environment in which they may be trapped and that encourages more open communication (Binger *et al.,* 1969; Cohen, Goldenberg, & Goldenberg, 1977; Krant *et al.,* 1976; Olsen, 1979; Sheldon, Ryser, & Krant, 1979; Vachon *et al.,* 1979; Wellisch *et al.,* 1978). It appears that families in which members communicate freely with one another are more likely to adjust to cancer effectively (Cohen *et al.,* 1977). Family counseling could increase the frequency and effectiveness of communication within families by providing training in communication skills and regular occasions in which to use them. In addition, exposure to other families could provide clarification of the problems associated with the disease. For example, family members could learn that their feelings of anger and guilt are normal under the circumstances.

In an article on a therapy program for couples in which the woman has had a mastectomy, Witkin (1975) describes a misunderstanding that is extremely common. Many husbands assume that they should not have sex or indicate a desire for sex until their wife suggests it:

> "One husband stated, 'I didn't have sex with my wife for a long time because I felt she really didn't want it, what with the operation and her breast gone. . . . I imagine I wouldn't feel like it after such an operation.' In his fear of early intercourse, the husband may be genuinely concerned about his wife and want to do what's best for her. What happens is the reverse: the woman interprets his abstinence as confirming her worst fears, that he is disgusted, sees her as half a

woman, can't stand looking at or caressing her, doesn't want her anymore [p. 300]."

Misunderstandings such as this can be headed off or cleared up through a family counseling program.

Peer Support Opportunities

A second implication is that it might be useful to increase cancer patients' access to others who have experienced cancer. This can be accomplished through support groups for cancer patients. Many types of groups exist in which cancer patients come into contact with other patients, but these groups vary in the emphasis they place on peer interaction. Self-help groups typically hold interaction among members as their primary goal (Adams, 1979; Cole, O'Connor & Bennett, 1979; Johnson, 1980; Parsell & Tagliareni, 1974; Peebler, 1975; Pellman, 1976), whereas other types of groups deemphasize this and have educational or psychotherapeutic goals instead (e.g. Ferlic, Goldman, & Kennedy, 1979). Still others include peer support as one of many goals (e.g., Foster & Mendel, 1979; Gustafson & Whitman, 1978).

There are many specific reasons why these groups can provide especially rich opportunities for clarification and support. First, they usually provide an ideal setting for open communication. Members are encouraged to share their problems and feelings in an atmosphere of understanding and support. Second, cancer patients can exchange factual information about such things as where to get a good price and fit on a prosthesis, how to minimize nausea from chemotherapy, how to go about making a will, and how to apply for disability benefits. Group members can also obtain advice and suggestions from one another about how to cope with specific personal problems. In trying to make decisions about such issues as what to tell people at work or how much to tell one's children, patients can profit enormously from learning about the experiences of others who have dealt with these problems. Third, interacting with similar others should help the patient make a more accurate attribution about the things happening to him or her. For example, by talking with other cancer patients, it may become evident that rejection or avoidance by others is a normal consequence of the disease, not a reflection of personal inadequacy and weakness. Finally, these groups offer an array of others from which an appropriate comparison person can be selected. In other words, it is possible to find another person with whom to compare experiences who is similar on such dimensions as age and type of cancer.

The few attempts that have been made to evaluate the effectiveness of groups for cancer patients suggest that they are beneficial (e.g., Bloom, *et al.*, 1978; Ferlic, *et al.*, 1979). Unfortunately, studies have not evaluated the peer interaction aspect of these groups as distinct from other aspects (e.g., dissemination of information). In fact, we are aware of no firm evidence that interaction with similar others is beneficial to people coping with major life events. Despite the popularity of self-help groups in recent years for people with a wide variety of life problems (Lieberman & Borman, 1979), and the many reasons mentioned above why they may be helpful, they may also be stressful or even harmful to participants at times. Many specific questions and issues about peer interaction are worthy of attention.

For example, when are cancer patients and others coping with misfortune receptive to interacting with similar others, and when do they prefer to avoid such contact? (McIntosh, 1977; Mitchell & Glicksman, 1977; Parkes, 1979a). At the earliest stages of the disease, people may be unreceptive to interactions with "similar others" because of the difficulty in accepting a new identity as a cancer patient. Moreover, some people with cancer may be hesitant to interact with other cancer patients at any time. For some, discussing problems with others is seen as a sign of weakness. These factors must be recognized in working with cancer groups.

Another question concerns the effects of variations in the degree of similarity between patients. Does the value of interacting with others in similar circumstances differ depending on whether they are doing better or worse, either psychologically or physically? Sanders and Kardinal (1977) have indicated that cancer patients often use others who are doing well as a yardstick to measure their own progress, but conceivably this social comparison might be distressing if the patient does not "measure up" favorably. Direct contact with other patients may also make it difficult to employ certain psychological defenses. For example, a patient who is coping with fear of recurrence by denial, thus believing that he or she is cured, may be made very anxious by encountering a similar cancer patient who has had a recurrence. In addition, the attitude of the comparison person may be a critical determinant of the value of an encounter. A study by Carey (1974) has suggested that the opportunity to talk openly and honestly with another dying person facilitates effective coping only when the dying person faces death with peace and equanimity. Talking with a person who was unable to accept his or her approaching death was negatively associated with effective coping. Brickman and Bulman (1977) have discussed the advantages and disadvantages of social comparison in general, highlighting that many comparisons can be disconcerting.

A related issue arises when family members participate in patient support groups. Is it always desirable for family members and patients to share their feelings in the presence of the other? Often it may be an important avenue for clearing up misunderstandings and facilitating further open communication. Sometimes, however, a member of the group may feel unable to express his or her concerns in the presence of their loved one. This hesitancy can stem from fear that particular concerns would hurt, worry, or upset the person. For family members these concerns might be intense personal grief, or personal problems stemming from the disease such as trouble at work. For the person with cancer, they might be new symptoms or fear of death. In our support group, we periodically divide into two smaller groups in such a way that the members of each particular family are not together. Then, these sensitive issues can more easily be brought up and the group participants can help decide whether they should be shared with the other person or not at that time. In these subgroups, the presence of both patients and family members is desirable (as opposed to dividing into one all-patient group and one all-family group) because their different perspectives can each be brought to bear on the discussion. For example, a family member who is worried about making plans for terminal nursing care may be advised by patients how this matter can be brought up with the person concerned. At the same time, other family members can indicate that these concerns are understandable and they are not something about which to feel guilty or embarrassed.

These and other major problems that may arise when cancer patients interact with other cancer patients have been discussed by Kleiman *et al.* (1977). Although we believe that contact with similar others is generally helpful, we feel this treatment should be utilized with care until further research has been conducted. Competent group facilitation can help to minimize the possibilities for problematic interactions. For example, we frequently need to remind members in our groups that their experiences, while generally helpful to others, are not necessarily applicable to everyone with cancer. Also, attendance at groups and participation in similar peer interaction programs should be strictly voluntary. Too often one hears of a newly diagnosed patient being visited by a volunteer who is a former cancer patient without having been advised or consulted beforehand; consequently, these visits are often perceived as distressing rather than helpful. Opportunities for peer interaction are highly desirable in our view, but they should be provided only with careful consideration of the individual patient's wishes and needs, and of the conditions under which the interaction will take place.

Hospice Care

In addition to family counseling and peer support groups, hospice environments can be a source of help for patients with advanced cancer. Hospices are typically places where dying patients can receive specialized physical and emotional care. Modeled after St. Christopher's Hospice in Sydenham, England, their goals usually include keeping the patient comfortable, free of pain, and alert if possible, and providing emotional support to patient and family. Hospice policies tend to encourage frequent and open interactions between patients and family members, between family members and staff, and between family members and other families (Parkes, 1979a, 1979b). This characteristic is in sharp contrast to the conventions and practices of most traditional hospitals.

In addition to encouraging open communication, hospices are likely to generate interaction between patients. The advantages of such contact are optimized by the similarity among patients with respect to the stage of the disease. In fact, empirical studies in hospices can provide useful information on the benefits and risks of contact between cancer patients. For example, Parkes (1979a) found that hospice patients were generally not upset by the deaths of other patients. Furthermore, hospices have been found to be preferred by patients over other inpatient care environments and to be beneficial to both patients and families (Hinton, 1979; Parkes, 1979b).

In summary, the most promising treatment interventions for cancer patients in helping them to meet their needs are suggested to be family therapies, peer support groups, and hospice care.

Guidelines for the Health Care Professional

From the time of diagnosis on, the health care professional is in a unique position to intervene on the patient's behalf. Through an awareness of the patient's needs for validation and support and of the destructive pattern of feedback that the patient is likely to receive from those in his or her social environment, health care professionals can take specific actions to help prevent or correct interpersonal problems. At a minimum, they can avoid relating to the patient in ways that exacerbate these problems.

One step that the health care professional can take early in the patient's treatment is to make available some information about the sensations, feelings, and possible emotions that are likely to accompany the disease or treatments.[3] As noted earlier, the literature has generally shown that information reduces the level of patient distress. Yet the available evidence suggests that such information is often not provided (cf. Messerli *et al.*, 1980; Mitchell & Glicksman, 1977; Morris *et al.*, 1977; Peck & Boland, 1977). For example, both Mitchell and Glicksman (1977) and Peck and Boland (1977) have conducted interview studies with approximately 50 cancer patients undergoing radiation therapy. In the study by Mitchell and Glicksman, the majority of patients indicated that they had received no information whatsoever from the referring physician about the nature of the therapy they were to receive. These results were corroborated by Peck and

[3] These recent publications by the National Cancer Institute (available free directly from the agency) may be very helpful to health care providers in providing information to patients, and in understanding the psychological aspects of the disease. *Coping with Cancer: A Resource for the Health Professional* N.I.H. Pub. No. 80–2080 September 1980, and *Coping with Cancer: Annotated Bibliography of Public, Patient, and Professional Information and Educational Materials*, N.I.H. Pub. No. 80–2129, May 1980.

Boland (1977), who concluded that patient beliefs regarding treatment were usually "inaccurate, pessimistic, and alarming [p. 181]."

Many physicians are reluctant to discuss the possibility of negative emotions or undesirable side effects with the patient even if the patient specifically requests this information. It is often believed that such discussions will increase the likelihood that the patient will experience the emotion or side effect in question. The interview study by Peck and Boland (1977), just mentioned, suggests that this is unlikely. Patients who had been informed about possible negative side effects of radiation appreciated this information and praised their physicians for providing it. None of the patients in the study complained because the physician had told him or her about a side effect that did not occur. However, patients who had not been warned about side effects that did occur were angry and disappointed with their physicians. Our experience in support groups has suggested that patients are often terrified by unexpected side effects and believe them to be evidence of metastasis. Interestingly, Peck and Boland (1977) also found that many patients assumed the worst about unexpected side effects and had difficulty accepting their physicians' explanations after the side effects had occurred.[4]

A second step that health care professionals can take at early stages of treatment is to inquire about the social support network that is currently available to the patient. Patients who lack social support may be in special need of time and attention from the health care staff. In cases where the patient's potential social support network is weak or underdeveloped, the health care providers may be able to play a role in mobilizing the support system (see Cobb & Erbe, 1978). For example, the likelihood that family members will provide support for the patient can be increased by involving them in the patient's care (Lewis & Bloom, 1978–1979). Family members who do not understand the nature of the disease or the medical procedures involved are not in a position to offer encouragement or support to the patient. A family member who is unaware of the side effects of chemotherapy, for example, may be annoyed rather than sympathetic with the patient's nausea and general tiredness.

Health care providers can also help by encouraging open communication, both in their own interactions with the patient and in the patient's interactions with family members. As noted earlier, available evidence suggests that the opportunity to discuss one's experience helps the patient reach an understanding of what is happening to him or her. Furthermore, misunderstandings and resentments can accumulate in settings where people are unable or unwilling to discuss their feelings about the disease (see,

---

[4] It is important to note that there is evidence for individuals differences in the desire for information and its effects (Christopher & Pfeiffer, 1980; Rice, 1982; Visser, 1980). However, a thorough discussion of these issues is beyond the scope of this chapter.

e.g., Glaser & Strauss, 1965). For example, a mother in our support group who was suffering from terminal bone cancer began drawing away from her children because she wanted them to learn to take care of themselves so that they would be prepared for the time when she would be gone. However, the children, who were unaware of her motives, were hurt and confused by this apparent rejection of them. In situations such as this, help from the health care provider in discussing the feelings behind specific behaviors can alleviate some of the patients' and family members' distress.

A final implication of this model for health care professionals is that it may help to explain why they often have ambivalent feelings toward their patients—patients whom they are supposedly trying to help. Past research has suggested that even a single encounter with a victim can be a powerfully distressing experience and can result in blame and derogation of the victim (Coates et al., 1979). In one study, nurses who worked on a new cancer care unit were found to have only slightly lower levels of stress, as measured on the Goldberg General Health Questionnaire, than new widows and considerably higher stress than breast cancer patients beginning radiation treatment (Vachon, Lyall, & Freeman, 1978). Since health care professionals frequently have repeated and intense interactions with people who are suffering, it is not surprising that ambivalent and negative feelings should develop.

Maslach (1976) has studied the phenomenon of burnout among professionals working in the helping fields. It is extremely common for such workers to come to think of their patients or clients in derogatory terms, and even come to believe that the clients deserve any problems they have. According to Maslach (1976), ''They lose all concern, all emotional feeling, for the persons they work with and come to treat them in detached or even dehumanized ways [p. 16].'' Many health care professionals believe that their negative reaction to their patients is a reflection of some personal failing (Maslach, 1976; Pines & Maslach, 1978). Research has suggested that burn-out rates are lower for professionals who can choose to minimize contact with patients or clients when the stress becomes too much for them and for professionals ''who actively express, analyze, and share their personal feelings with their colleages (Maslach, 1976, [p. 22]).'' (See also Vachon, 1978, 1979b; Vachon, Lyall & Freeman, 1979 concerning stress among those caring for the terminally ill and ways to alleviate it, and Edelwich & Brodsky, 1980; Freudenberger & Richelson, 1980; and Pines & Aronson, 1980 on burnout in general).

General Guidelines

When people have been alerted to the many things they are likely to do that disturb cancer patients, they usually wonder, ''Then what should I do in order to be helpful?'' A few implications for personal experiences with cancer patients can be derived from our analysis. Since each person and situation are different, however, and since research lags behind theorizing in this area at present, these guidelines ought to be considered tentative.

First, our discussion emphasizes the importance of permitting patients to talk about their feelings, if and when they wish to do so. Because many patients have learned that things go better if they keep their concerns to themselves, it may be difficult to initiate meaningful conversations. Yet, one can attempt to create an atmosphere of understanding with the patient in which open discussion is possible. A first step in this direction is to convey that one is receptive to hearing about the patient's concerns. For example, a comment such as ''it must be hard'' might signal to the patient that negative feelings are acceptable.[5] Pressuring the patient to ''open up'', however, would be inadvisable for at least two reasons. First, it is a counterproductive technique for fostering spontaneous and natural conversations. Such pressure is likely to lead to discomfort and superficiality rather than meaningful exchanges. Second, the need to express feelings is likely to vary considerably from patient to patient and over time for any given person. The most one can do, then, is to create opportunities for a cancer patient to ventilate while letting him or her determine when the time is right.

When a cancer patient is sharing his or her feelings, skillful and attentive listening is desirable. This entails attempting to understand but not evaluate or judge the person. It also involves restraining the typical impulse to react to every problem mentioned with a comment, piece of advice, or proposed solution. Common responses to the expression of others' woes are ''I know how you feel,'' or ''don't worry, it will be all right.'' These well-meant remarks are often unhelpful to cancer patients, we have found, because they minimize the person's problems and offer false reassurance. Merely to acknowledge that the person's concerns are being heard is probably a better response. In general, attentive listening constitutes a powerful and frequently overlooked means of support.

Another implication of the foregoing analysis is that one should try to be conscious of any cheerful or optimistic facades adopted in the patient's presence. Any attempts to cover up strong feelings of sadness, pessimism and anxiety are unlikely to be convincing; moreover, they can add to the patient's sense of confusion and bewilderment. In contrast, attempts to maintain a basically honest relationship with the person may be helpful. Such a relationship can serve as a source of strength at a time when others appear artificial. In addition to these reasons for questioning positive presentations, the difficulty of consistently acting upbeat if one feels low is a factor. This effort may take a considerable toll on family members and friends over time. We do not mean to imply that one should always admit or display negative feelings to the patient—only that continued efforts to cover them up are questionable in that they can be detrimental to everyone involved.

[5] This suggestion has been made by Elisabeth Kubler Ross in numerous talks she has given.

A related suggestion is to realize that these negative feelings are common among family and friends of cancer patients. If they are intense and persistent, it may help to take steps to manage or relieve them. Some of them might be shared with the patient in a sensitive and caring manner. For example, it might help to express a sense of helplessness about not being able to do more for the person or to share the emotional pain felt in watching the person suffer, but only if this can be done without imputing any blame. These admissions could potentially make it easier for the patient to express his or her feelings.

In many cases, however, it might be inadvisable to share negative feelings with the patient. For example, it would probably serve little purpose to tell a patient that one resents or feels angry with him or her for being ill. A better way to handle these feelings would be to discuss them with someone else who is less likely to be hurt by them. Along these lines, it could help to take advantage of support groups that are available for friends and family of those with cancer. Through this outlet for personal feelings, one may gain an ability to interact with the patient more confidently, as a better listener, and in a more genuine manner. In fact, sometimes the most helpful thing one can do for the patient is to recognize that one's own emotional needs deserve attention.

Perhaps the best advice on how to act in the presence of someone with cancer is from a patient. These words were spoken by a remarkably insightful woman who lived for eight years with lung cancer, and who was an inspiring and constructive force in the self-help groups in which both she and the authors took part: "What can you say to someone who has cancer? . . . All you can say is what you really feel. You can't upset us by telling us you're frightened or don't know what to say. We'd rather hear that than listen to someone say 'You're going to be just fine.' How can anyone know that? My doctors don't. I don't. I'm much happier when someone says 'I'd like to be your friend,' or 'I feel bad you have this disease' or 'I really give you credit for putting up a good fight.'"[6]

Cancer is undeniably prevalent; by statistical probabilities it will touch each of us in some way during our lifetimes. Very often, it will require difficult adjustment on the part of family and friends, and most of all, for the patient. This chapter is an attempt to examine the interpersonal dynamics of cancer. Both cancer patients' and others' perspectives have been consid-

[6] This quote is taken from *The Sky is Bluer Now: Thoughts on Living and Cancer,* a copyrighted booklet based on the memoirs of Anita Siegel and distributed by the Self-Help Center, 1600 Dodge Avenue, Suite S122, Evanston, Illinois 60201 for $1.00 to cover postage and handling. This is a useful source of information on the psychosocial effects of cancer. Also recommended is the N.C.I. publication *Taking Time: Support for People with Cancer and the People Who Care about Them,* N.I.H. Pub. No. 80–2059, September 1980.

ered, as well as the causal influences they exert on one another. Relevant research was presented when available, but since strong data do not currently exist on many issues raised, the reasoning in this paper is in need of further documentation. It is hoped that our endeavor to understand and articulate the social problems experienced by cancer patients, as well as their causes and consequences, will stimulate research and in some way help those affected by this disease.

ACKNOWLEDGEMENT

The authors wish to express their gratitude to Anita Siegel and the members of the Chicago Make Today Count chapters whose experiences provided a basis of information and a strong incentive for this work.

6

Sharon D. Herzberger
Deborah A. Potts

Interpersonal Relations during the Childbearing Year

The Siriono view childbirth as an easy, open process, in keeping with their relaxed sexual attitudes. Birth takes place in a communal hut and is a public event, witnessed by men as well as by women. The mother labors in a hammock while groups of women gather, gossiping about their own labors or wondering whether the baby will be a boy or a girl. They give no help to the mother during a normal labor. She ties the childbirth rope over her hammock to pull during contractions; she digs the earth under the hammock to cushion the baby's fall. Grunts and groans of labor appear to bother no one. When the baby is born, it slides over the edge of the hammock and drops a few inches to the ground.

[Newton, 1970, p. 75, speaking of the Siriono Indians of Bolivia]

A little after 4 in the morning my Wife call'd Me up by her extreme pains prevailing upon her and changing into signs of Travail. I rode over to Deacon Forbush's and brought her [Mrs. Forbush] over as our midwife. Sister Hicks, old Mrs. Knowlton, Mrs. Whipple, Mrs. Hephzibath Maynard, Mrs. Byles and Mrs. Rogers were call'd and brought and stay'd all Day and Night.

[Ebenezer Parkman's diary for December 26, 1738, quoted in Walett, 1961, p. 4]

In contrast to these descriptions of the birthing experience, contemporary childbearing has largely become the province and responsibility of a technologically oriented medical community. Although most professionals would argue that increased intervention has produced physically healthier mothers and infants, the concentration upon physical health can mean that the psychological health of the mother, father, and infant is dramatically overlooked. This chapter will examine an important determinant of psychological health during pregnancy, labor and delivery, and the early postpartum period—the social support available to expectant and new parents from medical professionals. We will discuss the means by which medical personnel can provide support to the couple and the likely consequences of receiving or failing to receive social support at various times throughout the childbearing year.

101

OVERVIEW

Much has been written about pregnancy and early parenthood as a time of "crisis" for the couple. Sociological theory suggests that the birth of a child inaugurates a process of disintegration of the family structure followed by a period of reintegration (Kirkpatrick, 1963; LeMasters, 1957). Other theorists (e.g., Holmes & Rahe, 1967) suggest that pregnancy is a major life change that when coupled with other life changes may be detrimental to one's health. Although the universality and intensity of the crisis experience has been questioned (Hobbs & Cole, 1976; Jacoby, 1969), much empirical research suggests that stresses are common during the childbearing year.

We can define a stress or stressor as an event or situation that the individual perceives as threatening or harmful (cf. Spielberger & Jacobs, 1978). There are many events during the childbearing year that may be seen as threatening by expectant and new parents. For example, changes in the woman's body or her emotional state during pregnancy may threaten her self-esteem and self-identity. Labor and delivery may be perceived as potentially harmful or, at least, painful. The arrival of the infant may upset the couple's financial stability or the woman's career. When events such as these are perceived as threatening, the individual may experience a variety of stress responses. Stress responses may be emotional, such as anxiety or depression; physiological, such as headaches; or social, such as increased argumentativeness or withdrawal.

Social support seems to reduce the impact of stressful situations, including those that couples encounter during the childbearing years. Social support has been conceptualized in varied ways (Cobb, 1979; Kahn, 1979). Most conceptualizations include *emotional* support, defined as expressions of liking and concern for another, and *esteem* support, referring to the communication that one is valued. Social support may also entail the provision of *assistance* or aid and the provision of *information* in terms of advice, reassurance, or appraisal of one's behaviors or beliefs. The different types of social support, although defined distinctly, often cannot be distinguished from one another in practice. For example, an individual who receives information or assistance from another may also feel emotionally supported by the act.

Recent formulations have attempted to understand how social support affects the recipient's physical or psychological well-being. Social support may directly enhance well-being because it meets basic human needs for social contact, security, approval, and affection (House, 1981). Social support may also assist individuals in coping more effectively: As supportive relationships lead to improved self-confidence, the individual may seek to modify or control the environment in a manner that leads to less stress (Cobb, 1976). Social support, particularly in the form of new information or appraisal of current behaviors and beliefs, may also "inoculate" the individual against the effects of stress (Janis, 1965). When an individual is provided with information about impending stressors, the individual develops realistic expectations about events that are likely to occur. A realistic outlook enables the person to "work through" his or her anxiety prior to the event and to prepare adaptive coping responses. It might also be argued that informational support provides the individual with a knowledge base by which to derive competence, confidence, and plans for action. Emotional and esteem support then provide the motivation and encouragement to pursue appropriate actions and to strive for or maintain well-being.

Throughout the childbearing year couples come into contact with various medical professionals and allied personnel. In addition to physicians, nurses, and sometimes midwives, couples often encounter such care givers as childbirth-education instructors, parenting educators, and leaders of breast-feeding support groups. Each of these persons focuses upon goals that may not be directly "psychological" or interpersonal in nature. Medical professionals, for example, are primarily concerned with maintaining the physical health of the woman and her child during pregnancy and the postpartum months. Childbirth educators are dedicated to reducing the discomfort of the laboring woman, and La Leche League facilitators are concerned with increasing the likelihood of successful breast-feeding. Each health care professional, however, has opportunities to provide social support to expectant and new parents and to promote an environment in which couples may obtain social support from other sources. Furthermore, as we shall see, the provision of social support may facilitate the achievement of the health professionals' primary goals.

THE NEED FOR SOCIAL SUPPORT

Expectant and New Mothers

During pregnancy, women often feel marked anxiety and insecurity. As many as 80% of expectant mothers, for example, feel some worry when they learn that they are pregnant (Caplan, 1964). This ambivalence occurs even among women who strongly desire a child. Disappointment and anxiety may be a result of nausea, bodily changes, and pains that she does not understand. Furthermore, the expectant woman may experience excessive fatigue and irritability that disrupt her normal routine and strain her relationships with others. Fears of having an abnormal infant and fears concerning their own physical well-being are also common among expectant mothers (Leifer, 1977), especially as the date of delivery approaches. In addition, pregnant women often worry about their ability properly to care for and rear a child and about the changes in identity and lifestyle that parenthood entails (Leifer, 1977; Rossi, 1968).

The consequences of anxiety during the prenatal months can be detrimental to both the expectant mother and the developing child. Sustained emotionality and stress can upset the mother's epinephrine–norepinephrine balance and affect adrenocortical and thyroid functioning (cf. Ferreira, 1965). These changes may affect, among other things, uterine contractibility and fetal oxygen supply. Although the exact causes are unclear, women who experience a stressful pregnancy are more prone to difficult labors, complications during delivery, and, as retrospective studies have shown, premature births (cf. MacFarlane, 1977; Sameroff & Chandler, 1975). They are also more likely to deviate from the dietary or behavioral recommendations of their physician during the prenatal months (Ferreira, 1965).

Once labor beings and the woman enters the hospital to prepare for her delivery, another set of concerns prompts the need for social support. Women often report that they feel a loss of identity during a hospital delivery (Ratner, 1977). They are typically deprived of familiar possessions and clothing, made to labor in bland, austere surroundings, and may be cleansed and shaved in preparation for birth. During labor women worry not only about their health and the health of their child but also about "doing a good job" (Danziger, 1979). They may feel pressure to suffer quietly through labor and delivery, to refrain from asking too many questions, and to subjugate their own wishes in order to conform with standard hospital procedures. Women also feel disappointed with themselves if they are unable to meet their prelabor goals about having a vaginal or nonmedicated delivery or if they lose control over their breathing and relaxation regimens.

The initial postpartum months are thought by many to produce the greatest need for support. Although postpartum depression or psychosis is rare (Pugh, Jerath, Schmidt, & Reed, 1963), some experts (cf. Rickel & Atkinson, 1979) estimate that 40–80% of new mothers experience the "baby blues." The birth of a child entails an abrupt change to immediate and complete responsibility for the child on the part of his or her parents. The shift in responsibility is particularly difficult for first-time parents (Cohen, 1966; Sumner & Fritsch, 1977), especially those with little or no experience with child care while growing up (Shereshefsky & Yarrow, 1974), and for women who have stopped working outside the home to become full-time mothers (cf. Parlee, 1980). Since time for personal-need fulfillment declines following the birth of a child, the mother periodically becomes frustrated and feels a need to escape from parenting responsibilities (Rossi, 1968). She may then suffer guilt feelings for being "selfish" and not living up to her image of the ideal mother (DelliQuadri & Breckenridge, 1978).

In short, women are likely to experience a variety of stressful events throughout the childbearing year. However, mothers are not alone in their anxiety. Although less research attention and intervention has been directed toward expectant and new fathers, they also experience stresses that warrant the support of others.

Expectant and New Fathers

In numerous cultures and throughout history, expectant fathers have exhibited the "couvade" syndrome, in which they engage in ritualistic behaviors and imitate some of the characteristics of pregnancy. Similarly, in Western society some men experience nausea, loss of appetite, and other gastrointestinal difficulties during their wife's pregnancy (Larsen, 1966; Richman & Goldthorp, 1978). These difficulties are particularly likely to emerge around the time of "quickening" (i.e., when fetal movements are first detected) and as childbirth approaches. The father's symptoms are variously interpreted as identification with the expectant mother, ambivalence about impending fatherhood, and expressions of latent feminism (e.g., Coley & James, 1976; Miller & Brooten, 1977). In addition to physical symptoms, expectant fathers often express distress with the demands created by their wives' increased dependency and emotional lability (Larsen, 1966) and with the economic and emotional demands that fatherhood will entail (Lynn, 1974).

During labor and delivery the father experiences new stresses. He may be called upon to attend to his wife's needs during a lengthy childbirth under unfamiliar and frightening circumstances. Although the mother's role in labor and delivery is defined, the father may feel that he is a guest at these proceedings, and he may not be entirely confident of his rights or sure of his responsibilities. As Richman and Goldthorp (1978) report, the father in the delivery room "is surrounded by the institutional rhetoric of the language and apparatus of medicine . . . birth sequences are governed by foetal, mother, medical, and institutional ties and exist largely outside of his experience. He can be uncertain where to stand or put his hands [p. 167]." A father who does not accompany his wife in the delivery room or who has been sent away because of a medical emergency may spend time in the waiting room worrying about the health of his wife and child.

Following childbirth, the new father will need to adjust to the demands created by the presence of a young infant. New fathers often experience jealousy at the attention given to the infant by the mother, (Kirkpatrick, 1963). If the mother breast-feeds, the father may feel left out and less powerful (Lerner, 1979). Furthermore, because breast-feeding mothers are likely to experience sore nipples or poor lubrication of the vaginal canal, the resumption of sexual relations following childbirth may be delayed (Wal-etzky, 1979). In addition, many fathers suffer from the same feelings of fatigue, insecurity, and loss of freedom as do their spouses.

The consequences of paternal stress are largely unknown. Psychoanal-ytic writers (e.g., Coley & James, 1976) warn of the likelihood of sexual act-ing out (having an affair or pursuing homosexual liaisons) among expectant fathers. Gelles (1975) reports an inordinate number of cases of wife beating during pregnancy, perhaps due to the stresses of the transition or to un-conscious efforts to destroy the unborn child. An increase in disagreements and resentment has also been noted among couples with young infants (Wainwright, 1966). We might further postulate that a father who is ex-periencing stress may not be able to perform a supportive role for his wife. The expectant or new father's anxiety also may be noticed by the wife, thereby serving to increase her anxiety. Thus, anxiety experienced by the father can interfere with his own enjoyment of new or impending father-hood and can create problems in the couple's relationship.

THE PROVISION OF SUPPORT

Many of the fears, anxieties, and concerns experienced by couples dur-ing the childbearing year may be alleviated by social support. Health care professionals are in an ideal position to provide support because of their contact with expectant and new parents and because of their expertise. In this section we will examine ways in which doctors, nurses, and other health professionals may play a supportive role during pregnancy, labor and delivery, and the initial postpartum months.

The Prenatal Months

Support during Routine Office Visits

The pregnant woman may be bothered by a wide range of concerns about her health, the health of the fetus, and impending motherhood. Medical professionals—physicians, nurse practitioners, or midwives—can en-courage their patients to discuss their worries and to ask questions. In many cases, during regular office visits, the professional will be able to eliminate the expectant mother's anxiety by explaining the origin of an ache or pain and by reassuring her that her pains or her emotions are common and no cause for alarm. Also, professionals can suggest ways of coping with the events of pregnancy. For example, the physician or nurse can recommend naps to reduce fatigue and exercises to alleviate back pain and other aches. By responding in such a manner to the fears and questions voiced by the pregnant woman, the professional demonstrates both emotional and informational support to his or her client.

Communicating a supportive, sensitive attitude may not be easy for the medical professional. The harried physician or nurse who closes the medical folder, heads toward the door, and asks whether there is anything else the client wants to discuss is unlikely to communicate sincere concern or to stimulate questions from the client. A pregnant woman, like other patients, is conscious of the professional's busy schedule and status.[1] Although she may have saved the many questions that arose throughout the month for her routine office visit, the expectant mother may hesitate to take "more time than absolutely necessary." Thus, unless the professional explicitly conveys an attitude of caring both verbally and nonverbally (cf. Friedman, 1979a, 1979b), the woman's questions and concerns are likely to remain unresolved.

The sensitive physician or nurse not only will address the questions and concerns raised directly by the client but also will be alert to the underlying implications of comments and actions (Stone, 1965). Questions about sexual relations during pregnancy, for example, may be motivated by more than a desire to know medically accepted rules. The client may want to discuss her declining interest in sex or fears concerning her partner's lack of interest. Similarly, unrealistic expectations about the benefits of childbearing (e.g., "this baby is going to save our marriage") may indicate difficulties that warrant professional concern and possible intervention. By listening to the client's overt and subtle communications, the professional demonstrates that he or she values the woman and thus provides emotional support.

Throughout conversations, however, the professional must recognize that the client may hesitate to discuss emotional issues out of fear for the type of intervention that the professional will make (Stichler, Bowden & Reimer, 1978). A woman who is experiencing stress due to her husband's failure to provide emotional support may desire the consolation and advice of her doctor or nurse, but she also may fear that the professional will discourage the husband's attendance at the delivery. In order to convey support and simultaneously to maintain the confidence and openness of the woman, the professional may need to listen and then respond in a nonjudgmental manner. In extreme cases the professional may want to refer the client elsewhere for help.

One type of intervention that will almost always be welcomed by the pregnant woman and her spouse is the provision of information. When the professional ensures that the couple knows about the physical and emo-

---

[1] The rising interest in midwife deliveries is attributed partly to the midwives' supportive, attentive attitude. Perry (1980) found that many women preferred midwives over physicians because of the midwives' enthusiasm and their willingness to answer questions and spend more time with clients.

tional changes that often occur during the childbearing year, he or she decreases the couple's anxiety and increases their ability to cope with the events of pregnancy, childbirth, and new parenthood (Brown, W. A., 1979). For example, by explicitly noting that the pregnant woman is likely to experience mood swings and fatigue, the professional prepares the couple for possible events and legitimizes their occurrence. Thus, the woman and her spouse are less likely to attribute these incidents to a weakness in the woman's character or to neglect on the part of the husband.

The expectant couple may be more receptive to different kinds of information at different times during the prenatal months. Both informal contact with pregnant women (Rubin, 1970) and formal interview studies (Leifer, 1977) have shown that women typically focus attention on infant care and infant development during their first or second trimesters of pregnancy and on labor and delivery in the third trimester. Although there is no evidence that couples will best learn information pertinent to topics of current concern, the professional who attempts to supply information that meets the expectant parents' immediate needs may be perceived as especially supportive. Individualized supportive treatment may increase the expectant mother's confidence that she will receive competent health care and increase the likelihood that she will comply with the professional's medical suggestions (cf. DiMatteo, 1979).

The medical professional also increases emotional support to expectant parents by encouraging the husband to participate in prenatal medical activities (Stichler et al., 1978; Wente & Crockenberg, 1976). When the wife visits the physician or nurse alone during pregnancy, the father may feel that he is left out, that pregnancy is not his concern, and that the relationship of real importance is between the expectant mother and the professional. By encouraging the husband's attendance at prenatal physicals, the professional explicitly recognizes that pregnancy is a shared experience and encourages the development of a supportive relationship between husband and wife. In addition, the professional communicates that he or she is interested in the husband's well-being. Joint attendance also permits the professional to address both members' concerns about the ensuing events of pregnancy, labor, and the postpartum months and to stress the importance of mutual support.

Childbirth Education

Although physicians, midwives, and nurses may provide some information about the process of labor and delivery, intensive preparation for childbirth usually falls within the province of the childbirth educator. Although numerous varieties of childbirth education are practiced, two of the most common methods, Dick–Read and Lamaze, are based upon similar philosophies and techniques (Beck, Geden, & Brouder, 1979; Miller & Brooten, 1977). Both methods depend upon respiratory exercises and relaxation techniques to control pain perceptions and to reduce tension during childbirth. The woman who is educated for childbirth is likely to require less analgesic medication, have fewer obstetrical complications, and experience less anxiety during labor and delivery (e.g., Hughey, McElin, & Young, 1978; Yang, Zweig, Douthitt, & Federman, 1976). Prepared mothers also express more enjoyment of the birth process (Charles, Norr, Block, Meyering, & Meyers, 1978) and greater maternal satisfaction (Chertok, 1967; Enkin, Smith, Dermer, & Emmett, 1972; Zax, Sameroff, & Farnum, 1975). Furthermore, since mothers who have undergone childbirth education require less medication, their infants tend to be more active and alert following delivery, a result that has both physiological and social benefits (see discussion later in this chapter; cf. Brackbill, 1979; Klaus & Kennell, 1976).

The exact mechanisms by which childbirth education produces these effects are probably multiple and interactive. The relaxation and breathing techniques taught by childbirth educators inhibit muscle tension that would otherwise contribute to the transmission of pain cues and distract the woman, preventing her from attending to pain (Miller & Brooten, 1977). Furthermore, the informed preparation that results from training may inoculate the laboring woman: The knowledgeable laborer is less likely to misinterpret a normal event or an offhand comment by medical personnel. She will understand how long each event is expected to last and can anticipate subsequent occurrences.

In addition to informational support, couples gain emotional support through participation in childbirth classes. The childbirth educator listens to expectant parents' concerns, answers their questions, and provides reassurance—often in a more relaxed manner than the busy physician or nurse. Since both spouses typically attend childbirth preparation classes, the educator also has an opportunity to encourage the development of a supportive relationship between husband and wife by providing tasks that require joint involvement, cooperation, and communication (Hahn & Paige, 1980). Couples may also derive support from other members of the childbirth education class (cf. Wortman & Dunkel-Schetter, 1979). Interaction with other couples helps expectant parents to realize that they are not alone in their fears and anxieties. Furthermore, other couples often serve as sources of additional information and as models with respect to husband–wife communication, affection, and supportive interaction.

Childbirth education classes, however, may not benefit all couples. First, interaction with other members of the class may serve as a source of reinforcement and comfort only when the couple perceives itself to be doing as well as or better than other couples across various domains. If, for example, a woman notices that other husbands provide more aid and affection to their wives than does her husband, she may grow more anxious and angry than she was prior to class attendance.

Second, childbirth education may not suit the personality styles of every expectant parent. Childbirth education classes, at least those teaching Dick-Read or Lamaze techniques, prepare the couple for active involvement in labor and delivery and for sharing decision-making power with the medical staff (Seiden, 1978). Whereas some couples relish the responsibilities of this role, others prefer to place complete trust in the professional's judgment and to accept more passive involvement for themselves (Colman, 1969; Willmuth, Weaver, & Borenstein, 1978).

Third, childbirth may be most pleasant when parental expectations for involvement during labor and delivery are similar to the expectations held by the couple's physician or midwife. Some medical professionals are resistant to the husband's presence during delivery. This may be due to a concern that the father will contaminate the surroundings, that he will faint or be in the way of medical personnel, or that he will closely monitor and evaluate the medical procedures (Hahn & Paige, 1980). Furthermore, some professionals do not appreciate the level of involvement and control over labor that a woman may desire after completing childbirth education classes. When the physician's and couple's expectations for the conduct of labor and delivery do not match, the couple is bound to experience disappointment and anxiety. Therefore, the couple that plans to take an active, involved role in the birth should seek a physician who will sanction and support their involvement.

In sum, medical professionals can alleviate much of the anxiety of pregnancy by including the father in prenatal activities, by providing information and encouraging discussion of parental concerns, and by remaining sensitive to the couple's often unexpressed needs.

Childbirth

In most cases childbirth in a modern hospital is very different from the more social experience of our ancestors. Although some hospital delivery rooms are opening their doors to the friends and family of laboring women and many delivery rooms admit husbands, the woman is still reliant upon the medical staff for much of her social support during childbirth. Childbirth can be either a painful and disappointing experience or a "peak" experience for couples, and the medical staff may be largely responsible for determining the outcome. Whereas many professionals argue that creating pleasant, supportive conditions for the couple is an important goal to be pursued for its own sake, evidence suggests that the benefits of support are numerous and varied. These benefits will be discussed as we elaborate the role that medical professionals play in providing support during childbirth.

One important source of support for the laboring woman and her husband is the delivery room attendant. Attending nurses, as well as physicians or midwives, can offer emotional support by praising the parents for their performance and encouraging them with their tasks. They can alleviate parental anxiety and fear through simple means such as smiling, informing the couple that labor is progressing normally, and avoiding untranslated medical terminology. They can also provide support by monitoring the couple's physical comfort. By offering suggestions that relieve the woman's pain or pressure and by attending to her need for warmth, sustenance, or rest, the attendants aid her in coping with labor. Furthermore, the staff member who ensures that the father has a comfortable chair, pillow, and the opportunity to rest helps him maintain his stamina during a lengthy labor and communicates that his welfare is important.

Although numerous books and articles attest to the benefits of direct social support provided during labor by the medical staff, empirical evidence is rare. Solicitous care from labor and delivery attendants is believed to promote maternal feelings toward the infant (Newton & Newton, 1962). Furthermore, observations of high-risk patients (Haverkamp, Thompson, McFee, & Cetrulo, 1976) suggest that the consistent presence of a reassuring nurse during labor positively affects the infant's health.

Unfortunately, however, solicitous care and a reassuring presence are not universal in hospital delivery rooms (e.g., Blair & Mahoukis, 1980). One-quarter of the women interviewed by Larsen (1966) complained about a lack of interaction and support from the nursing staff, physicians, and husbands, and 12% mentioned feelings of loneliness and uncertainty.[2] Many fathers who accompany their wives during childbirth report that they are ignored and that their needs are "considered last, if at all" (Shannon-Babitz, 1979). During observations of labor and delivery, Danziger (1979) found that nurses and doctors often expect couples to exhibit "normative" and "proper" birthing behaviors. For example, a husband who objected to

---

[2] The introduction of electronic fetal-monitoring equipment has often exacerbated women's feelings of lack of support. Starkman and Youngs (1980) report that women, except those who have experienced a previous fetal death, respond negatively to the use of the equipment, feeling that staff members, and even husbands, direct their attention to the monitor rather than to the woman herself. Furthermore, the sights and sounds of the monitor tend to increase the mother's anxiety. Given evidence that the use of electronic fetal monitors may unnecessarily increase the incidence of Caesarean deliveries (e.g., Haverkamp *et al.,* 1976), professionals and researchers are questioning the benefits of this intervention.

the use of a drug to stimulate his wife's labor was told, ''Well, she's putzy-ing around.'' Furthermore, information was often withheld on the assumption that more information would be stressful to a woman already ''in a state of anxious arousal.'' In addition, parental requests for special treatment (e.g., for a Leboyer delivery) were often acknowledged vaguely and then ignored or forgotten by the staff. Throughout labor, Danziger (1979) reports, ''the parent's perception of the situation remains unexplored, ir-relevant to the course of labor. It is as if the woman's views have no effect upon the physiological events [p. 899].'' Thus, if these observations reflect common experiences, the conduct of delivery is often at variance with the positive intentions of the medical staff (cf. Miller & Brooten, 1977; Swanson, 1978).

In recognition that parents do not always receive the individualized attention and support that they desire during delivery, some professionals have advocated changes in procedures that are likely to foster more support (cf. Sumner & Phillips, 1981). Since consistency of treatment may be important to the childbearing couple, some hospitals have implemented ''on-call'' systems for obstetric nurses, whereby a nurse stays with the couple throughout labor and delivery rather than working designated hours (Clausen, Flook, & Ford, 1977). Some obstetric nurses also meet with couples during prenatal visits so that clients will be familiar with the person who will guide them through most of their labor. Hospitals may also permit private-duty nurses to be hired by the couple to provide uninterrupted care during childbirth and the initial postpartum hours (Carlson & Sumner, 1976; Freeman, 1979). The importance of a continuously present, in-formed supporter is evident in the following comments provided by a couple who had been accompanied throughout labor by a nurse ''monitrice'' (Sumner & Phillips, 1981):

PAT: *Even though we had been extremely well prepared in our class, there were still some things we forgot or didn't anticipate. She [the monitrice] offered sugges-tions . . .*

JIM: *I think her role was almost that of a coach. We were the players and she made suggestions . . . . The coach can make suggestions after having been there or having experienced these things at least one time before.*

Support of Husband's Participation

The busy and limited staff of most hospitals does not have time for ''special'' supportive care. Perhaps partly in recognition of this, more and more obstetricians are encouraging the husband's presence and participation during labor and delivery. Although the evidence is slim, the presence of a supportive spouse may have beneficial effects on women. Women whose husbands are present during labor and delivery are more likely to label childbirth as a "peak experience" and subsequently to report more confidence in their husbands than do women whose husbands are not present (Tanzer, 1967). Furthermore, accompanied wives perceive less discomfort and receive less medication during delivery (Henneborn & Cogan, 1975).

We can suggest a number of reasons why husband participation benefits the laboring woman. First, the husband may be more familiar with techniques to soothe and calm his wife than are attending professionals. And, since his time and attention are not divided among several clients or between responsibilities for medical and nonmedical care, the husband can provide more sustained support. The presence of the husband also provides a touch of familiarity and stability in an otherwise alien hospital environment. Since animal studies have shown that placement in an unfamiliar locale at the onset of labor may result in longer labors and more stillborn offspring (Newton, Foshee, & Newton, 1966), professionals have advocated the presence of familiar others as well as the creation of homelike birthing rooms (Interprofessional Task Force, 1978). Finally, it is possible that the father acts as his wife's advocate during childbirth, ensuring that her needs are met by the medical staff.

It would seem that fathers should also derive benefits from attendance at labor and delivery. Attending fathers are able to share the intense emotional experience of seeing their child born. Those who play an active role during childbirth may also experience a greater feeling of self-worth and confidence as a result of helping their wives.

Interestingly, however, there is little research support for the notion that participation in labor and delivery positively affects paternal adjustment or interaction with the child. One study (Greenberg & Morris, 1974) found that fathers who were present at delivery differed from absent fathers only in the frequency with which they felt they would *recognize their infants.* Although recognition is certainly one step toward building attachment, the two groups did not differ on more critical factors, such as feeling that "the baby was theirs," feeling "glad," being satisfied with the baby's gender, and desiring to share parenting experiences. Furthermore, no differences have been found between fathers who actively coached their wives during childbirth and those who merely attended in terms of adjustment to parenthood or satisfaction with the delivery experience (Wente & Crockenberg, 1976). Participation during delivery can even reduce the father's self-perception of being a supportive spouse. In one study (Richman & Goldthorp, 1978), 48% of the fathers who attended labor but not delivery were "pleased" with their ability to comfort and support their wives; only 35% of the fathers who attended both labor and delivery were pleased.

It has been demonstrated, however, that fathers who are more involved during delivery, who have contact with their infants sooner after delivery, and who spend more time with their infants following delivery report more attachment to their infants (Peterson, Mehl, & Leiderman, 1979). Thus, experiences during the delivery, and not presence at the delivery per se, affect the father. Attendance at childbirth is not enough to ensure a positive outcome. The father has a need to feel involved and useful, as well as to be supported in that involvement by the medical staff.

Support of Early Parent-Infant Interaction

In addition to providing social support directly and encouraging social support between spouses, the medical staff may also support new parents in their early efforts to establish a relationship with their infant. Most new mothers want to have contact with their child immediately after delivery and to remain with their child during the hospital stay (Scaer & Korte, 1978). Immediate contact with the infant may be rewarding and emotionally satisfying to the parent who has just labored and even suffered through childbirth. In addition, new mothers often wish to initiate breast-feeding within an hour after delivery. As we have seen, immediate and sustained contact also facilitates the father's attachment (Peterson et al., 1979). By permitting such open interaction with the infant the hospital staff is showing sensitivity to the new parents' needs. Permission to care for and make decisions about the infant also communicates the professional's confidence in the parents' ability, which may be especially important to the insecure first-time parent. Furthermore, since the unmedicated infant is particularly active, exploratory, and, hence, social during the initial postpartum hours, immediate contact with the infant is likely to promote a higher quality of parent-infant relationship (Klaus & Kennell, 1976; see also Brackbill, 1979). Although parents may become attached to a child at any time (Parke, 1979), there is evidence that immediate postpartum contact facilitates the attachment process.

Delay of nonessential medical procedures may further increase the support offered to the couple's interactions with the newborn infant. For example, unless medically contraindicated, the routine application of silver nitrate or achromycin ointment may be omitted or delayed until the infant is sleepy (Faxel, 1980; Sugarman, 1977). Since the chemical may create eye irritation and sensitivity to light, infants who receive this treatment immediately after birth may achieve less eye contact with parents during their initial interaction than do other infants. Furthermore, the routine feeding of supplementary formula or water interferes with maternal attempts to establish breast-feeding (Salomon, Schauf, & Seiden, 1977). In addition, circumcision of male infants during the initial postpartum days can increase infant irritability and restlessness, thereby creating more difficulties for parents who are attempting to learn how to interact with and care for a young child (Sugarman, 1977; Wallerstein, 1980).

Three kinds of supportive measures have been suggested as useful during childbirth: direct solicitous attention from medical professionals, the presence and informed participation of the husband, and efforts to facilitate early parent–child interaction. Such supportive measures increase the likelihood that the couple will derive satisfaction from the birth experience, and such measures foster a positive beginning to their new family life.

Support during the Postpartum Months

The postpartum period may bring with it the most need for additional social support from medical personnel or allied professionals. As the parents' needs for information and emotional succorance increase, many of the support systems that had developed during the prenatal months are withdrawn. The childbirth education class is over, although some instructors encourage their postpartum clients to keep in touch. Visitors who flocked to the family's side during the first postpartum days have settled back into their own routines. Furthermore, the husband often withdraws some of the additional support he had offered during pregnancy (Raush, Barry, Hertel, & Swain, 1974), and neither husband nor wife may have time or energy to fulfill adequately each other's needs for support.

Although it is evident that medical professionals cannot solve or even address all of the difficulties faced by new parents, some procedures may help to alleviate parental stress. First, physicians and nurses can offer direct emotional and esteem support during contacts with parents. Because they recognize the importance of providing support to new parents, some pediatricians urge parents to return for a well-baby visit at 2 weeks postpartum, rather than the typical 4 weeks. Although usually not necessary for the child's well-being, the early visit serves to support the parent. The physician can reassure the couple that their infant is healthy and that they are performing well as new parents. In addition, a sincerely expressed concern during the visit about "how things are going" provides the parent with a much-needed opportunity to ventilate his or her feelings and will convince the parent of the professional's interest and concern (cf. Brown, W. A., 1979).

Medical professionals may also provide informational support that leads to better parent–infant interaction. Preparation for parenthood varies widely, and many new parents lack knowledge about infant capabilities and behavior (Riesch, 1979; Snyder, Eyres, & Barnard, 1979). For example, when first-time mothers were asked when they would "start teaching things" to their infant, they estimated ages ranging from birth up to 1 year (Snyder *et al.*, 1979). Responses also ranged from birth to 1 year when the mothers were asked when the child would start to become aware of his or her surroundings, and from birth to 2 years when they were asked when it was important to talk to the infant. Furthermore, new mothers often fail to detect when their infant focuses attention on them (Riesch, 1979). As a consequence of lack of information about infant behavior, parents lose opportunities for social interaction and fail to experience the joy that ensues from recognizing the interactive quality of the parent–child relationship (cf. Stern, 1977).

Medical professionals sometimes direct parents to parenting or child-care manuals or to various parental support groups (e.g., La Leche League) in order to provide them with needed information and emotional succorance (Cronenwett, 1980; McGuire & Gottlieb, 1979; Silverman & Murrow, 1976; Turner & Izzi, 1978). Others attempt to build the parents' knowledge base through direct intervention during postpartum hospital or office visits. With the parent as observer, the professional can perform a complete test of neonatal abilities, drawing attention to the child's capabilities and addressing parental concerns (Riesch, 1979). Information that is imparted during office visits is likely to increase parental sensitivity to the child (Casey & Whitt, 1979), which in turn affects the child's development (e.g., Donovan & Leavitt, 1978; Osofsky, 1979).

Once again, during the postpartum months the father's needs for support are likely to go unmet. Although some hospitals or physicians offer new-father or couple support groups (e.g., McGuire & Gottlieb, 1979), most of the parenting organizations are directed toward helping the new mother. The father may also be less likely to come into contact with medical professionals than is the mother. There are a few ways, however, in which the father can be supported. First, the physician or nurse practitioner can solicit information about the husband's reactions to fatherhood during the mother's office visits and can suggest methods of coping with the difficulties he may be experiencing. The professional may also suggest that the father call to discuss his concerns. Second, some childbirth educators contact the family following childbirth to congratulate the parents and to inquire about the birth experience. Contacts should be arranged when both parents are available to offer their views. Third, the medical professional or others can encourage the couple to plan for and support the father's involvement with the child. Some women, perceiving themselves to be more knowledgeable about child care than their husbands, convey the message that he is not competent. Admonitions to ''not drop her'' or to ''hold his head carefully'' make the father feel inadequate and may cause him to withdraw from interaction with his child. The professional can inform women of the potential impact of these communications on their spouse. The professional can also guide parents in defining specific functions for the father to perform. Fathers are more satisfied when they have a role to play with respect to the child, regardless of the particular characteristics of the role (Fein, 1976). Thus, just as during the childbirth itself, fathers want to feel that they are needed and that they are contributing something of importance to the family's well-being.

CONCLUDING REMARKS

In this chapter we have suggested that medical and allied professionals should provide social support to expectant and new parents. Support may be in the form of information, assistance, and esteem and emotional comfort. As we have seen, professionals may offer support directly or may facilitate the supportive roles of others. Supportive care may buffer the effects of stresses that the couple is likely to experience during the childbearing year. It may also eliminate some sources of stress. Since the childbearing couple is dependent upon the professional for their health needs and for guidance, a warm, sensitive, concerned professional will build the couple's confidence and trust and put them at ease. In contrast, nonsupportive professionals not only will fail to help couples with the problems they are experiencing but also will contribute to these problems. The professional is thus well positioned to aid the couple during the childbearing year.

Throughout this chapter it has been evident that the family is a complex social system, wherein each family member affects and is affected by the other. For this reason, we have suggested that professionals may best support each family member by regarding the events of the childbearing year from the perspective of both husband and wife. Including the father in prenatal, perinatal, and postnatal activities increases the likelihood that the father's real and legitimate needs will be met. A father who receives support may then provide better support for his wife, which in turn may affect the well-being of their child.

It is clear that more careful research is needed to specify the exact role of social support during the transition to new parenthood. Enough preliminary work has been done, however, to convince professionals that their affective and behavioral relationship with clients is of consequence. Thus, professionals who are primarily concerned with maintaining the physical health of the childbearing couple must necessarily monitor the couple's psychological health as well. Such monitoring may contribute to building a positive foundation for family development.

7

Nancy E. Adler

The Abortion Experience: Social and Psychological Influences and Aftereffects

All medical procedures can be examined from a social psychological perspective in terms of the interaction of the care giver and patient. Some of the more serious and/or chronic health problems and their associated treatments also involve patients' broader social networks of family, friends, and sometimes coworkers. Among medical procedures, abortion is unusual in that it not only involves this level of interpersonal interaction but also is enmeshed in a broader social context involving legal, political, economic, theological, and moral issues, which impinge on the experience of the individual woman undergoing the procedure.

The most dramatic effects on the nature of the abortion experience have resulted from shifts in the legal restrictions on the procedure. The legal definitions of abortion, in turn, are a reflection of political, economic, and religious concerns. The United States had virtually no federal or state strictures on the performance of abortions prior to the 1820s. States began to pass statutes regulating the practice of abortion beginning in 1820 and lasting through the end of the century. By 1900 restrictive abortion laws existed in every jurisdiction. Mohr (1978), a historian who traced the evolution of abortion laws, documents a variety of pressures for the enactment of these statutes. The first laws, enacted between 1821 and 1841 reflected not

119

opposition to abortion per se but concern about the safety of the procedure. These laws were passed as part of general revisions of criminal codes and were intended to protect women against poisoning. However, pressure arose in the 1840s against the practice of abortion itself. Mohr attributes this pressure to three trends: the greater commercialization and visibility of abortion, the increased use of the procedure, especially by married, native-born Protestant women, and the growing awareness by "establishment" males that abortion was, in fact, becoming more common among these women. These three trends contributed to a concern among lawmakers that the use of abortion could threaten the population balance in the United States by reducing the number of babies born to middle- and upper-class women. At the same time, physicians were bringing pressure to bear on legislatures to limit the practice of abortion. Most of the abortions were being performed by "irregular" doctors who were in economic and ideological opposition to the more scientifically trained physicians. In their attempt to professionalize and control the practice of medicine, in 1847 the latter founded the American Medical Association, which was committed to outlawing abortion. The physicians' campaign was eventually successful in changing abortion laws. However, Mohr notes that although the laws were changed, public opinion was still quite favorable to the practice. Moreover, most other groups and organizations, including religious groups, did not become involved in the campaign.

The abortion laws that were passed in the latter part of the nineteenth century remained virtually unchanged until the 1970s. These laws were either prohibitive or extremely restrictive. States that permitted abortion generally did so only upon proof that continuation of a pregnancy would pose a threat to a woman's life or health. In a few states, threat to health was interpreted to include mental health, and most legal abortions were granted on these grounds. In the 1960s and 1970s there arose organized opposition to restrictions on abortion. In contrast to the earlier campaign for more restrictive abortion laws, the medical profession was vocal in its opposition to restrictive legislation. Given changes in economic and social realities, health care providers were now most aware of the terrible costs of illegal abortions in terms of maternal morbidity and mortality. In addition, the decriminalization of abortion would bring the procedure into the sphere of legitimate medical practice.

Although some changes in the availability of abortion occured through legislative actions in states such as California and New York, the greatest change occurred as a result of the United States Supreme Court decision of 1973 that legalized abortion on a national level. The Court declared that a woman has a constitutionally protected right to obtain an abortion, a right that is derived from the right to privacy. However, there are limitations on this right. In its decision, the Court asserted that the state has no compelling interest during the first trimester; in this period the outcome should be left totally to the decision of the woman and her physician. Beyond the end of the first trimester the state has a reasonable concern about protecting the health of the woman and can impose restrictions designed to protect her safety. Commencing with viability (which has been placed at the beginning of the third trimester), the state "in promoting its interest in the potentiality of human life may, if it chooses, regulate and even proscribe abortion except where necessary in appropriate medical judgment for the preservation of the life or the health of the mother [Holman, 1973, p. 216]."

Following the Supreme Court decision, abortion technically was legally available everywhere in the United States and was equivalent to any other medical procedure in that respect. However, there is a good deal of evidence that abortion has not been treated like other medical procedures. There are many areas in which abortion simply is not available. In 1976, 34% of all women needing abortion services (over 600,000) were not able to obtain them (Forrest, Tietze, & Sullivan, 1978); in 1978, 26% (over 479,000) of women in need were unable to obtain these services (Forrest, Sullivan, & Tietze, 1979). Abortion services are not well distributed; they tend to be concentrated in large urban areas and in states that had relatively permissive abortion laws before the Supreme Court decision (Richards, 1978). For example, approximately 40% of all abortions performed in the first quarter of 1974 occurred in California and New York, which have about 20% of all United States women of reproductive age, whereas several states (e.g., Louisiana, Mississippi, and North Dakota) reported almost no abortions (Weinstock, Tietze, Jaffe, & Dryfoos, 1975). By 1977 this had changed somewhat, but 9% of abortion patients still had to travel out of state for the procedure, and identified abortion providers could be found in only 23% of United States counties (Forrest *et al.*, 1979).

In addition, abortion services are not organized along the lines of most medical services. Nathanson and Becker (1980) note that the

> mode of delivery of abortion services that has evolved in the United States since the U.S. Supreme Court legalized abortion in 1973 is markedly different from the pattern characteristic of other minor surgical procedures: tonsillectomies, routine D & C's and most deliveries occur in hospitals, but six out of 10 abortions are performed in freestanding nonhospital clinics [p. 26].

In fact, between 1976 and 1977 the average number of abortions per hospital actually dropped, whereas procedures done in clinics or private offices increased (Forrest *et al.*, 1979).

Despite the fact that abortions have not been treated as have other minor surgical procedures, following the Supreme Court decision there were significant changes in the availability and status of abortion. In the years following this decision there has been a tremendous increase in the availability of legal abortions, a sharp decline in death rates associated with illegal abortions (Center for Disease Control, 1978), and a shift in public opinion toward more favorable attitudes. This shift was particularly sharp immediately following the 1973 Supreme Court decision and became gradually more positive since then (Arney & Trescher, 1976; Gallup, 1978). At the same time, organized opposition to abortion began to grow and set the stage for recent legislation banning the use of federal money for abortions except in specifically defined situations. A 1977 Supreme Court decision on abortion ruled that states are not required to provide abortions for women who cannot afford them. In addition to legislative conflicts in individual states over whether abortions for poor women will be paid for with state funds, lobbying is underway for a federal constitutional amendment prohibiting abortions altogether. There also has been an increasing number of anti-abortion demonstrations, including sit-ins and violence directed against clinics across the country.

AFTEREFFECTS OF ABORTION

It is not surprising that research on abortion has mirrored the social and historical trends that have been noted in the preceding discussion. Research from the 1940s through the 1960s generally concluded that abortion was a traumantic experience, one that was likely to lead to psychopathology (see, for example, Bolter, 1962; Ebaugh & Heuser, 1947; summary in Simon & Senturia, 1966, and discussion in Sarvis & Rodman, 1973). This research reflected the widely accepted belief that abortion was beyond the range of "normal" experiences. It was a taboo subject, and both researchers and laymen appeared to assume that it would not be possible to undergo such an experience without emotional trauma. However, the research on which these assertions were based was not an adequate basis for the conclusions that were reached. Serious methodological problems in sample selection often occurred. For example, samples were often chosen from populations of women seeking therapy, and the negative psychological states of these individuals were assumed to be representative of all women who had undergone abortion. In addition, the phenomenon of abortion itself was not clearly defined. Differentiations were not made between women who had undergone legal or illegal abortion, between women who had undergone first-trimester or second-trimester abortion, or between women who were or were not sterilized at the time of the abortion. Termination of pregnancy was seen as the single crucial event, and concurrent events, even if powerful, were not identified as important.

In addition to biases introduced by the nature of the research itself, the conclusions were frequently influenced by the beliefs of researchers and writers. Kummer (1963) noted that the frequent reference in medical literature to postabortion psychiatric illness was not based on statistical documentation. His review of literature from other countries and a survey of experiences of United States psychiatrists led him to conclude that the widely held belief in psychiatric problems following abortion was a myth resulting from the enforcement of a taboo against abortion. Although value biases are a problem in many areas of research, they seem to have been particularly strong in the early abortion research. This may have been because of the complexity of the subject and the difficulty of obtaining representative samples, as well as the strong emotional and social beliefs about abortion. Simon and Senturia (1966) reviewed the literature from 1935 to 1964 on psychiatric aftereffects of abortion and concluded that "deeply held personal convictions frequently seem to outweigh the importance of the data, especially when conclusions are drawn [p. 387]."

A dramatic shift in conclusions regarding psychological aftereffects of abortion occurred in the 1960s and 1970s. A study done in Scandinavia by Ekblad (1955) is often considered a turning point. This was the first large-scale, relatively well controlled study of legal abortion. It revealed few serious psychological problems following abortion. Since then, numerous studies on the effects of abortion have been conducted in the United States. The studies have almost unanimously concluded that strong negative reactions are rare (e.g., Brody, Meikle, & Gerritse, 1971; Osofsky & Osofsky, 1972; Patt, Rappaport, & Barglow, 1969; Peck & Marcus, 1966; Senay, 1970; Smith, 1973; Whittington, 1970). The predominant response immediately following abortion most often is relief (Ewing & Rouse, 1973; Monsour & Stewart, 1973; Simon, Senturia & Rothman, 1967); improvement in mood and functioning from the preabortion to the postabortion state has also been shown (Brody et al., 1971; Niswander & Patterson, 1967). However, negative effects have been observed as well, and some women report periods of regret, depression, and guilt following the procedure (Ford, Castelnuovo-Tedesco, & Long, 1971; Peck & Marcus, 1966; Smith, 1973); these are usually experienced to a mild degree and diminish over time.

Several studies have gone beyond mere description of responses to abortion to consider the characteristics associated with more positive or negative reactions. This research begins to shed some light on the nature of abortion and the influence of social psychological variables on responses to the procedure. These research findings will be discussed, and their implications for understanding the abortion experience will be considered next.

Demographic Variables

Age, marital status, and religion have frequently been found to be associated with postabortion responses. On the average, younger women react more negatively than do older; unmarried women more negatively than married; and Catholic women more negatively than non-Catholic (e.g., Adler, 1975; Bracken, Hachamovitch, & Grossman, 1974; Osofsky & Osofsky, 1972; Payne, Kravitz, Notman, & Anderson, 1976).

Demographic variables are not independent of one another: age and marital status, for example, are generally highly correlated since older women are more likely than younger to be married. However, research has shown that these variables can have independent as well as joint effects on postabortion responses (Adler, 1975).

Social Variables

The extent to which having an abortion is a woman's own choice, and the degree of support she receives for this choice from other people who are important to her, can play a significant role in her response to the procedure. The strongest negative reactions are likely to occur in women who did not themselves want to terminate their pregnancies but who were persuaded or coerced to do so by their partner or parents (Senay, 1970). In recognition of this, one major goal in counseling a woman seeking an abortion is often to establish whether the decision is the woman's own, and to give her an opportunity to discuss her choice with a neutral person.

A more common situation is one in which a woman herself wants to terminate her pregnancy, but significant others are opposed or disapproving, or would be if they knew. In some instances, the woman may not tell her partner or parents about the pregnancy or her intention to have an abortion for fear of opposition or of disapproval of the pregnancy and/or the abortion. Bracken *et al.* (1974) examined the relationship between social support from parents and partner and immediate postabortion responses. In cases in which parents did not know about the abortion, the women's estimate of their anticipated reaction was used. Postabortion responses were more positive when there was greater social support for the abortion, suggesting that one source of stress for a woman is known or anticipated disapproval of significant others. Not surprisingly, the reaction of the partner was more highly related to postabortion responses for women who were 23 years of age or older, whereas among the younger women parental support was more important than that of the partner. Bracken, Klerman, and Bracken (1978) found among a sample of never-married women that those who were continuing the pregnancy, as well as those who were terminating it, found the decision to be easier, and were more likely to accept and be satisfied with the choice, if the decision was supported by significant others.

The Abortion Setting

Remarkably little attention has been given to the effects of the social environment surrounding the abortion procedure itself. Abortions are performed in a variety of settings including hospitals, clinics, physicians' offices, and ''back alleys.'' It seems likely that a legal, safe abortion will have a markedly different impact on a woman than an illegal procedure. In the latter, the procedure is likely not only to be far more physically painful and traumatic, carrying a significantly greater risk of morbidity and mortality, but also to be done under clandestine circumstances. There has been no research on the differences in responses to abortion under these different circumstances, probably due in large part to the difficulty of obtaining comparable samples of women undergoing illegal versus legal abortions. However, the findings of earlier research that did involve women who had undergone illegal procedures include far more negative effects than do the more recent research findings on women undergoing legal abortions. Although some of this difference may arise from changes in methods, assumptions, and biases of researchers, some of the shift in findings regarding abortion undoubtedly is due to improvements in the conditions under which abortions are performed.

We also know very little about the effect of the delivery system for legal abortions. As noted earlier, abortion services have been organized differently from other services. Women undergoing abortions are likely to have their procedures in a special abortion clinic. This may cause problems for some women since it differentiates abortion from other medical procedures. The clinics may be seen as less legitimate places than hospitals and may increase the woman's sense that she is doing a socially stigmatized act. However, the clinics also serve some positive functions. They are designed for the specific needs of abortion patients. Women who have abortions in hospitals are frequently treated on the obstetrical floor and are surrounded by an environment geared for delivery of babies. Not only can the clinics separate abortion patients from obstetrical patients, but also clients of such clinics are likely to come in contact with other women who are undergoing the same procedure. This gives an opportunity for peer support. It may also serve to destigmatize the procedure. One woman who had recently undergone an abortion at a clinic reported to me that she had expected that the other women there would all be prostitutes or teenagers. She was amazed and relieved to find that many of the other patients seemed to be just like her and her friends. Thus, even without explicit peer support, the opportunity to see others like oneself undergoing the procedure may be beneficial.

Abortion Procedures

One cannot speak of abortion as though it were a single universally applied procedure. Although all serve to terminate pregnancy, there are many different techniques that are called abortion. They range from a dilation and evacuation (D & E), which takes only 10–15 min and can be done with local anesthetic, to saline abortion, which involves injection of a saline solution into the amniotic sac, bringing about the expulsion of the dead fetus within approximately 24 hr. The abortion procedures used in the first versus the second trimester carry different rates of morbidity and mortality and involve quite different experiences. It is difficult, however, to compare the relative impact of early versus later procedures since women who delay until the second trimester differ in a number of ways from women who act more promptly to terminate an unwanted pregnancy. Differences have been found in demographic variables, such as age, race, marital status, and income, as well as in psychological variables, such as use of denial, ambivalence about the pregnancy and type of relationship with parents (Bracken & Kasl, 1976; Kaltreider, 1973; Kerenyi, Glascock, & Horowitz, 1973). Kaltreider, Goldsmith, and Margolis (1979) note that women undergoing second-trimester abortion are frequently ''young adolescents overwhelmed by a first pregnancy and older women who are ambivalent about the emotional and economic costs of an additional child [p. 238].''

Beyond differences in characteristics of women undergoing early versus late procedures, the experience of saline abortion used in later pregnancy is likely to be more stressful than procedures used for early abortion. Bracken et al. 1974) note that the saline procedure ''performed after quickening when fetal movement may already have resulted in some psychological investment in the fetus, culminates in the delivery of a dead fetus. Intuitively one would expect this to result in more serious psychological sequelae than the relatively innocuous early pregnancy suction procedures [p. 154].'' Research findings support their hypothesis. Kaltreider (1973) conducted interviews with women a few days following their abortions. Whereas women who had undergone an early abortion reported a sense of relief and a desire to take up life where they had left off, the mid-trimester group described more mixed feelings or tried to continue coping by the use of denial. They described themselves as empty and having lost a ''child,'' a feeling not reported by women aborted in the first trimester. Osofsky, Osofsky, Rajan, and Sptiz (1975) also found greater difficulty among saline patients than among first-trimester patients or those aborted by D & E at 14–17 weeks.

The use of D & E in the second trimester has recently been expanded, and its application poses some difficult problems. It appears to be safer physically, is experienced as less painful and stressful, and is associated with more positive psychological outcomes for the patient than is the saline procedure (Kaltreider et al., 1979; Osofsky et al., 1975). At the same time, it is a far more emotionally draining experience for the physician performing the procedure and ''shifts some of the emotional problems of the abortion away from the woman and onto the physician [Kaltreider et al., 1979, p. 235].'' The difficulties associated with second-trimester D & E compound the already-growing problem of professional staff reaction to participating in abortions, which will be discussed later.

Treatment by Staff

The reactions of health care providers who come in contact with abortion patients may affect patients' responses to the procedure. Walter (1970) notes that "a critical factor in mild, immediate guilt is the actual physical setup of the clinical situation and the attitude of the people caring for the patient [p. 284]." Marder (1970) similarly comments that "hostility and resentment toward the patient by staff and nursing personnel have been responsible for some of the emotional disturbances experienced by patients [p. 1236]." Evans and Gusdon (1973) also attribute patient responses to the treatment received from staff, who sometimes communicate their disapproval of abortion both verbally and nonverbally.

Negative treatment of abortion patients by staff may be subtle. Wolff, Nielson, and Schiller (1971) compared hospital records of 50 abortion patients, 25 nonpregnant patients undergoing D & C (dilation and curettage), and 25 vaginal hysterectomy patients. The charts of the abortion patients differed from the others. Although abortion patients may, in fact, have behaved differently than did other patients the nature of the differences in chart content and tone suggest some problems in staff reaction. The material in the abortion patients' charts was often confused and overly elabortated, seemingly reflecting a sense of uneasiness about the patient and the abortion. Such uneasiness may well be communicated to the patient and increase her sense of shame or guilt over the abortion.

Interpersonal treatment is not the only way in which staff behavior can affect postabortion reactions. Another important variable is the medical treatment received by the patient. Bracken (1978) found that a patient's anxiety following abortion was related to how much pain she reported experiencing during the procedure. The report of pain was found to be a function of the skill of the physician performing the procedure as well as of the woman's anxiety prior to the abortion.

Counseling

Unlike preparation for other procedures, women who are in the process of obtaining an abortion are likely to receive counseling from a person other than the health care provider. Such counseling may range from an in-depth exploration of a woman's situation and feelings to a brief information-giving session (Baldwin, 1973; Goldsmith, Potts, Green, & Miller, 1970; Spaght, Kenan, & Torrington, 1973). The typical counselor is likely to be similar to the patient. One survey of counselors found the vast majority to be sexually active women of childbearing age. Many were volunteers, and none received special training in abortion counseling outside of the setting in which they provided their services (Dauber, 1974).

There are a number of purposes of counseling that reflect different aspects of the abortion experience. One purpose is to give each woman the opportunity to discuss her decision with a neutral person. This is done in recognition that the procedure is elective and that the woman may be under conflicting pressures to make one or another decision. Most counseling is designed to assure that the woman is not being coerced into having the procedure and that she understands the choices she can make and the possible outcome of these choices. Unfortunately, some organizations that provide counseling do not do this. Rather, they have a general position on abortion and add their own pressures for one or another resolution.

A second purpose of counseling is to prepare the woman for the procedure so that she understands what will happen to her. Because of the legacy of illegal abortion, which was often painful and dangerous, women may be particularly fearful about it. In fact, some women decide against abortion because of their fear of the procedure (Swigar, Breslin, Pouzzner, Quinlan, & Blum, 1976). The procedure is, in fact, rather simple (though it can be painful), and accurate information should reduce anxiety.

A third purpose of counseling is to provide information on birth control. Most providers take the position that the need for abortion reflects a failure of adherence to a recommended regimen of contraception. Contraception is stressed in order to avoid the need for a repeat abortion.

The effects of counseling have not been systematically evaluted. There is some anecdotal evidence that it does prepare women better for the procedure. Some physicians have said that when they perform abortions they can tell which patients have received counseling and which have not by how tense or relaxed the woman is. Tension, in turn, affects the difficulty of performing the abortion and the degree of pain the woman experiences.

Bracken, Grossman, Hachamovitch, Sussman, and Schrier (1973) found that most women who received counseling felt it was beneficial. They compared reactions of women who had received three different types of counseling: (a) group orientation, in which groups of four to eight women received a description of the procedure and information regarding birth control but had no discussion; (b) group process, in which a similar number of women received the same information but also engaged in a discussion of social and psychological problems; and (c) individual counseling, in which the patient met alone with a counselor and discussed her attitude toward abortion, her own situation, and birth control (but to a lesser extent than in group situations). Follow-up was conducted in the recovery room after the abortion. The greatest satisfaction with the counseling experience was expressed by women given individual counseling, but the women who had been given either of the group treatments actually showed more favorable responses to the abortion (i.e., they felt calmer and happier and experienced less pain). There was an interaction of treatment and age. Younger women reacted better to the abortion after receiving group rather than individual counseling. Older women showed more favorable responses to abortion when counseled individually.

It also appears that counseling may be effective in encouraging women to return for postabortion checkups. Dauber, Zalar, and Goldstein (1972) found that 94 of 99 women who received counseling returned to the hospital for a checkup, whereas only 60 out of 99 uncounseled patients returned. Return for follow-up is particularly important since it can reduce the incidence of complications as well as provide further information and encouragement for contraceptive use.

That counseling has been a major part of abortion services and absent in other medical services underscores the unique aspects of abortion. There are many other procedures where counseling could be as important but where it is not stressed. In other elective surgery, (e.g., cosmetic surgery, gastric bypass) individuals may be confused about the right decision and may be under pressure to undergo a procedure. Although they may receive some counseling from the provider, there is usually no requirement or encouragement for separate counseling before the provider is contacted or the service is provided. Similarly, there are other procedures (e.g., hysterectomy, breast biopsy and mastectomy) that are equally or more stressful than abortion and for which women receive little additional preparation beyond that given by individual providers. That counseling is frequently a part of the process of obtaining an abortion may be because many of the services grew up outside of traditional medical settings. Individuals (frequently nonphysicians) who had been dealing with women in need of abortion services and were already involved in referral for services were frequently instrumental in the planning of abortion clinics and included counseling as a necessary component. Beyond this, however, the inclusion of counseling may also reflect the effects of the abortion taboo and the belief that women need careful counseling before taking such an abnormal act as terminating a pregnancy.

The fact that counseling has been provided for abortion patients and not for others should not be taken to mean that counseling should be eliminated for the former. Rather, it may argue for the inclusion of counseling in other medical services. As abortions have become more widespread and as research has shown that serious aftereffects are relatively rare, the use of counseling has diminished. Proponents of counseling are frequently asked to justify its need, and particularly to document its cost-effectiveness. Bracken (1977) has pointed out that although abortion does not appear to leave women in an adverse psychological state, this does not imply that they approach the procedure without stress and anguish. Unfortunately, there are few studies that one can use to judge the efficacy of counseling in terms of either immediate or long-term effects other than the ones already cited. It would be useful, for example, to study procedure-related variables for women who have and have not received counseling. One could examine the effects of counseling on variables such as pain perception, amount of analgesia required, and time taken to perform the procedure. The last two variables would have clear cost implications. In addition, studies to determine later effects of counseling are needed. If the results of Dauber *et al.* (1972) hold up, one could also justify counselng in terms of its positive effect on follow-up, which could reduce complications and incidence of repeat procedures.

Individual Variables

Individual women undergoing abortion under seemingly similar circumstances vary widely in their responses. Payne *et al.* (1976) identified seven factors that predicted difficulty in working through the conflicts associated with unwanted pregnancy and abortion: (*a*) prior history of mental illness; (*b*) immature interpersonal relationships; (*c*) unstable, conflicted relationship with one's partner; (*d*) history of a negative relationship with one's mother; (*e*) ambivalence regarding abortion; (*f*) religious or cultural background hostile to abortion; and (*g*) single status, especially if one has not borne children. Ewing and Rouse (1973) also found that prior psychiatric history was associated with more negative aftereffects. It should be noted that these characteristics are associated with *relative* risk and should not be considered contraindications for abortion. These same variables may predict problems following any decision. There is no stressfree solution to the occurrence of an unwanted pregnancy, and many of the variables seem to reflect possible problems of adjustment to stress. Abortion may be the best choice among the various alternatives. Payne *et al.* (1976) noted that, at the 6-month follow-up, women in even the most vulnerable groups reported, almost without exception, that the decision to have an abortion was the right one. Ewing and Rouse (1973) similarly concluded that although women with psychiatric histories were at higher risk, abortion was still therapeutic for them and that the actual incidence of emotional symptoms was low.

As noted earlier, age is associated with differences in negative effects. Age not only is a demographic variable but also reflects differences in psychosocial development. Schaffer and Pine (1972) argue that pregnancy in adolescent girls involves a conflict between being mothered and being a mother. Postabortion adjustment was found to depend in part on whether the girl's identification was more with the infant or with her own mother. Those who identified more with the former tended to become passive, letting their mother take charge, and to establish regressive ties with the mother. Those who identified with the mothering role were more able to care for themselves and coped more successfully with the abortion. Hatcher (1976) identified varying response patterns in the different stages of adolescence: early (12–15 years), middle (15–18 years), and late (18–21 years). The role and nature of significant other people in the abortion decision, the adolescent's defensive style, and her reaction to abortion all varied by stage. Consistent with other research, the older adolescents generally showed the most positive responses. They were more realistic about the pregnancy and were able to anticipate some of the sense of loss. On later follow-up, they felt more matured by the experience than did younger adolescents. In contrast, early adolescents dealt with both the pregnancy and the abortion with denial. Continuing a pattern of denial following the abortion, they were the hardest to study and avoided returning for follow-up. Middle adolescents were most concerned about autonomy during the decision-making stage. They experienced more postabortion depression than they had anticipated. On later follow-up, they were disappointed that they had not achieved independence with their pregnancy and that their parents had not changed. This group was more likely than others to experience repeat pregnancy.

Pregnancies are terminated for a variety of reasons, and the reasons behind seeking an abortion will be likely to influence the emotional aftereffects. Prior to the availability of abortion on demand, legal abortions were granted on one of three grounds: medical (continuation of the pregnancy would pose a threat to the life or health of the mother), eugenic (there was a good possibility of fetal deformity), or psychiatric (continuation of the pregnancy would pose a threat to the mental health of the mother). Several studies have revealed varying aftereffects among women aborted for these different reasons. Peck and Marcus (1966) found more frequent reports of depression among women who had undergone abortion on medical grounds than among those aborted on psychiatric grounds. No significant differences in amount of reported guilt were found between the groups. Simon et al. (1967), however, did find differences in reported levels of guilt. Moderate to marked guilt in a 10-year period following the abortion was reported by 25% of the women aborted for psychiatric reasons, 33% of those aborted because of rubella exposure, and 50% of those aborted on medical grounds. Niswander and Patterson (1967) also found a relatively greater frequency of unfavorable responses among women aborted for physical reasons than among those aborted for psychiatric reasons.

The differences in responses to abortion probably reflect differences in the extent to which women in each group wanted to continue their pregnancy and in the extent of loss experienced. Women in the psychiatric group may have experienced the least loss; if the pregnancy was a threat to their mental health, it would have been experienced as psychologically burdensome, and its termination, although representing some loss, would also have been likely to bring about psychological relief. Pregnancies terminated on medical and eugenic grounds were more likey to be pregnancies that the women wanted to continue had it not been for the threat to their health or the likelihood of deformity. Thus, one would expect a greater sense of loss. The sense of loss may be particularly great among women in the medical group, since their future childbearing may be more threatened than that of women in the other two groups.

In recent years, the introduction of amniocentesis to identify genetic abnormalities has led to another category of women who are terminating their pregnancies. These women are generally carrying a wanted pregnancy that they would physically be able to carry to term but that is terminated because of the negative outcome of amniocentesis. In addition, the amniocentesis cannot be performed until the fifteenth week of gestation, so that these women must undergo the more stressful second-trimester abortion procedures. The women may also experience feelings of shame or guilt for having produced a "defective" baby. One study (Blumberg, Golbus, & Hanson, 1975), which followed 13 families in which the woman had terminated her pregnancy following amniocentesis, found evidence of depression among the majority of both men and women; the incidence was much higher than in comparable samples of women undergoing elective abortion. One woman in the sample who had previously had an abortion on psychosocial grounds stated that the postamniocentesis abortion was far more upsetting and difficult. Although more research is needed comparing the responses of women undergoing abortion on different grounds, it appears that women who are terminating their pregnancies because of genetic abnormalities may be at particularly great risk for negative reactions to the experience.

THE EXPERIENCE OF ABORTION

The preceding discussion has considered the relationship of individual variables to reactions to abortion. However, abortion is a complex event. Responses are not determined by a single variable or set of variables. The manner in which any woman responds to the procedure will be a joint function of her psychological state and the social and physical environment in which the abortion occurs. Thus, it seems most appropriate to view abortion in a relatively broad perspective. In addition, although the individual woman is most involved and has rightly been of predominant concern to researchers, one needs also to consider the effects of the experience on other participants.

Comparison of Abortion with Other Procedures

Abortion is an elective procedure, and the individual must decide whether she should or should not have it. However, compared with other procedures, the outcomes are relatively clear: If one has an abortion, the pregnancy will end, and if one does not, she is likely (though not certain) to give birth in a certain number of months. In the abortion decision the major concerns are more frequently psychological and social than medical. The relevant parties to the decision are more likely to be family, partner, and friends and less likely to be medical personnel, as compared with the situation in other surgeries. As has been noted, the woman is far more likely to receive counseling regarding her decision for abortion from someone other than the health care provider than are individuals deciding on other elective procedures. In addition, the decision has consequences not only for the individual woman but also for her partner or family. Thus, the woman frequently has to consider and arbitrate among differing opinions and pressures.

Abortion not only is a surgical procedure but also ends a pregnancy. In this way, it shares with miscarriage the experience of loss. However, abortion is the result of a conscious choice and terminates a pregnancy that is less likely to be wanted. The issue of choice brings with it questions about the beginning of human life and concerns about the moral and religious implications of a decision to have an abortion. Further, abortion has been socially stigmatized so that even a woman who herself believes it to be a morally neutral act is subjected to social pressures that suggest that she is deviant. At the same time, abortion in a single woman acts to end another state that is also socially stigmatized: out-of-wedlock pregnancy.

There is no one procedure that is comparable to abortion. The difficulty of defining an appropriate comparison can be seen in the absence of comparison groups in most research. A few studies have compared reactions of women to abortion with those of women who have carried to term. Fleck (1970) has noted that compared with postpartum blues, postabortion blues are briefer and milder. Athanasiou, Oppel, Michelson, Unger, and Yager (1973) compared women who were matched on various socioeconomic and demographic variables and who underwent early abortion, late abortion, or term delivery. Few differences were found between women terminating or completing their pregnancies. Burnell et al. (cited in Osofsy et al., 1975) compared abortion patients with women who delivered and who placed their infants for adoption and with women having normal term deliveries. Both groups with unwanted pregnancies (abortion and adoption) had more severe psychological problems during pregnancy than did the normal pregnancy group. At follow-up, the abortion group showed much better adjustment and felt less negative about their experience than did women who had delivered and given their babies for adoption.

Interpreting Responses to Abortion

There is some controversy over the relative importance of social and psychological variables with regard to abortion. Early research tended to ignore social variables. Though not often explicitly stated, the assumption underlying the research appears to have been that abortion itself is such a critical event that the effects of other events or of the surrounding circumstances should be negligible. More recent research has focused on situational variables as well as on individual differences in responses to abortion. Some disagreement about the relative impact of social and intrapsychic varibles derives from debate over the appropriate level of analysis.

It is difficult to reconcile data from studies of the conscious and unconscious levels since research focusing on each is generally done within different frameworks, using different methods and utilizing different criteria for evidence. Robbins (1979) notes that women who have undergone an abortion report regret on subjective measures but that long-term changes in psychological state reflected in objective measures are generally positive. Robbins's research showed no relationship between reports of regret and willingness to repeat the abortion under the same circumstances on the one hand, and scores on clinical scales of the Minnesota Multiphasic Personality Inventory (MMPI), on the other. Kent, Greenwood, Nicholls, and Loeken (1978) argue that research using questionnaire data ignores the intrapsychic meaning of abortion. They found more negative responses from clinical data than from self-report.

It is difficult to obtain reliable and valid measures of intrapsychic or unconscious conflict. Most of the evidence derives from clinical case studies that introduce a self-selection bias since the women have sought therapy. No studies to date have shown that legal, safe abortion leads to intrapsychic conflict in general samples sufficient to interfere with normal functioning or to the kinds of emotional or psychological changes that can be detected on diagnostic tests such as the MMPI (Brody *et al.*, 1971; Niswander, Singer, & Singer, 1972).

Nonetheless, abortion is generally experienced as a stressful event. Much of the stress is associated with the discovery and acknowledgment of an unwanted pregnancy and the need for a decision about whether to continue or to terminate it. Additional anxiety may be generated for women who are not sure if they will actually be able to obtain an abortion (a situation that will become more common with increasing restrictions on abortion). Women generally report that the time of greatest distress is between the discovery that they are pregnant and the abortion. Thus, the psychosocial aftereffects of abortion must be viewed not only as reactions to abortion per se but also as reactions to the experience of having had and terminated an unwanted pregnancy.

Abortion as Crisis

Payne *et al.* (1976) argue that unwanted pregnancy and abortion can best be understood in terms of a model of crisis and crisis resolution. As with other crises, it holds the potential for psychological maturation for women who master the experience successfully.

What is the nature of the crisis associated with abortion? Some ideas can be drawn from a factor analysis of emotional responses in a 3-month period following abortion (Adler, 1975). The first of three factors from this analysis consisted of two positive emotions: relief and happiness. Although these positive emotions were experienced most strongly by women following abortion, reactions to abortion are not unidimensional. Women are most likely to experience relief and happiness afterward, but they may also feel regret, guilt, or anger. The negative emotions themselves separated into two factors. One factor consisted of the emotions of guilt, shame, and fear of disapproval and reflects the social stigma and norm violation associated with unwanted pregnancy and abortion. Not surprisingly, several demographic variables that reflect the extent to which social disapproval was likely to be encountered were found to correlate with this factor. Younger women, single women, and women who attended church more frequently experienced these ''socially based'' emotions more strongly. The other factor included regret, anxiety, depression, doubt, and anger. It appears to reflect a second source of stress associated with the abortion, deriving from a sense of loss. Many women are at least somewhat ambivalent about ending a pregnancy. In addition to the important and often compelling reasons that a woman has for wanting to terminate her pregnancy, there may be conscious or unconscious reasons for wanting to continue it. Abortion eliminates the positive potential the pregnancy may have held. The woman may experience a sense of loss and undergo a mourning process, as reflected in the emotions in the second negative factor. This may be particularly likely in second-trimester abortion, when there has been more acknowledgment of the existence of a potential child. The ''internally based'' emotions were not related to any demographic variables except age; younger women experienced these more strongly than did older women. Younger women may have more hopes for what a pregnancy and child could bring them (such as adolescents' hopes for autonomy, noted by Hatcher, 1976), whereas older women may be more realistic about the possibilities of their pregnancy. It is interesting to note that the difficulty of the decision to have an abortion (measured beforehand) was significantly related to the internally based emotions. Those who reported more difficulty in decision making later experienced these emotions more strongly. The difficulty of the decision was not, however, related to either the socially based emotions or the positive emotions experienced afterward.

The abortion experience varies in the amount and kinds of stress it produces. The extent to which it creates a crisis for a woman depends upon several factors. One is the meaning the pregnancy holds for a woman: for example, whether it is wanted, what it represents to the woman, and what her feelings are about the pregnancy and its termination. A second is the nature of the social environment surrounding the abortion process: for example, whether significant others support the woman's decision, whether she is able to obtain a legal abortion in a safe, medical environment, whether she is treated with respect and support by the medical staff, whether she receives counseling, whether she is a member of a religious or cultural group that opposes abortion. A woman's response will also depend on the resources she brings to the situation. Women with more adequate coping abilities will likely experience few serious problems. Each woman probably deals with the crisis in terms of her usual defensive and coping strategies. Women who generally tend to use denial and avoidance, for example, are likely to deal with the pregnancy and abortion in the same manner. Women with a prior history of psychiatric problems, which may indicate more difficulty in coping with stress in general, also may have a more difficult time dealing with the abortion.

Effects on Other Participants

This chapter has considered the effects of abortion on the patient. However, there are other participants in the abortion experience who may also experience negative effects and who may be in need of psychosocial interventions.

As mentioned earlier, there has been growing concern about the effects on health care staff of participating in abortions. Several studies have shown differences by profession in feelings about abortion. Of professionals involved in working with abortion patients, social workers are generally the most favorable and nurses the least, with physicians in between. Social workers generally have more contact with the patients, understand the reasons for the abortion, and identify more with the woman than with the fetus. The roles of nurses and physicians, in contrast, tend to involve them very little with the woman as a patient (or as a person) and more with the fetus. Research has found that nurses tend to overidentify with the fetus and are disturbed by participation in abortion procedures (Char & McDermott, 1972; Kane, Feldman, Jain, & Lipton 1973; Rosen, Werley, Ager, & Shea, 1974). Specifically, their participation frequently leads to hostility toward patients (which could influence patient care) and toward doctors because of perceived lack of support. They also experience identity crises regarding their medical roles. Some physicians have also reported an aversion to performing abortions. Kane *et al.* (1973) found that physicians dreaded the days they were to do abortions, experienced depression on those days, and found themselves engaged in rumination about the rights and wrongs of the procedure.

Physicians and nurses have particular concerns about performing midtrimester abortions. The procedures used after 12–14 weeks gestation are most stressful for the staff as well as for the woman. However, the different procedures used at this point in pregnancy carry with them implications for nurses different from those for physicians. Saline abortions involve little physician involvement. Physicians do the initial induction, and it is the nurses who generally care for the patient when the dead fetus is later expelled. It is not surprising that nurses working on a gynecology service view saline abortion procedures as their most upsetting experience (Kaltreider *et al.*, 1979). In contrast, the use of dilation and evacuation in the second trimester requires the physician to be directly involved with the removal of the fetus and requires much less contact for nurses. This procedure, which is far better for the patient in terms of relative safety, expense, time, and psychological effect, is much more upsetting for the physician, and many providers appear hesitant to perform it (Kaltreider *et al.*, 1979; Rooks and Cates, 1977).

Some of the reactions to abortion work reported by medical staff resemble symptoms reported by Maslach (1979) to be indicative of the "burn-out" syndrome. This syndrome occurs in a wide range of settings in which professionals work under emotionally stressful circumstances. It involves physical and emotional exhaustion "in which the professional person no longer has any positive feelings, sympathy, or respect for patients or clients. A very cynical and dehumanized perception of these people often develops in which they are labeled in derogatory ways and treated accordingly [p. 113]." Several of the suggestions Maslach gives for counteracting burn-out could be effectively implemented among health staff involved in abortion work. Peer support may be particularly important. Presently, the taboos surrounding abortion appear to exert an influence. Doctors and nurses participating in abortions may not only lack the support of their colleagues but also encounter hostility and resentment of those not participating in the provision of abortion services. They may also experience criticism and loss of status from their own patients or the public at large. Educational efforts could be directed at the public to remove some of the pressure from abortion providers. In addition, providers could give greater support to one another. There may be little discussion and mutual support among health professionals who are involved in abortion work. When group meetings have been held in which nurses are given the chance to share feelings and doubts about their work, they have often been quite successful in raising morale and increasing willingness to take part in abortion procedures. More attention needs to be paid to providing support for these health personnel, for both their own benefit and the good of the patients.

Finally, a participant in the abortion experience who is often ignored is the male partner. In some instances the partner may not know about the pregnancy and abortion. In other instances he is actively involved. A case study by Wallerstein and Bar-Din (1972) documented the influence of an abortion on both members of a couple as individuals as well as on the dynamics of their relationship. Blumberg *et al.* (1975) found evidence of depression among most of the husbands as well as the wives following an abortion for genetic indications. Thus, in addition to continued research and intervention to reduce negative effects and encourage psychological growth for women undergoing abortion, and to reduce burn-out among health professionals involved in abortion services, work is called for on the possible need for services for male partners who are involved in the abortion experience.

SUMMARY

Abortion is a unique medical procedure. Most medical procedures are performed to cure or ameliorate a disease state. The "disease state" that abortion cures is pregnancy, whose definition as a positive or negative event depends on the situation or perspective of the patient. Thus, more than most medical practices, abortion involves social meanings and poses a number of dilemmas for all participants.

Although many procedures are influenced by the interpersonal context in which they occur as well as by their symbolic meaning for the patient, these factors are particularly salient in abortion. As with any procedure, the doctor–patient interaction can affect responses to the experience. In this instance, however, the physician is unlikely to have a personal and continuing relationship with the patient and may have ambivalent feelings about the services he or she is providing. Both of these factors can contribute to impersonal and rejecting treatment. Nurses, also, may communicate disapproval to abortion patients. They play a central technical role, especially in saline abortions where they are likely to care for the patient at the time the fetus is expelled. At the same time that abortion patients may receive treatment from medical personnel less supportive than that given to other patients, they are more likely to receive attention and help from counselors and social workers. It is interesting to note that counseling is more routine for abortion than for other procedures, such as hysterectomy, where the physcial and emotional stress would seem to be as great or greater. Abortion is also more likely than other procedures to involve and affect other people. The male partner and parents frequently participate in decision making, and their actual or anticipated reactions can influence a woman's emotional responses. Further, more than any other procedure, social norms exist concerning the appropriateness of its performance, and postabortion reactions may be affected by both the immediate and the larger social context within which the abortion occurs.

Research on abortion has not yet dealt with the complexity of the experience as a whole. Most research has investigated a single influence on responses to the procedure. Research is complicated by the rapid shifts that have occurred in the legal status and availability of abortion, which have serious ramifications for the experience. It is also complicated by the strong moral and emotional feelings about abortion to which researchers, respondents, and society as a whole are subject. Abortion is a controversial and important issue that is affecting the lives of millions of women, of health care providers, and of others. There is a need for continuing research on the effects of abortion and for interventions designed to diminish negative effects for all concerned.

III

EXPECTATIONS, PAIN, AND THE NATURE OF ILLNESS

Many medical students experience symptoms that they ascribe to some serious pathological process. These "medical-student illnesses" can occur at any point in training and generally share a number of precipitating factors: The students are experiencing anxiety or fear in their medical training; they are being exposed to vivid examples of patients with serious or exotic diseases; they are learning hundreds of specific labels for symptom collections; and they are establishing emotional relationships of various sorts with patients who may deteriorate or die.

These students are temporary hypochondriacs; eventually their symptoms disappear on their own, and the disease labels are shed. Their condition is easily understood. They are in the classical attribution situation, first detailed by Schachter and Singer (1962), in which unexplained bodily arousal must be interpreted in terms of external, situational cues. Students account for their state of emotional arousal by assuming any of the convenient labels to be found in their pathology texts. In many ways, the medical students' syndrome is a microcosm of the whole health care system. Patients detect symptoms—usually nebulous symptoms like pain or weakness—and impose a meaning on these symptoms with the help of health care professionals. At every step of the way, the process is influenced by the social context.

A useful distinction is sometimes made between the terms *disease* and *illness*. *Disease* refers to a biological disorder in an organism; it involves physical or organic deterioration. *Illness,* on the other hand, involves a subjective judgment that an individual is not healthy. Disease often leads to illness, but sometimes it does not (if it is not detected). Illness is often due to disease, but sometimes no organic basis can be found, and sometimes the illness is purely psychological—"mental illness." The health care system is geared to treating illness: people generally seek health care when they are not feeling well and leave the health care system when they feel a sufficient improvement. Disease is only rarely of primary importance, as, for example, in a tuberculosis screening program conducted by a public health service. Yet, paradoxically, although the health care system is constructed around illness, health practitioners are oriented and trained to focus on disease. Too little attention is generally paid to the pervasive influence of the social milieu as it affects interpretations of bodily states.

In this part, we focus on the social nature of illness. It becomes quite clear that the patient's perception of illness, the practitioner's approach and diagnosis, and the patient's recovery from and coping with illness are all heavily influenced by the social context. In contrast to the previous part's emphasis on social interaction, the present part focuses on the cognitive variables of expectations and perceived control. But rather than considering these matters in the abstract, as social psychology has done in the past, the following three chapters deal directly with the medical situation, with a particular emphasis on pain.

Pain is a central but understudied concept in health care. Pain is typically a key factor in the patient's decision to seek medical care and in the practitioner's search for a diagnosis. Yet the phenomenon of pain itself has not been adequately defined, and the relationship of pain to the social aspects of illness is often ignored. Furthermore, the processes and mechanisms by which psychosocial factors influence pain are not well understood; undoubtedly they are very complex. At least two major processes are involved. First, psychosocial factors influence daily activities, which in turn influence the individual's well-being. For example, our social environment influences whether we eat healthy foods, drink, smoke, exercise, rest, and so on. Second, psychosocial factors influence a person's physiology. Placebo effects are well documented in medicine, especially in the area of pain control. Placebo effects arise from therapies or pills that have no specific effects on the condition being treated; they can be very powerful, however. Their possible physiological basis in natural opiate-like substances called endorphins is now being investigated. Thus, psychosocial (interpersonal) factors such as expectations can bring about physiological responses.

Relatedly, concerning the physiological basis for the psychosocial control of pain, there is increasing evidence in support of a "gate-control theory" of pain. This theory posits a brain-controlled ''gate'' in the spinal column that can block pain impulses. This control gate is influenced by feelings and thoughts, which can arise from social relationships and interactions. Thus, social psychology is directly relevant to pain control. These and other challenging issues in the forefront of health care are discussed in the following three chapters.

8

Russell A. Jones

Expectations and Illness[1]

The models we have of disease process—the beliefs and expectations we hold about the nature of disease—determine the kinds of data we look for in our fights against disease (Eisenberg, 1977a). Phenomena become "data," in fact, precisely because they appear relevant to particular models or conceptions of the nature of disease. If our model is that heart disease is hereditary, for example, we are unlikely to pay attention to information about recuring patterns of behavior among the coronary prone (Jenkins, Zyzanski, & Rosenman, 1976). Thus "models act to generate their own verification by excluding phenomena outside the frame of reference the user employs [Eisenberg, 1977a p. 18]."

The variable that we shall explore in this chapter is one that has usually been excluded from discussions of disease causation, even with the growing recognition of the importance of social, psychological, and behavioral factors in health and disease. Specifically, we shall look at the role of expectations and argue that expectations are implicated at every point—from the likelihood of contracting a disease and defining oneself as ill, through the

[1]The writing of this chapter was supported in part by National Institute of Mental Health Training Grant MH15730.

145

diagnostic process, to recovery and prevention of further diseases. We begin with a brief look at the nature of disease and illness in modern society in order to gain some perspective on where expectations might come into play.

EXPECTATIONS AND ILLNESS IN MODERN SOCIETY

Differences among social classes in the incidence and prevalence of diseases can usually be explained by differences in sanitation facilities, congestion of living conditions, adequacy of nutrition, and stressfulness of work. However, there is evidence that even *within* homogeneous social groups, disease and illness are not randomly distributed. During the early and middle 1950s Lawrence Hinkle and his colleagues (Hinkle, 1961; Hinkle, Pinsky, Bross, & Plummer, 1956; Hinkle & Wolff, 1958) investigated the frequency and distribution of illness episodes in a number of different homogeneous populations. In each of these studies, regardless of the method of data collection and regardless of the particular population examined, the results were essentially the same. Within each group, during the 2 decades of young adult life, 25% of the individuals experienced approximately 50% of all illness episodes, and another 25% experienced less than 10% of all illness episodes. Further, those experiencing the greater number of illness episodes were found to have more different major and minor syndromes involving more different organ systems and falling into more different etiological categories. Thus, it appears that even within homogeneous social groups some people have a greater general susceptibility to illness than others. The question is, Why?

There are many possibilities, including genetic influence and the fact that illness episodes are not independent—having one disease increases the probability of subsequent disease via purely physiological mechanisms. Even so, there have been numerous speculations, suggestions, and anecdotes in the literature that implicate expectations as contributing factors in general susceptibility. Engel (1968), for example, suggested that a psychological giving up of attempts to cope with one's problems often preceded the onset of illness. The idea that the perceived inability to obtain valued goals in life could somehow result in physiological changes that increased one's susceptibility to illness seems to run through much of the psychosomatic literature. Before looking at the evidence for that link, however, let us be a little more specific about the kinds of diseases that afflict life in the twentieth century.

It is true, of course, that the threat posed by infectious diseases has decreased dramatically in the last century. In 1900 the leading causes of death in the United States, were, in order, influenza and pneumonia, tuberculosis, and gastroenteritis. By 1976 these infectious killers had been replaced by diseases of the heart, cancer, and cerebrovascular diseases as the leading cause of death. In fact, in 1976 diseases of the heart accounted for 34.5% of all deaths in the United States, and cancer for 21.1%, with the two combined accounting for over 55% of all deaths (USDHEW, 1978, p. 38). Thus, if we want to make a case for the importance of expectations in disease and illness, the primary interest must be in how expectations might play a role in those chronic, debilitating diseases that have come to be called the "new morbidity" (Eisenberg, 1977a) and the "diseases of civilization" (Dubos, 1971).

Stress and Life Change

In the last few years, several people have proposed conceptual models in which stress is the main mediating mechanism between social psychological variables and disease (e.g., Cohen, 1979; Jenkins, 1979; Mechanic, 1978; Selye, 1976). These models vary in many particulars, but all have in common the idea that reactions to psychosocial stimuli can include physiological changes that if prolonged can lead to disease. This idea is made explicit in Levi's (1974) model, presented in Figure 8.1. As may be seen in the model, the relationships among the various components form a cybernetic system with continuous feedback. Thus, the hypothesis underlying the model is that social psychological stimuli, which include expectations, can act as stressors that, in predisposed individuals, may lead to disease.

To help make the model concrete, consider one example. There is evidence that genetic predispositions may play a role in the excessive retention of salt and water that increases blood plasma volume and, in turn, cardiac output and the peripheral resistance that produces hypertension (Boyle, 1970). Excessive salt intake, promoted by an acquired taste for salt early in life, may have the same effect (Kaplan, 1978a). Of interest here, however, is the physiological pathway outlined by Kaplan (1978b) by which stress, of psychological origin, may also produce hypertension. There is a fair amount of evidence that people in stressful occupations, such as air-traffic controllers (Cobb & Rose, 1973), or those subjected to sustained environmental stressors, such as noise (Jonsson & Hansson, 1977), develop hypertension more frequently than do comparable people not subjected to such stressors. Kaplan (1978b) points out that such psychogenic stress increases the activity of the sympathetic nervous system, thus increasing vascular reactivity, narrowing the arterial lumen, increasing peripheral resistance, and, consequently, increasing blood pressure. Repeated or prolonged occurrence of such activation could result in permanent hypertension.

As for the evidence bearing on the model, it is now well established (Oken, 1967; Selye, 1976) that such psychosocial stressors as high-pressure

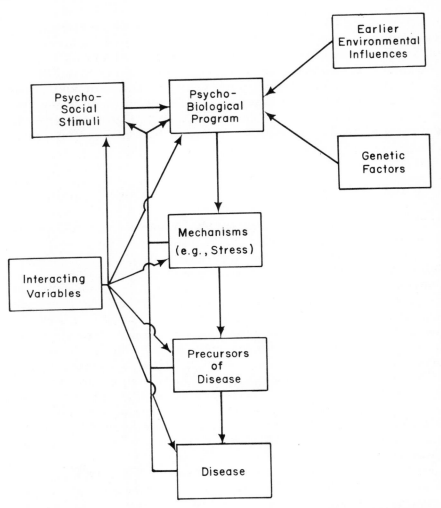

Figure 8.1. This conceptual model shows the relationship between psychosocial stimuli and disease (Levi, 1974, p. 10; Copyright by Charles Thomas).

work situations or anticipation of danger (Rubin & Rahe, 1974) trigger in humans the types of physiological and endocrine responses that if prolonged are literally deadly. The body's adaptive capabilities are called into play whenever one experiences a change of any sort—whether it be the invasion of a microbe, walking up a flight of stairs, or divorcing one's spouse. If we consider one's general susceptibility to illness to be inversely related to the state of one's adaptive reserve at any given point in time, it follows that the more change one has recently experienced, the greater one's susceptibility to illness will be. Emphasis on life events and life change as links in the chain leading to disease has long been a theme of psychosomatic medicine (Cleghorn & Streiner, 1979; Hinkle, 1961; Holmes & Rahe, 1967; Meyer, 1912; Wolff, Wolf, & Hare, 1950).

The best known of the attempts to relate life change to disease is the work of Holmes and Rahe. Their intention was to develop an easily understood and scorable instrument for quantifying the amount of life change—and, by inference, stress—that a person had recently experienced. To accomplish this, Holmes and Rahe (1967) requested a large heterogeneous sample of subjects to rate a number of life-change events, such as divorce or a change in residence, in terms of the amount of readjustment that would be necessary if they were involved in this event. The ratings were made by assigning marriage an arbitrary value and asking each subject to assign a number to each event on the basis of whether it took more or less readjustment than marriage. The rank order of 43 such events and the mean values of perceived readjustment necessitated in relation to marriage are given in Table 8.1.

Following the development of the Schedule of Recent Experience, the name given to one of the questionnaire formats used to solicit information about which of the life-change events respondents have experienced, Holmes and Rahe and their colleagues, plus numerous other investigators (cf. Dohrenwend & Dohrenwend, 1974; Garrity, Marx, & Somes, 1978) have carried out a multitude of both retrospective and prospective studies relating life change to illness. As an example, in one of the most frequently cited prospective studies, Rubin, Gunderson, and Arthur (1971) administered the Schedule of Recent Experience to navy enlisted men prior to their embarking on an extended cruise. Upon the ships' return to base some months later, the health records were obtained from the ships' infirmaries, and illness episodes experienced during the cruise were related to total life-change events experienced in the 18 months prior to the beginning of the cruise. Those subjects with higher total life-change units at the start of the cruise tended to have more illnesses during the cruise.

Although the life-change–illness literature has been subjected to some serious, and well-deserved, criticism (cf. Rabkin & Struening, 1976), the basic relationship seems fairly well established. Consequently, recent research has been less concerned with continued demonstrations of the link between life change and susceptibility to illness and more concerned with refining the meaning of "life changes." That is, are there particular kinds of life changes that are more likely to lead to an increase in one's susceptibility to illness? If so, what are the defining features of these events?

Perceived Control and Coping

Consider the life events listed in Table 8.1. It is immediately obvious that these events differ in a number of ways in addition to the magnitude of readjustment necessitated by their occurrence. Although 13 of the events are

TABLE 8.1
Rank Order and Mean Ratings of Readjustment
Necessitated by Forty-three Events

Rank	Life event	Mean value
1	Death of spouse	100
2	Divorce	73
3	Marital separation	65
4	Jail term	63
5	Death of close family member	63
6	Personal injury or illness	53
7	Marriage	50
8	Fired at work	47
9	Marital reconciliation	45
10	Retirement	45
11	Change in health of family member	44
12	Pregnancy	40
13	Sex difficulties	39
14	Gain of new family member	39
15	Business readjustment	39
16	Change in financial state	38
17	Death of close friend	37
18	Change to different line of work	36
19	Change in number of arguments with spouse	35
20	Mortgage over $10,000	31
21	Foreclosure of mortgage or loan	30
22	Change in responsibilities at work	29
23	Son or daughter leaving home	29
24	Trouble with in-laws	29
25	Outstanding personal achievement	28
26	Wife begin or stop work	26
27	Begin or end school	26
28	Change in living conditions	25
29	Revision of personal habits	24
30	Trouble with boss	23
31	Change in work hours or conditions	20
32	Change in residence	20
33	Change in schools	20
34	Change in recreation	19
35	Change in church activities	19
36	Change in social activities	18
37	Mortgage or loan less than $10,000	17
38	Change in sleeping habits	16
39	Change in number of family get-togethers	15
40	Change in eating habits	15
41	Vacation	13
42	Christmas	12
43	Minor violations of the law	11

Source: From Holmes & Rahe, 1967, p. 216. Copyright 1967
by Pergamon Press, Elmsford, N.Y. Reprinted by permission.

clearly unpleasant, most of the events could be either pleasant or unpleasant, desirable or undesirable. The events also differ in the extent to which they are under the control of the person involved. For example, one usually has no control over such events as the death of a close friend or a change in health of a family member, whereas one is usually able to exert some influence over such events as marital reconciliation or a change to a different line of work. The question, thus, is whether there is any evidence that perceived control over events reduces the stress of those events.

There is, in fact, a good deal of experimental research with animals that bears directly on the issue. Weiss (1971, 1972), for example, reports an experiment on stress in which some rats could avoid or escape an electric shock (the stressor) by performing a wheel-turning response while other rats experienced the same amounts of shock but could not escape or avoid it. The main dependent measure in Weiss's experiment was the length of gastric ulcer lesions that were produced by these conditions in the lower, glandular area of the rats' stomachs. The results revealed two things of particular interest. First, animals that could avoid or escape the shock ulcerated significantly less than the no-escape animals. The latter experienced exactly the same shocks in the same sequence but could not do anything to avoid or escape the shock. Secondly, the predictability of the shock (in some conditions a signal was given prior to each shock) reduced its stressfulness for both the avoidance-escape and no-escape rats. Thus, both controllability and predictability of aversive stimulation ameliorate its ulcerogenic effects. Similarly, Sklar and Anisman (1979) have found that the perceived ability to cope, to control aversive events, may play a role in tumor development.

The evidence that is available repeatedly implicates perceived ability to cope (the expectation of being able to "handle" things) as a major factor in reducing the deleterious effects of stressful events. Paykel (1974), for example, in summarizing a series of studies that employed variations on the Schedule of Recent Experience (Table 8.1) reports that he distinguished "those events which were at least partly under the respondent's control and could be initiated by him from those outside his control and found that the uncontrolled events were perceived as more stressful [p. 152]." The problem of course, is that those events outside one's control may indeed have been more stressful. The perception of ability to control may have been confounded with amount of readjustment necessitated.

There is, however, a fair amount of experimental research with humans indicating that the perceived ability to control can, in itself, reduce the effects of stressors. For example, in two studies by Hokanson, DeGood, Forrest, and Brittain (1971) subjects' systolic blood pressures were recorded as they worked on a complex matching task. Some subjects were given "control" in that they could choose when to take breaks during the task, whereas other subjects were simply told when to take their breaks. The main result of interest here is that over the entire course of the experimental session the subjects lacking control exhibited a significantly higher systolic blood pressure level than did the subjects who perceived they could control their time-outs from the aversive task.

There is another result of interest in the second study reported by Hokanson *et al.* (1971). In the latter experiment, essentially the same task was used as in the first, but all subjects were allowed to take rest periods whenever they chose. However, in order to take a rest, subjects had to indicate that they wanted to do so 30 sec in advance, by depressing a switch with their free hand while they continued to work. Thus, a brief anticipatory period occurred prior to each rest period. The results indicate that a reduction in systolic blood pressure occurred during these periods when the subjects were anticipating a rest. Further, the reduction in systolic pressure occurred even though there was no detectable relaxation in their work rate on the matching task.

These results are consistent with Lazarus's (1966) theoretical notion that the perceived availability of coping responses, a rest period in this case, over which one has control or believes one has control, should diminish stress reactions. Further, Hokanson *et al.* (1971) point out that the higher systolic pressure of subjects who lacked control over their rest period is ''at least reminiscent [of the] . . . feelings of time urgency, a sense of unrelenting external demands, and behavioral patterns of compulsive activity to ward off impending harm [p. 681],'' which have been identified as characteristic of those most likely to develop coronary problems (Friedman & Rosenman, 1974).

More recently, Gal and Lazarus (1975) have suggested that merely being engaged in activity—as opposed to being passive—is preferable when one is in a stressful situation and may, in fact, be highly effective in reducing perceived threat and the effects of stress. In particular, they suggest that it is activity that is functionally related to the threatening situation that is most efficacious, since such ''activity implies a sense of control over the threatening conditions—which itself has, in many instances, stress-reducing effects [p. 13].'' Activity does other things, of course, in addition to implying a sense of control. It may divert one's attention from the source of threat, for example. Also, Weiss (1972) suggests that unless activity is followed by feedback indicating that it is being effective in removing or reducing the stressor, continued activity will increase, not decrease, the amount of stress experienced. The key may be the amount of ambiguity in the situation. As long as one can reasonably convince oneself that the activity is somehow relevant to reducing, removing, finding, destroying, or just living with the source of threat, it may indeed imply a sense of control and, thus, actually reduce the amount of stress experienced. On the other hand, if the ambiguity is so great that one cannot decide what to do, both actual and perceived control are impossible, and successful coping and stress reduction unlikely (Shalit, 1977).

In the course of development many people come to believe that the events they experience are *generally* contingent on their own behavior, that is, they develop a belief in internal locus of control (Rotter, 1966; Wallston, Wallston, Kaplan, & Maides, 1976). As Strickland (1978) points out, the evidence suggests that such people are likely to take steps to change aversive life situations—because they expect to be able to do so. Such expectancy-induced activity can be quite effective, of course, in preventing disease and maintaining health. People with a belief in internal locus of control have been found to be more likely to engage in preventive health measures of all sorts, from gathering information about disease threats to wearing seat belts to participation in voluntary exercise programs. A benign circle is thus set up. Belief in the ability to maintain health leads one to engage in activities that not only help prevent accidents and disease but also maintain one in better physical condition to withstand the stress of disease, should it occur.

On a more general level, Moss (1973) has suggested that illness and immunity are systematically related to the social networks in which we find ourselves immersed. Specifically, his idea is that as long as the information received from our social networks appears congruous with the way things "really are," our general susceptibility to illness is relatively low. We are under little stress. However, the perception of incongruity produces physiological arousal and an increased susceptibility to illness. Incongruities, of course, make us uncertain about how to respond and undermine our sense of being able to "handle" things. It follows that members of modern heterogeneous societies who belong to multiple reference groups and overlapping social networks would have higher susceptibilities to illness because of the increased likelihood of encountering incongruities among the informational and value systems of their various sets of associates. In addition to playing such a role in sheltering one from and/or exposing one to informational incongruities, the expectations and beliefs derived from our social or cultural milieu play a major role in the labeling process by which we define ourselves as ill.

Cultural and Social Influences on Definitions of Illness

Every culture includes a set of widely shared beliefs about the nature and causes of both physical and psychological disorders. Even though such beliefs may appear irrational to outsiders—such as the Hindu prohibition of eating beef or the Jewish and Moslem prohibitions on pork—there is evidence that they are, in fact, usually quite logical within the given cultural context (Harris, 1974). Further, such beliefs about the causes of disease are constantly, albeit circularly, reinforced by the very "reality" that gave rise to the beliefs. For example, we now know that tuberculosis is an infectious disease that usually requires prolonged contact with an infected person for its spread. This bit of reality, in eighteenth- and nineteenth-century Europe, gave rise to the belief that tuberculosis was hereditary. This belief, of course, was reinforced by the fact that tuberculosis tended to run in families, that is, where there was "prolonged contact", the very datum that gave rise to the beliefs in the first place (Dubos & Dubos, 1952).

Knowledge about disease and illness must fit into the general knowledge structure and belief systems of a society. There are obviously strongly felt needs to make sense of how diseases are spread, who is likely to be taken ill, and what can be done to stay healthy. The beliefs that develop to answer these needs—even when they turn out to be incorrect—help reduce the threat posed by disease. Historically, this has produced some genuinely odd medical theories. For example, McMahon (1975) points out that, for a long time after the death of Descartes, medical practitioners believed that only physiological explanations could suffice to account for bodily afflictions. Descartes had proclaimed that the mind and body were separate entities. Thus, psychosomatic causation was simply ruled out as a possibility. Things began to get a little difficult, however, as a result of the large-scale hostilities and wars of the early nineteenth century. Bodies of dead soldiers on which no physical cause of death could be ascertained were repeatedly found on the battlefields. One of the most remarkable hypotheses put forward to explain such deaths, and one that was seriously discussed for a number of years, attributed the deaths to "the wind of the cannon ball." Elaborate variations of this hypothesis were put forth—the vacuum caused by a cannon ball passing in front of the stomach was supposed to produce intestinal hemorrage, a ball passing in front of the eyes was said to produce blindness. Deductions were even made about the effects of different directions of rotation of the ball as it passed near the body.

Now, of course, we consider "the wind of the cannon ball" a ridiculous hypothesis, but it was wholly consistent with the prevailing mechanical, physiological model of disease causation at the time. The prevailing "models," the cultural belief systems of any society at any given time and place, dictate the nature of acceptable explanations. Caporael (1976), for example, makes a serious case that convulsive ergot poisoning, a condition resulting from eating contaminated rye bread, was the source of the fits that afflicted a number of young girls in Salem, Massachusetts, in 1692 and eventuated in the executions of dozens of witches. The good villagers of Salem knew nothing of the pharmacologic effects of ergot. Witchcraft, however, was something they could "understand" and deal with.

There are other ways in which expectations influence self-definitions of illness. It is common knowledge that many people ignore, or define as normal, symptoms that induce others to seek medical assistance (Kirscht, 1974). In fact, the results of multiphasic medical screenings and required periodic health examinations imply that most people, most of the time, are experiencing clinically identifiable physical symptoms for which no help is being sought. Schenthal (1960), for example, found that over 90% of the "well" patients participating in a multiphasic screening had at least one disease or clinical disorder, and, yet, they were not defining themselves as ill. Part of the explanation for such apparent anomalies is that the physical and psychological states experienced by many individuals—states that an outsider would use as an index of diseases—are often expected concomitants of the individuals' lifestyles. One whose lifestyle is such that tiredness is to be expected and, hence, explained in terms of the lifestyle (working full time, going to school at night, tending house) is unlikely to be able to or willing to test the validity of that explanation by changing his or her way of life. Thus, the symptom will be tolerated because its meaning is "understood," and as Banks and Keller (1971) point out, "The meaning of the specific symptom as perceived by the respondent is a key variable [p. 502]" in the decision to seek aid.

On a general level, an expanded version of Schachter's (1964, 1971) theory about the interaction of cognitive and physiological determinants of internal states may provide the most parsimonious explanation of how expectations influence self-definitions of illness. The principal parts of Schachter's theory are the experience of some altered physiological state and the presence or absence of an apropriate explanation for it. If the individual does not have an appropriate explanation, evaluative needs arise, and he or she is likely to seek an explanation. If the individual has an appropriate explanation, evaluative needs will not arise. The most likely source of appropriate explanations for what one is feeling is, of course, one's recent experience and/or lifestyle. Chronic fatigue, difficulty going to sleep, back pain, and headaches are the early symptoms of several dread diseases including cancer, diabetes, and hypertension, but they are also symptoms that can reasonably be expected to occur as a consequence of certain, unfortunately common, life and work situations. Individuals with such symptoms are likely to believe they have appropriate explanations for what they are experiencing. Hence, the symptoms are likely to be tolerated, and no need will be felt for an informed medical opinion. The evidence seems to indicate that only when such symptoms begin to interfere with normal functioning (Mechanic, 1966) are they defined as indexes of illness.

Pseudoappropriate explanations for altered physiological states, explanations that delay the decision to seek medical aid, may also be a function of what is normal or expected within one's subcultural group. DiCicco and Apple (1960), for example, found that among a sample of elderly persons living in a low socioeconomic district of Boston there was a widespread belief that aches and pains and physical limitations are simply part of being old and that nothing could be done about them. As a result, of course, nothing was done about them. Zola (1975, p. 545) cites several other examples where various pathological conditions are explained away or ignored because of cultural beliefs that the symptom or condition is "to be expected," that is, simply a fact of life.

Thus expectations play a part both in the production of various somatic disorders and in the likelihood that those disorders will be labeled as worthy of medical care. As we have seen, the expectation of being able to cope, of being in control of stressful situations, reduces their deleterious effects. Further, we have seen how both cultural expectations about what are appropriate explanations for bodily states and individuals' expectations about the consequences of their particular lifestyles play major roles in self-definitions of illness. However, once the decision to seek medical aid has been made, the problem becomes even more complex and the influence of expectations even more problematic.

EXPECTATIONS AND THE DIAGNOSTIC PROCESS

The diagnostic process involves several steps, the major ones being obtaining information from (and about) a patient concerning the nature of his or her symptoms and the use of that information to formulate a "best guess" about the disease process underlying the patient's symptoms. For the practicing physician, diagnosis can be an exciting, problem-solving activity. Further, diagnostic accuracy is the single most important factor determining the likelihood that the patient will receive quality medical care. An accurate diagnostic label does not, of course, ensure that cure-producing treatment will follow; there are still all too many diseases that can be diagnosed but not cured. However, an inaccurate diagnosis ensures, almost by definition, that the best available treatment for the patient's disorder will not be the treatment of choice.

There are a number of ways in which the physician's expectations may bias both the information obtained from a patient and the decision based on that information. It does not stop there, however. As we shall see, there is reason to believe that expectations continue to influence the manner in which information about the patient is processed even after a diagnosis has been made.

Expectations and the Diagnostic Interview

According to Reiser (1979), diagnoses at the end of the eighteenth century were being made primarily on the basis of the patient's description of his or her symptoms and the physician's observations of the patient's general condition. One of the few diagnostic techniques available at the time was percussion, the practice of striking the body to generate sounds that could serve as clues to the states of various internal organs. But, for several reasons, percussion was not widely accepted, and it remained for René Laënnec in 1816 to introduce the stethoscope, the first generally accepted diagnostic aid. The promises held out by the stethoscope and by the many subsequent diagnostic aids—from X-rays to lab tests to computers—were that they would free the physician of dependence on the patient's verbal reports of symptoms and put the physician in direct communication with the patient's body. But, these "new and more dependable techniques" have not been able to do away with the need for verbal communication with the patient. The diagnostic interview is still the key to medical practice and is likely to remain so for the foreseeable future.

There are, however, ways in which expectations can get the diagnostic interview off on the wrong track, with serious consequences for everyone concerned. Research on medical problem solving suggests that physicians typically generate hypotheses, or expectations, about a patient's illness quite early in the intake interview (Kassirer & Gorry, 1978). Such initial hypotheses often appear based on little more than a combination of the patient's general appearance and one or two presenting complaints. To the extent that the patient and physician perceive the same additional physical sensations and symptoms to be associated with the presenting complaints, the initial hypotheses generated by the physician are likely to increase the ease and accuracy of communication in the interview. The presenting complaints—whether they be pain in the joints and ringing in the ears or sore throat and headache—serve the physician as bases for inferring a host of additional concomitants of the hypothesized disease. Such inferences can then be spot-checked by questions to the patient or by laboratory tests and, if confirmed, allow a much more direct "homing in" on the most likely diagnosis.

On the other hand, if the patient and physician associate different additional sensations and symptoms with the presenting complaints, the physician's initial hypotheses are likely to lead the content of the interview away from what the patient has been experiencing. The physician's attempts to confirm the presence of a syndrome that he or she has inferred on the basis of one or two complaints will then be unsuccessful. Or, more seriously, given the ambiguity of many bodily states (Schachter, 1971) and the fallibility of patients' memories (Ley, 1979), the physician's attempts to confirm an inferred syndrome may lead patients into providing information that, erroneously, is taken as confirming evidence for the presence of the syndrome.

There is, in fact, an ongoing debate about whether it is better for physicians to entertain hypotheses early in the diagnostic interview or history taking or to suspend judgment entirely until some minimum amount of information has been obtained from the patient (Elstein, Schulman, & Sprafka, 1978; Weed, 1971). Elstein *et al.*, for example, advocate early hypothesis generation, but apparently for no reason other than that the physicians in their research did generate hypotheses early in the simulated diagnostic interviews employed. Weed, in contrast, believes that early hypothesis generation increases the probability that the physician will miss or ignore a number of patient problems because the initial hypotheses result in premature closure on one or two lines of questioning in the interview. Weed's argument is compelling. As he puts it, in medicine today complete histories and physicals are routinely expected but only rarely obtained. The consequences are that problems are missed, symptoms instead of diseases are treated, and patients die unnecessarily. Further, as Dubos (1971) points out, as exposure to carcinogenic agents in the environment becomes more common, complete and detailed history taking will become more rather than less important for the practice of medicine.

Thus, the tendency to formulate hypotheses quickly and pursue specific lines of questioning can seriously affect the quality and breadth of information obtained in the medical interview. There is, however, a more general way in which the physicians' expectations almost ensure that information will be missed in the interview. Although the precise percentage varies, depending on the location and the socioeconomic status of the patients, surveys of medical practitioners suggest that the vast majority of problems that patients bring to them are minor and self-limiting (Mechanic, 1978). Gross (1966) notes that the attitude that this leads to among physicians was captured some years ago by a cartoon in the *Medical Tribune* in which a smiling physician was pictured beneath a sign that proclaimed, "You'll Live." Of course, in the long run, we will not, but it is easy to see how a few years of practice filled with such an enormous volume of minor aches and pains and functional-psychiatric disorders and general "problems of living" (Szasz, 1961) could produce some insufficiently cautious physicians.

The purpose of the information obtained in the diagnostic interview is to provide the physician with the raw material for a reasoned clinical judgment about the most likely cause of the patient's problem and the most efficacious treatment regimen available. As we have seen, that information may be seriously distorted by the initial hypotheses that the physician entertains or by the expectation that the patient's problem is probably minor. Unfortunately, there is reason to believe that even if the information obtained in the interview is perfectly accurate and the patient is able to make himself or herself understood completely, the physician's subsequent clinical judgment may still reflect the deleterious effect of expectations.

There is seldom a one-to-one relationship between the symptoms expressed by a patient during the medical interview and a particular disease. A headache, for example, may be the result of sinus trouble, psychological stress, too much coffee, a brain tumor, a ruptured blood vessel, or a hangover. This causal ambiguity surrounding the typical symptom has several consequences. First, it is the source of the physician's search for syndromes during the medical interview. Since most disease states produce more than one symptom, the presence of specific concomitants with the presenting complaint narrows the range of diagnostic possibilities. A headache accompanied by a shuffling gait, both of which began at approximately the same time, casts some doubt on a diagnosis of sinus trouble. A second consequence of the probabilistic relationship between individual symptoms and diseases is that it provides an opening for the physician's expectations to play a role in clinical judgment.

Consider the dilemma of the physician at the end of a diagnostic interview when no clear diagnosis has emerged. It could be assumed that the patient is simply a hypochondriac who has been overly attentive to a diffuse set of bodily states that bear little relation to one another. However, Scheff (1966) points out that one of the most salient norms in medical practice is that it is better to diagnose a well person as sick than a sick person as well. The assumptions underlying the norm seem to be that: (*a*) diseases are usually progressive and if untreated will eventually endanger life; and (*b*) the act of medical diagnosis itself is relatively harmless, with reversible effects should it later be demonstrated to be in error. The physician confronted with an ambiguous syndrome, no clear basis for a differential diagnosis, and pressure from both the norms of the profession and the patient to decide is thus in the position of assessing probabilities. That is, what is the likelihood of someone with this syndrome, or with one or more of the components of this syndrome, having, say, conversion hysteria as opposed to multiple sclerosis—two diagnoses that can, in fact, be easily confused by physicians (Elstein *et al.*, 1978).

According to Tversky and Kahneman (1974), when people attempt the task of assessing such probabilities they rely on a limited number of heuristic principles that reduce the complexity involved. Although these principles are generally quite useful, reliance on these heuristics can sometimes lead to severe, systematic errors. For example, probability judgments are often based on what appears to be a simple law of repetition: The more frequently an event has occurred, the stronger the associative links to that event are. Strength of association to the event is later used as an aid or clue in making judgments about the probability of the event. The ease with which instances of a particular class of events can be brought to mind has been termed *availability* by Tversky and Kahneman (1973), and it is generally a valid clue for making probability judgments because frequent events are usually easier to recall or imagine than infrequent ones. There are things other than repetition, however, that affect the availability of a particular class of events. Anything that makes a particular class more salient or distinctive than related classes will make the class more available. Since, in general, frequent events are more available in memory than infrequent ones, bias occurs when the frequencies of related classes do not correspond to the ease with which those classes can be retrieved from memory. As Elstein *et al.* (1978, p. 80) point out, there are several reasons why particular diagnostic categories might be more salient to a physician than their actual probabilities would warrant. For example, a recent rare or particularly dramatic case or simply knowledge of "what's going around" may make the pertinent diagnostic categories more prominent than they should be.

One might expect that diagnostic errors based on such inappropriately salient categories would be quickly discovered by either the patient or the physician, but, as we have seen, most problems brought into the physician's office are minor and self-limiting. Consequently, even if misdiagnosed and treated, chances are that the problem will go away, the patient will get better, and the diagnosis will be perceived to have been correct. It is rare, of course, that a diagnosis is based on a single symptom or presenting complaint. The major purpose of the medical interview is to get a more complete picture of the patient's condition, to see if the symptoms that the patient has focused on are part of a syndrome that can be used for a differential diagnosis. Medical interviews, however, are rarely complete and detailed. It seems to be the case, in fact, that the typical examination interview is less than 10 min in length (Balint & Norell, 1973). With such cursory examinations it is quite possible that the presence of a syndrome will be inferred on the basis of the identified presence of only one or two of its component parts.

Thus, expectations play a role in the information obtained from patients and in the judgments based on that information once it has been obtained. As we have seen, there are several ways in which expectations may make clinical judgment somewhat less rational than we would like—norms that favor action over inaction, biases in the way alternative diagnostic categories are considered, and failures to register inaccurate diagnoses. It does not stop there, however. Once a diagnosis has been made, expectations continue to play a part.

Theoretically, a diagnosis should be a tentative working hypothesis. It appears, however, that diagnoses are sometimes treated as conclusions about patients, and there is evidence that premature conclusions about a person can interfere with appropriate utilization of new information about the person. For example, in a series of experiments, Dailey (1952) asked subjects to read autobiographical sketches written by others and to predict how those others would respond to specific items on a personality inventory. The criterion in each case was how the other person had actually responded. Some subjects made predictions after reading half an autobiography and again after reading all of it. Other subjects made predictions only after reading all the information. The latter group was significantly more accurate. As Dailey puts it, "Premature conclusions on the basis of a small amount of data can apparently prevent the observer from profiting as fully from additional data as he would without the premature decision [p. 142]."

The ideal situation for diagnosis and treatment evaluation is one in which the physician has continuing, or at least periodic, contact with the patient so that repeated observations can be made over time to assess the course of treatment. However, according to D'Andrade (1974), situations in which one makes repeated observations and evaluations of the same persons over time are "subject to a specific effect analogous to that of an illusion: an effect in which there is a reliable and systematic distortion in judgments [p. 161]." D'Andrade's argument is that when an observer relies on his or her long-term memory in making assessments of a number of different people, each of whom have a number of different characteristics (or symptoms), the characteristics and symptoms that the observer considers to be related are likely to be recalled as applying to the same person. If such a bias exists, and the evidence seems to indicate that it does (cf. D'Andrade, 1974; Shweder, 1977), it would present serious difficulties for physicians. Physicians have clear expectations about syndromes, sets of related symptoms, and are constantly in the position of making repeated observations on many different patients over time. The diagnostic labels applied to patients may be fleshed out by the sort of memory distortion D'Andrade has identified. The patient who exhibits only two or three components of a syndrome may sometimes be recalled as having had the full-blown syndrome if several other patients exhibited the missing components. Such an error, of course, would inappropriately reinforce the diagnosis and leave the physician less open to other possibilities. Thus, applying a diagnostic label may affect a physician's subsequent behavior in several ways.

HOW EXPECTATIONS INFLUENCE RECOVERY AND PREVENTION

According to Mechanic (1966, p. 11), medicine has several tasks: to understand the origins of disease, to recognize its presence, to cure, and to promote healthful living conditions. We have seen how expectations are important variables in the first two of these tasks. Let us briefly examine some of the ways in which expectations play a part in cure and prevention.

Placebos

A number of medical historians (e.g., Houston, 1938) have pointed out that up until the late nineteenth century nearly all medicines and therapeutic procedures were, in effect, placebos. It was rare that the physician's prescription contained a pharmacological agent with a specific effect on the malady at hand. Despite prescribing such useless medications and, often, carrying out actively harmful procedures such as bloodletting, physicians have generally enjoyed respected positions in society. How can that be? It appears that they took credit for what we now recognize were spontaneous recoveries and remissions, self-limiting diseases, and placebo effects. Of the cures produced by these various means, the only ones for which physicians may have deserved at least part of the credit were the placebo effects. By convincing patients that they could be cured, by shoring up patients' faith that it was possible to recapture health, by leading them to expect that this little bottle of "Tail-of-Mouse-with-Honey" would soothe and heal, physicians may indeed have promoted the healing process. There is now a considerable body of evidence that the belief or expectation that a particular substance will produce psychological and physiological change can actually bring about such change. Further, in the practice of medicine the source of expectations about particular medications and procedures is usually the physician; when the physician firmly believes in the efficacy of a particular treatment and communicates that conviction to the patient, the treatment quite often works. Conversely, when the physician loses faith in the treatment and communicates that to the patient, the treatment may turn out to be less than optimal.

As an example of this cyclical effect of expectations, Benson and McCallie (1979) have documented the extent to which placebo effects have been implicated in the history of treatments for angina pectoris. They point out that the diagnostic criteria for angina pectoris and the evaluation of its severity have not changed much since the late eighteenth century. Recommended treatments, however, have changed constantly, and there seems to be a discernible pattern to treatment changes. For example, a vasodilator called Khellin was introduced as treatment for angina pectoris in the mid-1940s, and research indicated that 80–90% of patients responded to treatment with marked subjective (pain relief) and objective (exercise tolerance) improvement. In the early 1950s, reports that Khellin was not effective in pain relief began to emerge, and by 1954 reports of the use of Khellin for angina pectoris had ceased to appear. Benson and McCallie trace a similar trajectory for four other treatments for angina, including two surgical procedures that were still being used in the 1960s and 1970s. The pattern has repeated itself many times.

One possible limitation imposed by the use of research on angina pectoris as an example of the influence of expectations on placebo effects is that it might be argued that the indexes of patient improvement in such research are primarily subjective—pain relief, exercise tolerance, and self-reported need for medication. However, the evidence seems to support the proposition that placebos can produce objective, physiological change and that the expectations that such change will occur are crucial to its occurrence, whether the change be constriction of the nasal air passages (Strupp, Levenson, Manuck, Snell, Hinrichsen, & Boyd, 1974), decreased blood pressure (Blackwell, Bloomfield, & Buncher, 1972), or the electrical conductivity of the skin (Loftis & Ross, 1974).

An issue of some importance in connection with placebo effects is whether there are stable individual differences among patients in the tendency to show positive reactions to placebos. The value of being able to identify placebo reactors versus nonreactors has been clearly demonstrated in various studies of reactions to drugs. For example, in a study of postoperative pain, Beecher, Keats, Mosteller, and Lasagna (1953) found that among patients whose pain was decreased by ingestion of a placebo, there was no reported difference in pain relief from aspirin as opposed to morphine. However, among patients for whom the placebo was not effective, aspirin was significantly more likely to give relief than morphine. Similarly, Jellinek (1946) found consistent and reliable differences in pain relief for three headache remedies only among patients whose headaches were not relieved by a placebo. Thus, placebo reactions can mask genuine pharmacological reactions, and it would be of value to be able to identify a priori those patients who are likely to show strong placebo reactions. However, the attempts to identify such patients with tests of suggestibility or intelligence or other personality and/or demographic factors have generally been unsuccessful or inconsistent (Shapiro, 1971; Shapiro & Morris, 1978).

If it is true that placebo effects are a function of patients' expectations, the failure to identify stable groups of placebo reactors versus nonreactors should not be surprising. If placebo effects are really dependent on the patient's expectations or faith or hope or anticipation of improvement or relief, then those expectations and anticipations are likely to be specific to certain situations. What inspires faith in one situation for one patient and leads to improvement may be missing in a second situation or perceived differently by a second patient in the same situation. Research on central nervous system activities, such as the production of endorphins (a natural internal opiate-like substance), which may differentiate reactors and nonreactors, is still quite new but promises more finely grained analysis of the mechanisms underlying placebo effects. As Levine, Gordon, and Fields (1978, p. 657) note, there is little to be gained by simply continuing to record behavioral manifestations of placebo effects. Rather, it would be nice to know what variables increase or decrease endorphin activity.

Self-Efficacy

The evidence is clear that many of the major health problems of today are caused by factors that are, or could be, under the contol of individuals. Sexton (1979) points out that for 9 of the 10^2 leading causes of death in the

[2]The exception is "diseases of early infancy." Even in this case, there is reason to believe that the *mother's behavior* during pregnancy is a contributing factor.

United States, there is research suggesting that specific behavioral factors contribute to the magnitude of the death rate. Diseases of the heart, for example, have been linked to inadequate exercise, excessive smoking, and overeating. Cancer has been tied to smoking and a variety of other behaviors including insufficient fiber in the diet. One occasionally detects a tendency to blame the victims that is not quite justified by the data, but it does seem to be the case that many of our mental and physical health problems are of our own making.

Usually, we know that. If we simply quit smoking or quit drinking or ate less or got more exercise or were more pleasant to the boss, many of our problems would vanish. We know what behaviors will produce the desired outcomes. The problem is that we are often unsure of our abilities to carry out those behaviors. We lack what Bandura (1977) terms *efficacy expectations,* convictions that we can successfully execute the behavior required to produce those desired outcomes. The absence of such efficacy expectations detrimentally affects both the initiation and persistence of attempts to cope with any given situation. More, lack of perceived self-efficacy may even lead people to avoid altogether situations that they believe call for skills beyond their abilities. The avoidance, of course, ensures failure and confirms the lack of perceived self-efficacy. Conversely, the stronger the perceived efficacy is, the more effort one will expend, the longer one will persist, and, should failure occur, the more likely one will make renewed attempts to produce the desired outcome. But, what produces feelings of self-efficacy? Bandura suggests there are four principal sources: past performance accomplishments, vicarious experience, persuasion by others, and monitoring of emotional responses to situations (high arousal implies fear and poor performance).

These sources of perceived self-efficacy differ in effectiveness. Bandura, Adams, and Beyer (1977), for example, found that among patients with severe snake phobias, a mastery-based treatment in which the patient actually goes through a series of specific steps—looking at, touching, holding a boa constrictor—was more effective in raising feelings of self-efficacy than was merely observing a therapist perform the same graduated set of activities. Further, the stronger the feelings of self-efficacy, the more likely patients were to generalize their approach behavior to a different snake. Bandura *et al.* (1977) note that treatments such as their series of gradual approach behaviors reduce physiological arousal and improve performance "because they raise expectations of personal efficacy rather than by eliminating a drive that supposedly instigates defensive behavior. The social learning perspective thus places greater emphasis on the informative function of physiological arousal than on its automatic energizing property [p. 137]."

A number of others have suggested that variables similar to Bandura's *perceived self-efficacy* are crucial to the initiation and persistence of behavior.

Jones (1977), for example, uses *subjective probability of success* in a manner very similar to feelings of self-efficacy, and one's subjective probability of success is postulated to be a function of, among other things, past performance accomplishments and social comparison (vicarious experience). Seligman's (1975) concept of learned helplessness is also related, although it refers only to one end of the continuum. With any of these concepts it is easy to see how they apply to such overt health-relevant behaviors as smoking, eating, and drinking and various preventive health activities such as obtaining chest X rays and brushing one's teeth. But what about those internal physiological activities that are produced by the frustrations of daily life, those insidious changes that may lead to hypertension, stroke, heart disease, kidney failure, and death? Is there any reason to believe that notions such as perceived self-efficacy are relevant to the control of what Claude Bernard referred to as the *milieu intérieur?*

At first glance the answer appears to be no. There has, in fact, been a great deal of research in the last 2 decades predicated on the idea that we are very poor discriminators of our internal states. Hence, it is difficult to see how one could control or manipulate things one cannot perceive. Ordinarily we make no such attempt, of course. Our attention is directed outward, and we pay little attention to our internal physiological processes until something goes wrong. However, for many years there have been reports of various Yogas and Eastern mystics reputed to be able to increase or decrease their heart rates at will and of occasional circus performers who could so relax their throat muscles so as to "swallow" swords. Houdini, for example, taught himself to swallow and regurgitate keys so he could free himself from locked chains and trunks submerged in water and perform other "miraculous" escapes (Ornstein, 1975, p. 210).

In the last few years, it has become apparent that we can indeed learn to perceive and then control a great deal more of our internal processes than was once imagined. Although often requiring the use of sophisticated electronic equipment to detect and signal to the individual when certain internal changes are occurring, biofeedback has blossomed as a field of inquiry and clinical application. There is evidence now that people can learn to control their blood pressure, heart rate, skin temperature, and a variety of other responses once thought to be beyond the realm of voluntary manipulation (Shapiro & Surwit, 1979). A note of caution is in order, however, because there is reason to believe that biofeedback may have been oversold at this stage of its development. The extent to which people have been able to decrease blood pressure via biofeedback, for example, has been relatively small and of uncertain long-term clincial significance. Even so, as Shapiro and Surwit (1979, p. 49) point out, biofeedback holds out the promise of selective control of specific responses, a promise that may turn out to be of tremendous importance in the management of certain physiological symptoms and disorders.

Although there is some controversy about precisely how biofeeback works, it seems reasonable to view the electronic gadgetry as simply an aid that helps the individual learn to perceive when certain internal physiological changes are taking place (Brener, 1977). The feedback, often in the form of a light or a sound, signals the individual to attend to his or her visceral responses at that instant. With increased awareness of both the visceral responses and their antecedent conditions, control is facilitated and specific states can eventually be produced at will. Biofeedback training, in short, teaches one that certain internal processes and states can be perceived and changed, thus imparting a feeling of self-efficacy over the internal milieu.

The experiences of pain and illness and the anticipation of an untimely death are so unpleasant for most people that the incentive to behave in ways that will prevent disease and prolong life is powerful. As Bandura (1977) points out, "Given appropriate skills and adequate incentives . . . efficacy expectations are a major determinant of people's choice of activities, how much effort they will expend, and of how long they will sustain effort [p. 194]." It is clear that we have the skills to prevent many of our own health problems but unless we believe we can, we are unlikely to try.

SUMMARY

Expectations may influence the experience of stress, and it appears to be the case that the perceived ability to cope with stressors can reduce or ameliorate their effects. In addition, expectations, in the form of culturally shared beliefs and beliefs about the consequences of one's particular lifestyle, influence self-definitions of illness and play a role in the decision to seek medical aid.

Examination of the diagnostic process that follows the decision to seek aid reveals a number of ways in which expectations detrimentally influence the outcome. Physicians generate hypotheses about a patient's problems quite early in the diagnostic interview, hypotheses that may result in premature closure on one or two lines of questioning. Further, physician's expectations that most of the patients they treat will have benign, self-limiting problems may also result in problems being missed. The physician's expectations may also influence the attempt to formulate a reasonable clinical judgment by making certain diagnostic categories more salient than is warranted. Once a diagnosis has been made, expectations continue to play a role. Diagnosis may interfere with the ability to utilize new information about a patient for purposes of revising the diagnosis.

Finally, expectations may influence recovery and prevention. Placebos appear to have existed since the dawn of medicine and have been demonstrated literally to work wonders. The influences of the enthusiasm of physicians in prescribing particular courses of treatment and patients' expectations that the treatment will cure were illustrated with the example of angina pectoris and a series of ''cures'' for this malady that have since been demonstrated to produce nothing beyond a placebo effect. Expectations, in the form of feelings of self-efficacy, also appear to play a role in the willingness of people to attempt to carry out behaviors necessary for the maintenance of health and prevention of disease. It appears that biofeedback can be conceived of as the attempt to extend feelings of self-efficacy to the internal environment.

ACKNOWLEDGMENTS

I would like to thank Phil Berger, Robin DiMatteo, Joseph Engelberg, Howard Friedman, Tom Garrity, Howard Leventhal, Robert Moore, John Silvestro, Robert Straus, and Jean Wiese for their comments on an earlier version of this chapter.

9

Sonia Blackman

Social Psychological Perspectives on Pain

Mr. M., age 27, has chronic back pain. He injured his back while working for a restaurant as a fast-food cook. After three months of bedrest, which did not result in pain reduction, further medical diagnostic tests were conducted. Mr. M.'s physician, an orthopedic surgeon, decided that surgery should be performed because Mr. M. was suffering from a slipped or herniated disc. Although the surgery was considered a success by the physician, Mr. M. was still in a great deal of pain.

Mr. M. has been in continuous pain for 7 years, and he has been unable to work for that entire period of time. He receives Social Security Supplementary Income (SSI) benefits rather than regular disability benefits, because he had not accrued enough work credits before becoming disabled. He has gained 80 lbs, and he now weighs 250 lbs. He estimates his daily pain is 80–90% on a scale of 1–100% (1 = no pain at all; 100 = pain so unbearable that one would commit suicide). Most of Mr. M.'s day is spent lying down watching television, and he only leaves the house for appointments with his doctor. He takes 1/2-grain tablets of codeine eight times daily; when analgesics do not alleviate his pain, he drinks beer for additional pain relief.

Mrs. M. has one child from a previous marriage, 8 years of age, and one child, 6 months of age, from her present marriage to Mr. M. She has had to take a part-time job delivering newspapers, because SSI payments do not cover all their expenses. She is fearful that when she leaves the house something might happen to her baby and Mr. M. would not be able to rescue the child. Consequently, she rarely leaves the house except to go to work or to shop for food. Although she is supportive of her husband, she

169

expresses some dissatisfaction with having him "lying under foot all the time." John, the 8-year-old, is angry because Mr. M. cannot play with him, and because he always has to be careful and quiet in the house so he will not upset his father. He wishes "daddy would be like other fathers."

Mr. M. is severely depressed and feels that there is no hope for his future. He resents the welfare existence and the requirement that he have annual medical checkups to "prove" that he is completely disabled. He fears that his children will not love that "log on the floor watching television" and that his wife will leave him. If he were pain free his greatest dream would be to attend "chef's school." His greatest desire used to be that "someone would fix it."

Mrs. G., age 67, has chronic pain. She injured her shoulder while working in the garden. She has had two surgeries, but neither operation resulted in pain relief; in fact, she now has more pain than when she originally injured herself. She has been in continuous pain for 5 years and finds it difficult to sleep through the night. She has raised three children and has seven grandchildren who live in close proximity. Her hobbies were gardening and weaving, both of which she has been unable to do since her injury. She estimates that the pain is 65–70% on a scale of 1–100%; most of the day she spends trying to find a comfortable position and daydreaming. She takes eight 10-mg tablets of Valium and four 1/2-grain tablets of codeine daily; each night she takes a sleeping pill. Consequently, her speech is slurred, and she has great difficulty concentrating.

Mr. G., aged 70, is a retired nurse whose work was solely in emergency rooms. He has taken over all of the household duties and does not feel it is safe for Mrs. G. to "even boil water." He does not have any hobbies but feels that taking care of his wife is a full-time job. He does not resent her condition but wishes she would not try to do things occasionally as it "only makes her worse."

Mrs. G. is depressed and disoriented. She would like to get back to her household duties and plant a new garden. She feels badly because she gets jumpy and irritable when the grandchildren are around. Consequently, she discourages anyone from visiting, as she might not "feel well." Although resentful of her husband's help, she concludes she "just couldn't manage without him." Her concluding daily thoughts are, "I wish someone would fix it."

In addition to chronic pain, both Mr. M. and Mrs. G. are experiencing severe disruption in the social and psychological spheres of their lives. They are depressed and have no hope; they continue to feel badly about themselves due to diminished capacities. Each views his or her body as some type of a machine that has broken down and hopes that someone will "fix it." Neither leaves the house except for physician appointments, and they both have several doctors. They are overusing medications. Their social lives have become so restricted that they only spend time in the company of their spouses. Their children feel alienated and annoyed with them because of their irritable moods. They are angry with their physicians and their families and feel that no one understands them. They spend a great deal of time dwelling on the organic explanations of their problem and current symptoms, fearing that people will think, "It's all in their heads."

UNDERSTANDING PAIN

The scientific study of pain, dolorology, is fairly recent (Bonica, 1976). Historically, pain has been seen as the meaningless and random sport of an evil spirit, or a punishment inflicted upon mortals by offended deities. Treatments such as herbs for the alleviation of pain have been found on ancient Babylonian clay tables (Bonica, 1976).

Despite theoretical and empirical research on pain, there is no one truly adequate definition of pain. A definition that often satisfies researchers is the following: "Pain is an unpleasant experience which we primarily associate with tissue damage or describe in terms of tissue damage or both." This definition is not complete because it does not cover many of the paradoxes found in the study of pain (Melzack, 1976). Sternbach (1968) provides a more delineated definition: "Pain is an abstract concept which refers to 1) a personal sensation of hurt; 2) a harmful stimulus which signals current or impending tissue damage; 3) a pattern of responses which operate to protect the organism from harm [p. 12]."

Pain is a subjective experience, and it is private. These two components serve to make the measurement of pain difficult because self-report of the person experiencing the pain must be relied upon (Sternbach, 1978; Wolff, 1978). Indeed, pain is dependent on the consciousness of the person (Ripley, 1953). Pain is often a signal or symbol of something physically wrong, implying that there is tissue damage. But this signal of tissue damage is just one function of pain. It is not only intrapersonal, in that it alerts the person who is experiencing pain that something is wrong, but also interpersonal or communicative in function. The expression of pain (wincing, moaning, etc.) can serve to elicit aid from others (Szasz, 1957).

Another major issue in the study of pain, beyond its definition, is the search for an adequate theory to explain the phenomenon of pain. This area is complicated by the tendency of each theory to use concepts and terms that are particular to the professional describing pain (Sternbach, 1968). Degenaar (1979) argues that pain is a real entity that refers to many phenomena. He suggests that pain be approached from three domains: (a) the body or neurological approach consisting of specificity, pattern, and gate-control theory; (b) the mind or psychological approach, which deals with the emotional, conscious dimension (concerning the total ongoing experience; for example, the condition of suffering and distress that a pained person experiences); and (c) the philosophical domain or social domain (it can include examinations of disrupted social systems due to pain or concerns over the finiteness of life; for many, pain means we can die [Bakan, 1968]).

One of the major drawbacks of this breakdown of the categories of pain domains, and indeed of other categories (Sternbach, 1970), is the lack of utilization of or concern for a social psychological perspective in either the laboratory or the clinical setting. This social perspective is necessary. Pain is a private phenomenon that must be communicated in a social context; there is no material entity such as "pain" in the sense, for instance, that there is a tumor. This social perspective is especially important in the medical therapeutic relationship. It is necessary to integrate the theories and belief systems of individuals with a neurological orientation (usually medical personnel) with the individual patient's experience of pain and the meaning it has for him or her. Often patients' attributions concerning pain are in direct conflict with those of the physician. Social psychology can provide avenues for integration of these views.

In this chapter, the neurological perspectives will be presented first—the primary orientation of medical personnel. Psychological theories of pain are then discussed in the subsequent section because they serve to facilitate an understanding of the social variables that serve to alter the perception of pain. Then, a broad social psychological perspective that contrasts with existing approaches will be proposed for the study and treatment of pain.

THE NEUROLOGICAL APPROACHES TO PAIN

Specificity Theory of Pain

One of the earliest theories of pain, and one which has been most influential in the history of medicine, is the specificity theory of pain. This theory proposes a specific pain system in which specialized pain receptors carry a message of pain to a specific area in the brain (Melzak, 1973). These pain receptors or nerves carry specific information and are only receptive to certain ranges of stimuli (Bonica, 1974). Specific nerve endings are specifically sensitive to one of the four major cutaneous modalities: touch, warmth, cold, and pain. In other words, in this theory there is a one-to-one relationship between types of receptors, fiber size, and the quality of experience. The location of a pain center in the brain is still debated by specificity theorists, and anatomical and psychological research does not support this theory (Bakan, 1968). For example, cornea and teeth, which have only pain receptors, can also give rise to the sensation of touch. (Currently, there is a very qualified view of specificity of pain: it primarily concerns the neuronal level [Basbaum, 1978; Liebeskind & Paul, 1977; Sternbach, 1968].)

Pattern Theories of Pain

Several pattern theories of pain have been proposed. For example, one theory proposed that stimulus intensity and a central summation of signals are the determinants of pain. This means that no one stimulation results in pain but that many pain signals summate to produce the experience of pain. An example of such an instance is that pain is sometimes still experienced up to 45 min after noxious stimulation has ceased. There has not been a great deal of empirical support for pattern theories of pain; in laboratory studies and in clinical work, where there has been a neurosurgical lesion of the spinal cord, pain is often not abolished. In addition, if the pain is abolished after this type of surgery, it often resumes after 6 months to 1 year (Melzack, 1973; Sternbach, 1977).

The Gate-Control Theory of Pain

Although this theory is included with neurological approaches to pain, it is unique in providing an inclusion of psychological contributions to the experience of pain that is not provided in the preceding theories. An adequate theory of pain must account for several empirical findings about pain. First, it must incorporate the specialization of receptor fibers and their pathways in the central nervous system (specificity theory). Second, it must account for temporal and spatial patterning in transmission of the pain as explained by pattern theories of pain. Third, it must be able to explain the influence of psychological processes on the perception and response to pain. For example, suggestion and attention can alter the perception of pain. Last, it must account for the phenomena of summation, the spread of pain, and the persistence of pain after healing. Melzack and Wall's gate theory of pain addresses these four areas of empirical findings. Although there are many physiological questions still unanswered about this theory, it has generated a substantial body of research on pain and has greatly influenced the clinical treatment of acute and especially chronic pain. The theory suggests a hypothetical "gate" that can disrupt or facilitate a pain sign before the signal reaches the central processes (Liebeskind & Paul, 1977; Melzack, 1973; Weisenberg, 1977). In other words, the gate can cancel an adequate pain signal before it reaches consciousness (Sternbach, 1977), or it can serve to intensify a weak pain signal (Clark & Hunt, 1971).

This theory also proposes that the gating mechanism can be affected by and can affect central control mechanisms. This component of the theory serves to integrate many pain anomalies that appear to be due solely to psychological variables. For example, soldiers' reactions to wounds (due to the meaning of the injury) are much different from those of individuals who have sustained the same amount of tissue damage due to surgery (Beecher, 1956). The differences in their attributions mattered considerably. Injury meant the soldier would be sent home, but tissue damage to the patients meant that something was wrong in their bodies. Thus motivational and affective systems may exaggerate or initiate pain. Reductions in fear and uncertainty and increases in affective factors can decrease pain. For example, when subjects are given correct information about the particular sensations and pain they are going to experience, they experience less pain than if they were given no information or information that is not relevant to their experience (Egbert, Battit, Welch, & Bartlett, 1964; Johnson, 1973; Staub & Kellett, 1972; Taylor, 1979). Hypothetically, when people know what to expect in terms of what will happen to them, their fear is reduced. This results in a decrease in pain. A classic example of the influence of motivational factors is the professional athlete who continues to participate in sports events even after he or she has sustained a substantial injury (Ryan & Kovacic, 1966). In addition, affective factors such as depression can cause or exaggerate the experience of pain (Delaphaine, Ifabumuji, Mersky, & Zarfas, 1978).

The possibility of a gating mechanism engaged by central control processes and motivational and affective processes has proved to be fertile ground for both psychological research and treatment.

THE PSYCHOLOGICAL APPROACH TO PAIN

Learning Theories

The most prominent psychological theory of pain is that the perception of pain is a function of learning. Individuals must learn to experience pain (Mersky, 1970) through a developmental learning process. Pain is seen as those *behaviors* that an individual exhibits while in pain (Fordyce, 1974). For these theorists, pain is a hypothetical construct in that it must be inferred by behaviors. One cannot observe pain, but it is possible to record reports of pain, nonverbal expressions of pain (wincing), or bodily movements (limping). Although these behaviors may have originally been elicited through antecedent events, such as a broken leg, they soon come under control of consequent events, such as escaping from work or receiving sympathy while on crutches. In fact, by 4 months of age a person's reaction patterns to painful stimuli have been modified by the environment (Poznanski, 1976). Pain has intrapsychic, interpersonal, and societal significance.

Zborowski (1952) also views the experience of pain as a result of a learning process. However, he focuses on sociocultural learning. He sees pain as involving attitudes; pain expectancy and pain acceptance are two of these attitudes. Expectancy is the likelihood of experiencing pain in a given situation. Acceptance is the willingness to experience the pain. This orientation is most concerned with cultural attitudes. For example, two cultures may expect that being involved with war will entail pain, whereas only one may accept the pain. This acceptance may manifest itself in injured soldiers' disinterest in analgesics. Various cultures have different norms for the members of their group in relation to specific pain experiences.

Most of the psychological theories view pain as a subjective experience that manifests itself in pain behaviors (Fordyce, 1976b; Fordyce, Fowler, Lehmann, De Lateur, Sand, & Treischmann, 1973; Sternbach, 1974). Theorists who view pain behaviors as developing as a consequence of some type of learning usually cite Melzack and Scott's (1957) study with Scottish terriers. These animals were reared in an isolated environment in which they experienced restricted perceptual experiences. They were then compared with litter mates raised in an ordinary environment or in homes. These restricted animals were found to tolerate noxious stimuli, such as candle flame, even to the point of tissue damage. They had not learned appropriate pain responses, but they did show reflex avoidance to pinpricks, so there did not appear to be peripheral nerve damage or atrophy of nerves.

In conclusion, regardless of whether the pain experience is innate or due to learning, it is agreed that pain behaviors come under specific control of some type of learning. For example, pain may be a consequence of learning to attribute some type of meaning to symptoms. Initial instances of noxious stimulation, such as an infant falling, may be experienced as diffuse sensations. Because of responses of other individuals in the environment, such as, "Did baby make an ouch?" these sensations are labeled as pain. Eventually, pain behaviors may occur solely because of their consequences without any internal experience (Fordyce, 1976b). This approach to pain has implications for the treatment of chronic pain behaviors. These theories can also be used as explanations for many of the differences found between groups of individuals, such as various cultural groups.

The Psychological Measurement of Pain

There are five experimental pain parameters. Occasionally the terms for different parameters are used interchangeably, causing confusion over reported results. The first is the pain *threshold*. This is the point at which pain is just perceived. It is also called the minimal pain level. Theoretically, pain threshold should not vary across subjects. With good experimental controls, and trained subjects, the threshold for a given level of stimulation is at about the same level for most subjects. But, Sternbach and Tursky (1965) found that subjects trained in different laboratories revealed different threshold levels. The second measure is the *just noticeable difference*. This is the smallest discriminable interval between successive pain intensity levels. This parameter is not usually reported. Third is pain *tolerance*. This is the point at which the pain is no longer tolerated. It is also referred to as distress level, motivated threshold, voluntary withdrawal, and maximum pain level. It is the most frequently reported pain parameter. Fourth is the *pain sensitivity range*. It is the difference of interval between threshold and tolerance. Although this parameter is used infrequently, it appears more often in clinical research. Last, there is *sensation*. This is measured by asking subjects to report their perceptions of the intensity of the stimulus. Pain threshold and tolerance are the most frequently used pain parameters in clinical and experimental research. Care must be taken in reading the literature on pain because these terms are occasionally used interchangeably but do not really refer to the same phenomenon.

THE SOCIAL PSYCHOLOGICAL APPROACH TO PAIN

The social psychological approach is an integration of the various theoretical viewpoints that were discussed in the preceding sections. In addition, it will also include the pain patient's perspective. This latter perspective is important because even though the majority of all patients in medical clinics report pain symptoms, patients enter into a situation where others are utilizing differing definitions and theories of pain.

A Cross-Cultural Perspective

Several factors influence response to chronic as well as to acute pain. A very important factor is culture.

Zborowski's study (1952) on pain responses of different cultural groups is one of the most often cited cross-cultural studies. His comparisons were among Yankees (several generations of Anglo-Saxon), Italians, and Jews. All subjects were males. Data were collected by interviews with patients, patient observation, discussion with medical care professionals, and (in selected cases) interviews with patients' families. In doctors' opinions and by observation, Jews and Italians manifested similar pain reactions. Examination of further data indicated differing attitudes underlying these similar behaviors. Italians wanted immediate pain relief but were contented once the pain was alleviated. On the other hand, Jews were interested in the meaning and the future implications of the pain symptoms. They were reluctant to take analgesics, fearing that they would become addicted or that medication would mask important symptoms. Home and hospital behavior also differed for these two groups: Italians complained less at home, and Jews complained less in the hospital. Yankees, on the other hand, tended to remain aloof and unemotional about their symptoms, and they withdrew socially when they were in pain. They tended to be optimistic and future oriented and to view the body mechanistically. They were relieved once they were receiving treatment.

Sternbach and Tursky (1965) supported Zborowski's hypotheses in a laboratory study using Jews, Italians, and Irish as subjects. Both Jews and the Irish had significantly higher tolerance levels than did the Italians. The

Jews did not respond as they had in Zborowski's study, probably because there was no fear of the future meaning of the pain. Laboratory pain was clearly defined, and there were no health-consequence fears; hence, they had greater pain tolerance.

In sum, similar behavioral reaction patterns do not necessarily indicate similar attitudes about the meaning of the pain. In addition, similar pain behaviors may serve different functions for different cultural groups. Symptom presentation may also differ in different settings. In other words, one must examine the person's attitudes and behaviors in relation to specific social situations.

Zola (1966) examined patients' presentations of symptoms and the sphere of disruption that those symptoms caused in the patients' lives. The sample of 181 subjects was drawn from outpatient clinics. They were new patients and ranged in age from 18 to 50 years. They were matched on standard measures, such as education, social class, and occupation, and on diagnosis. Data collection, via interview and questionnaires, was taken prior to seeing a physician. The three ethnic groups that were compared were Irish Catholics, Italian Catholics, and Anglo-Saxon Protestants. The results indicate that the Irish reported less pain and that their symptoms were situated in more specific body locations. They also expressed fewer complaints and saw these symptoms and complaints as having less effect on other spheres in their lives. In other words, they viewed their symptoms specifically and locally and expressed complaints with little elaboration. Italians, on the other hand, were much more expressive in general. These findings may be indicative of the way in which these two groups approach life in general. The Italians may overexpress as a means of dealing with anxiety; the Irish, who tend to view life as hard, may use denial. In other words, patients' manner of self-presentation in a medical setting is similar and in accordance with their general self-presentation.

In a 4-year longitudinal study of patients (Woodrow, Friedman, Siegelaub, & Colleen, 1972) it was found that: Caucasians had the highest pain-tolerance levels, blacks had intermediate tolerance levels, and Orientals had the lowest tolerance levels. Racial differences were more marked between males. Differences in age were consistent for all races and both sexes. Pain-tolerance levels decreased with age for all races and both sexes. Other studies have also found this decreased pain tolerance with age (Harkins & Chapman, 1976). It appears frm other research (Knox, Shum, & McLaughlin, 1977) that Orientals have lower pain tolerance than Occidentals even with acupuncture treatment. In terms of dental pain, Caucasians had the least avoidance, blacks the second, and Puerto Ricans the most denial and avoidance (Weisenberg, Kreindler, Schachat, & Werboff, 1975). These results, as with all cross-cultural differences, have important implications for patient presentation in a medical setting. For example, the elderly are more sensitive to pain and hence may be seen by others as being overdependent on physician visits. Patients and physicians should be aware that there are differences in pain tolerance, but tolerance should not have either a positive or a negative label.

Many factors could account for these cross-cultural differences: experiences, beliefs, and, most importantly, the social context. Pain is not a well-defined experience, and one needs to look toward the social environment for validation of appropriate behaviors (Weisenberg, 1977). Responses can differ depending on information about the referent group. Both Jews and Protestants increased their pain tolerance when told that their referent identity group had low pain tolerance (Buss & Portnoy, 1967; Lambert, Libman, & Poser, 1960). In addition, Lambert et al. (1960) found that the identity of the experimenter could make a difference in pain tolerance. If the experimenter was Roman Catholic, there were no differences between Roman Catholics and Jews; if the experimenter was Jewish, Jews exhibited a lower tolerance. In this case of social context, the experimenter's identity made the difference. When examining pain responses in the laboratory and in the medical clinic, the researcher must take into consideration all these social variables that influence self-monitoring and self-control.

The Medical Model

Traditionally, medical personnel view pain within the context of a medical model (Fordyce, 1974). They look to identify antecedent stimuli that elicit pain behaviors. They observe symptoms or illness behaviors, try to identify the underlying pathology, make a diagnosis, and treat by attacking that underlying pathology. The approach is similar to that of the mechanic, with the body analogous to a car to be fixed once the offending physical problem is identified. In other words, pain is seen as a symptom that something specific is wrong with the body. In this regard, medical personnel tend to utilize the neurological specificity theory: Pain is localized and refers to a specific pathology. The physicians are healers. Indeed their primary social function is often thought to be relieving pain (Szasz, 1957). In this view, if a physician is a good healer, the patient gets better.

The medical approach works well with acute pain. This is the situation in which there is: (a) tissue damage; (b) pain; (c) anxiety; (d) a seeking of help; and (e) then pain relief and reduction of anxiety after medical intervention usually involving drugs and/or surgery. Both the physician and the patient are comfortable with this way of understanding pain and its relief. In fact, patients learn these five steps as a coping mechanism for pain relief. The problem for both the physician and patient begins when pain becomes chronic. Chronic pain cannot be successfully treated by physicians adhering to the traditional medical view, and patients cannot recover utilizing their usual coping mechanisms. The medical model fails; a social psychological perspective is necessary.

The person with chronic pain is usually referred to as a "pain patient" (Sternbach, 1974, p. 3). This is the individual who seeks relief within the medical system for pain that persists for 6 months or longer. The pain is benign—it is not life threatening—consequently, the patient must learn to live with it. Chronic pain patients must also deal with physicians who cannot help them and with individuals in their social network whose lives are disrupted as a result of the pain.

The Patient's Perspective

Much of the information about patients and the view that physicians have of pain patients are based on research designed to detect differences between functional and organic pain. Organic pain is primarily due to tissue change, and functional pain is mainly of psychological origin.

Literature concerning chronic pain patients has concentrated on trying to find means for assessing how much of a patient's pain is functional or psychological. Another area of inquiry has been whether there are differences among patients whose pain is mostly organic. The general finding is that chronic pain patients tend to score two standard deviations above the mean on the Minnesota Multiphasic Personality Inventory (MMPI) on the subscales: hysteria, hypochondriasis, and depression (Fordyce, 1976b; McCreary, Turner, & Dawson, 1977; Sternbach, 1974; Sternbach, Wolf, Murphy, & Akeson, 1973). Others have found that those patients with pain of organic origin appear maladjusted (Woodforde & Mersky, 1972). It is not clear whether individuals with specific personality patterns are most likely to develop chronic pain, or whether being in constant pain causes personality changes. In addition, one must also examine what the results of these tests might mean for the patient.

The particular personality orientation shown by the MMPI may serve a function for the patient. For example, being depressed and concerned with one's body may be a measure for gaining aid. It could be a statement of, "See, I really need help." Sternbach and Timmermans (1975) examined MMPI scores after surgical intervention. They found that there were changes toward normality on personality scales. These results must be viewed tentatively since these changes were at the time of discharge. Greater changes may be found on at least a 1-year follow-up evaluation when patients have entered into more normal life patterns. Utilizing the Introversion–Extroversion scale, the degree of pain experienced is positively correlated with neuroticism, but complaint and receipt of analgesics is positively correlated with extroversion (Bond, 1971, 1973; Bond & Pearson, 1969; Bond & Pilowsky, 1966). In other words, the request for analgesics may not mean that the patient is a hypochrondriac, it may simply be that he or she feels comfortable in requesting analgesics. Others have found that both patient groups (organic and functional) scored similarly to neruotic patients with high neuroticism scores (Woodforde & Mersky, 1972). Patients with psychological disturbances use more pain descriptions, and these descriptions are most diffuse. They use more words to define their pain, and these definitions are less specific (Leavitt & Garon, 1979). It appears that even when researchers find differences between functional pain patients and organic pain patients, there is a large degree of overlap between the two patient groups (McCreary *et al.,* 1977). In addition, it is not clear whether chronic pain results in a more disturbed personality profile. It has been found that those with functional pain had more premorbid personality characteristics (Mersky & Boyd, 1978). On the other hand, it has also been found that although there may be a neurotic personality problem associated with chronic pain, individuals with newly developed chronic pain do not show the personality pattern (Crown & Crown, 1973). Personality change may take place as a function of prolonged chronic pain.

Personality changes may also be a result of social interaction in the treatment relationship. In a study of private patients and pain-center patients (Chapman, Sola, & Bonica, 1979), private patients were found to exhibit a less disturbed personality profile. They were less depressed, had less conviction of disease, scored lower on hypochondriasis, and had fewer affect disturbances. However, it may be that chronic-pain patients who are still being treated in a private practice have not been in pain as long as those that are seen in pain centers. These results also point out the problem of generalizing from patient populations seen in different types of treatment centers.

The Patient in Pain

Pain patients are decribed as living in a nightmare (LeShan, 1964). There are three major components to this nightmare. First is the perception of the lack of control. They are often told they will just have to live with the pain. Second, there is lack of definition of what they are experiencing; all previous experience has been with acute pain where relief is obtainable. (Pharmaceutical companies prosper because our daily expectations are that we will be pain free. It is not a matter of whether we will obtain pain relief, it is a question of how fast we obtain the relief.) Third, strange and terrible things are happening to them; the pain is unbearable, and no one seems to understand.

In order to gain a sense of control, patients search for additional treatment, they begin to restrict their physical movements, and they limit their involvement with outside social activities. In other words, they begin to exhibit what is referred to as a disturbed life pattern (Sternbach, 1974). Because of this they encounter prejudice from the medical profession. In their search for a cure or relief they are termed crocks or "low-back losers" (Sternbach, Murphy, Akeson, & Wolf, 1973) and are likened to the alcoholic (Sternbach, 1974). In the usual acute illness medical situation patients and physicians are usually united in a common enterprise (Szasz, 1957). Pain serves to give illness authenticity, and the physician's role is to provide the cure and hence stop the pain. For the patient, the concept of psychogenic pain does not exist; certainly the physician and the patient's family begin to suspect that there is nothing organically wrong with the chronic pain patient (Sternbach, 1968). This fits with the notion that observers tend to blame victims for their fate (Ryan, 1971). Observers—physicians and families—begin to feel that the patients' pain is self-created. In addition to being blamed for their own pain condition, patients may become what has been defined by Taylor (1979) as the "bad patient." They are not passive in their approach to health care professionals; they are demanding and argumentative. When labeled as such by medical staff, they are most frequently referred for some type of psychological help, and their complaints are seen by staff as being less serious than the complaints of those who are viewed as being good patients (Katz, Weiner, Gallagher, & Hellman, 1970; Lorber, 1975). What results is an escalation of tension and anger between the patient and physician. The physician increasingly disregards the patient as someone worthy of traditional medical help, and the patient sensing this disregard responds with anger and aggression—hence the label, a bad patient.

These negative reactions can serve to reduce the patients' feelings of self-worth (Wortman & Dunkel-Schetter, 1979). Many chronic-pain patients think in terms of Cartesian Dualism and believe that if the cause of the pain is not in the body or cannot be fixed, it must be in the mind and therefore unreal. The interaction that results is described by Szasz (1968) as "painmanship." Both physician and patient try to confirm their identity: the physician as healer and the patient as a person with a legitimate condition, often at the expense of the patient.

The lack of personal control that chronic-pain patients must face can lead to helplessness and depression (Seligman, 1975). In addition, lack of perceived control leads to an increase in suffering (Bowers, 1968; Greer, Davison, & Gatchel, 1970). When patients can control the stressor, they have increased tolerance (Staub, Tursky, & Schwartz, 1971) and are more willing to tolerate more pain. Patients usually try to develop modes of attempting to control their pain, but the behaviors they usually choose actually increase their pain perceptions. For example, chronic-pain patients tend to pay close and constant attention to all their symptoms. They decrease physical movement and restrict life behaviors so much that they ultimately cause more pain (Fordyce, 1976b; Sternbach, 1977). More pain leads to more preoccupation with pain and more life restrictions, and an unfortunate cycle is perpetrated. Mr. M., described at the beginning of this chapter, is a good case in point.

In this type of ambiguous situation, where patients remain convinced that something is wrong (they are receiving a pain signal) but are unable to obtain medical confirmation, they look to others to see how to act (Friedman, 1979a). This is a new situation in which their usual coping behaviors appear to be inappropriate or lead to failure. With proper pain-coping models, they may learn more successful positive behaviors. In addition, observing others may reduce the perception of pain (Craig, 1975; Kleck, Vaughan, Cartwright-Smith, Vaughan, Colby, & Lanzetta, 1976). Patients need more information, the impact of which may be twofold. Information may help to provide a source of appropriate behaviors, and it may help to reduce pain perception directly (Egbert, Battit, Welch, & Bartlett, 1964; Johnson, 1973; Langer, Janis, & Wolfer, 1975; Staub & Kellett, 1972). Information can also contribute to cognitive control (Averill, 1973), which serves to reduce pain. In addition, an information approach can function to inform the patient about what he or she may expect to happen. Hence, the individual may experience reduced pain in response to a reduction of unrealistic fears concerning the unknown.

Patients also need to understand how pain behaviors such as nonverbal expressions of pain can increase the perception of pain (Blackman, 1980; Lanzetta, Cartwright-Smith, & Kleck, 1976). It has been found that exaggerating or freely emitting nonverbal expressions of pain tends to increase the perception of pain. Suppression of nonverbal expressions of pain tends to decrease the pain. Thus, the utilization of the findings from the social psychological research literature can serve to reduce many of the factors that lead to an experience of increased pain.

The social system is also critically important in its effects on pain perception and behavior. This includes not only the family but also the other networks. The patient–physician relationship is not entirely confidential, for the physician may need to report to various insurance agencies who pay the medical bills (Sternbach, 1978) and to employers and state or federal agencies that aid the patient. The physician faces a dilemma. He or she may not be able to find an acceptable diagnosis for the patient, but one is needed in order for the patient to receive monetary compensations. Social Security and disability compensation programs pay not for partial disability, but only for total disability. So, definition of the latter must be made, and the diagnostic label serves to influence the patient's behavior. Thus, pain needs to be viewed not only from the patient–family and physician–patient relationships but also from that of the larger medical compensation network as well. The situation need not be hopeless, however. Researchers are examining the contribution of the family to the patient's condition (Blackman, 1981), and agencies such as Vocational Rehabilitation are working with Social Security to institute self-support programs.

The field of social psychology contributes to the understanding of chronic illness such as pain through controlled laboratory studies, field studies, and an individualized case-study approach. In addition, it brings a unique framework through which we might view the problem of chronic illness. The patient is seen not as a static unitary component to be studied in isolation, but as a changing dynamic variable that interacts (acts upon and is acted upon) with individuals and institutions in the environment.

TREATMENT OF CHRONIC PAIN

The patient who is in pain initially faces the feeling that something is wrong (Sternbach, 1974). After repeated reliance on the medical profession for interventions such as medication and surgery, the pain of the chronic-pain patient still persists, and so too does the belief that something is wrong. The pain tends to increase in intensity, and the patient's anxiety increases also. In about 6 months, the patient may begin to believe his or her pain is not treatable. He or she then tends to experience despair and hopelessness. The patient worries about the lack of proper diagnosis and develops bitter and resentful feelings toward physicians. These factors all need to be considered when assessing treatment methods.

Treatments

Treatment methods are usually based on the researchers' or clinicians' theoretical orientations or are developed on the basis of clinical experience.

Melzack and Chapman (1973) base their treatment on the gate-control theory of pain. They identify several psychological factors that contribute to pain perception: attention, anxiety, depression, learning, and social factors. They suggest two types of treatment based on their theory. They recommend an increase in large fiber output (which theoretically decreases pain and can be accomplished through acupuncture) or acupuncture plus electrical stimulation. They also recommend maximizing central control mechanisms for modifying pain such as gaining cognitive and behavioral control through biofeedback training, suggestions of no pain, relaxation for less anxiety, and training for the development of a sense of self-control. Both forms of treatment, fiber stimulation through mechanical means and central control processes (through psychological means), are used in many multidisciplinary pain clinics.

Fordyce, on the other hand, believes that the illness behavior should be observed, identification of consequence (reward) relationships should be made, and behavior should be changed by principles of learning. Since pain is a private phenomenon, one must rely on patients' behaviors in order to know that they are in pain (Fordyce et al., 1973). Those actions (cries, grimaces, and requests for medication) that were initiated by noxious stimulators may now be exhibited because of their subsequent consequences unrelated to the pain (e.g., attention from others). This does not mean that these actions are not initiated by preceding events or that there is no organic cause of pain. It is just that pain may now be a consequence of antecedent and subsequent actions.

When using operant (learning) treatment approaches with social components, the focus is not on whether there is a modification of specific neurophysiological pain responses. The treatment is geared to modifying only those pain behaviors having to do with daily functioning. If one wishes to increase a behavior, it is followed by a positive reinforcer; when one wishes to decrease a behavior, the reinforcer is removed or incompatible behaviors are reinforced. This type of treatment works well in an inpatient treatment center, but it is difficult to bring about generalizations of program results to environments outside the hospital. There is also the problem of determining the best means of structuring the home environment. Inclusion of the patient's family in the treatment program is one method of solving these difficulties. Family therapy could facilitate the use of this type of treatment on an outpatient basis (Caines, Thomas, Mooney, & Pace, 1976).

Progress may come from a multidisciplinary approach. Bonica (1974) feels that a well-coordinated team approach, utilizing such specialties as anesthesiology, neurology, psychology, sociology, and surgery, should be used. His program is in an inpatient facility. Before admission, all the patient's previous records should be received, and the patient should have completed a 2-week pain, activity, and medication diary. On the initial visit, the MMPI should be administered, a family and a pain history taken, a general exam as well as any necessary consulting exams completed, and a social evaluation taken. Weekly conferences should be held to discuss the patient's treatment. Behavior modification treatments are used in Bonica's facility.

Black (1975) emphasizes environmental management as part of a multidisciplinary approach. Environmental stress at home or work should be assessed, and the patient should be actively involved in this type of treatment. This can be in the form of explanations or utilization of community resources such as vocational rehabilitation. He emphasizes that major environmental changes should not be made casually. This type of approach can be included within an inpatient or outpatient facility. Unfortunately, the assessment of such a treatment program has not been made.

Caines *et al.* (1976) have reported on their multidisciplinary approach. In addition to those treatment factors included by Bonica and Fordyce, these authors recommend additional preadmittance evaluation questionnaires of multimedical indicators, such as the Cornell Medical Index and the stress index. They also emphasize the patient's need for control. This is accomplished by having the patient actively participate in the treatment program. Patients are responsible for maintaining their own schedules, and they graph their own activity and medication levels. If symptoms still persist after pain medication reduction, a full exercise program, a recreation therapy, and a behavioral modification program is begun. A total of 175 patients have gone through their program, which lasted 4–6 weeks. The researchers found that weekly therapy groups were essential in seeking appropriate alternative behaviors. Family members also attend conferences. Research data have shown that on follow-ups after up to 12 months, there were several changes: 70% of the patients experienced a decrease in pain and an increase in activity, 35% required less medication, 74% did not seek further treatment, and 75% were participating in rehabilitation programs or were working. Unfortunately, no control groups are usually used in the evaluation of pain clinics.

Swanson, Swanson, Maruta, and Floreen (1978) report a similar type of multidisciplinary program. They include an educational program, the use of biofeedback and relaxation, and the use of videotaping along with group treatment. The authors do not fully explain how they utilize the videotaped feedback material. It is assumed that it enables patients to become more aware of their own behaviors. As suggested by this, future research might be conducted that explores the effects of alleviating pain behaviors during videotaped group sessions, perhaps incorporating some of the findings of research on the nonverbal aspects of pain, described earlier.

Volkerts and Bookwalter (1978) also report a multidisciplinary program. Although this approach is similar in many ways to that of other treatment programs, it emphasizes lectures on holistic health concepts, group therapy focusing on family interaction patterns, and encouragement of family participation daily. This focus on family involvement is an important one. The patient may be able to make good progress in the hospital, but if it is not supported by family members, the patient is likely to return to pretreatment behaviors. For example, in the case of Mr. M., Mrs. M. as well as the 8-year-old child would participate in Mr. M.'s daily treatment. The family would meet with other patients' families to discuss the impact of pain on the family structure and how the family can be active in changing the patient's behavior in the home.

CONCLUSION

It appears from the literature that a multidisciplinary inpatient pain clinic brings about significant changes in the patient's life. These programs rely on extensive pretreatment evaluations and use behavior modification procedures to decrease pain behaviors (including the intake of analgesics) and increase well behaviors (activity). They also involve relaxation training and group, family, and individual therapy. Although several of the programs emphasize the need to assess the patient's social environment and to include the patient's family in the treatment program, social psychological variables have not been sufficiently used.

There is a need for the adoption of some of the laboratory findings from social psychology about pain. For example, different types of cognitions have been found to lead to lowered pain perception. One form of treatment could consist of identification and changing of pain cognitions. A patient may constantly tell himself when he moves, "That hurts, I need medication," and so on. These statements could be replaced by such self-statements as: "If I move I'll get stronger and feel better." Or, the patient could divert his or her attention to music. These types of cognitive therapies might be utilized in both inpatient and outpatient facilities as well as by individual practitioners and might be successfully combined with an emphasis on the individual's entire social network. More empirical research on all of these issues is needed.

Chronic-pain patients need not be medical pariahs. With education, medical professionals can seek alternate modes of viewing pain once it has been established that a patient's pain cannot be relieved by usual medical methods. The social psychological framework can help prevent the view of chronic pain as being a solely psychological problem ("It's all in your head"). Indeed, all pain is perceived by the head, but pain also has social consequences. Pain can be modified by the head, and social factors can contribute significantly to pain reduction.

10

Coping with Stressful Medical Examinations

Each year American citizens endure literally millions of painful and stressful invasive medical procedures. Invasive medical procedures require the "invasion" of the body, either through surgery or through the insertion of medical instruments into the body cavities.

Invasive medical procedures may produce both fear and anxiety among patients. For the purposes of this chapter, fear will be defined as an emotional reaction to a specific procedure. Anxiety refers to a more general unpleasant emotional state that is characterized by both physiological arousal and cognitive factors, such as apprehension or a sense of impending disaster. Stress is a feeling or reaction that occurs when a person is confronted with a situation that requires a response (Sarason & Sarason, 1980). Invasive procedures are also stressful for medical staffs, who frequently complain that situations that are more noxious for the patients are also more stressful for those who must subject the patients to them.

Most readers have experienced some stressful medical procedures in the past. As an example, consider the electromyograph (EMG), which is a common neurological procedure used to diagnose neuromuscular problems. If you were to experience this procedure, you would first receive a series of electric shocks of increasing magnitude. Small electrodes would be

187

attached to your wrist and elbow, and the physician would deliver shocks to your wrist and record the time required for the electrical impulse to reach the second electrode. Over the course of about 45 min, the voltage of the shock would gradually increase to about 250 millivolts! In many medical centers you may also receive a second examination to study voluntary muscle activity. This portion would require the insertion of long needles in several body sites. Although this procedure is often necessary to make a neurological diagnosis, the great majority of patients report that it is a very unpleasant experience. This chapter considers psychological interventions that may be useful for easing the burden caused by the EMG and other stressful medical exams.

Although many medical examinations are known to be stressful events, they also provide some unique opportunities for intervention. Unlike many other stressful events, medical examinations occur under well-controlled conditions. The stressor is clearly identifiable, and the patient is available prior to the aversive event. Under controlled conditions, patients can be given specific preparations, and the effects of these interventions can be observed.

There have been few studies on preparing patients for painful medical exams. However, this appears to be a promising field for the emerging specialty of health psychology. Considerable laboratory research has documented that brief psychological interventions significantly increase tolerance to experimentally induced pain. Since the painful stimulation used in laboratory studies is not dissimilar to the discomfort associated with common medical and dental procedures, it seems reasonable that effective laboratory interventions will also be effective in clinical settings.

In this chapter I will review research relevant to the preparation of patients for stressful medical examinations. The first portion of the chapter will review laboratory studies that identify potential interventions. After considering the laboratory studies, I will review demonstrations of the effectiveness of psychological interventions for helping patients cope with specific medical procedures. The data summarized in this latter portion of the chapter were obtained in actual medical settings.

LABORATORY STUDIES ON COPING WITH NOXIOUS STIMULATION

The perception of pain is a very complex phenomenon. Until recently, most of the emphasis was placed upon sensory discrimination. However, cognitive and emotional factors play a crucial role in the experience of pain (Melzack, 1974; Sternbach, 1968). Pain experiences are moderated by sociocultural background (Sternbach & Tursky, 1965; Wolff & Langley, 1968) and personality characteristics (Davidson & Bobey, 1970; Kendall,

Williams, Pechecek, Graham, Shisslak, & Herzoff, 1979; Petrie, 1967; Shipley, Butt, & Horwitz, 1979; Spear, 1967).

Pain is also moderated by cognitive factors, such as the meaning of the situation to the patient (Beecher, 1959; Lambert, Libman, & Poser, 1960), anxiety about the source of the pain (Beecher, 1959; Hill, Kornetsky, Flanary, & Wilder, 1952), attentional focus (Beecher, 1959; Blitz & Dinnerstein, 1971; Kanfer & Goldfoot, 1966), and the anticipation of pain (Hill *et al.,* 1952; Wolff & Horland, 1967). This extensive evidence on the cognitive mediation of pain suggests a variety of psychological interventions for helping people cope with unpleasant medical experiences.

Placebo, Suggestion, and Expectancy Effects

Much of the initial interest in psychological methods of pain control was stimulated by documented placebo effects in the medical literature. A placebo is a medication containing no known medically effective substances. After reviewing 28 *clinical* studies, Evans (1974) concluded that 35% of patients suffering severe pain obtained relief from placebo medications. Placebo effects in *laboratory* studies were observed less often, with only 16% of the patients obtaining pain relief. A number of differences between the laboratory and the clinical settings may account for these differences. For example, clinical patients may experience more anxiety and anticipate more pain or define pain differently (Turk, 1975). The role of anxiety in the placebo effect has been demonstrated by Beecher (1972), who reported that anxious patients gain greater relief from placebos than do clinical patients who are less anxious.

The placebo response may be augmented by a positive doctor–patient relationship (DiMatteo, 1979). For example, placebo effects depend upon the individual's prior experience with physicians, his or her belief and confidence that something is being done to ameliorate the pain, and an expectancy that relief will be obtained (Weisenberg, 1977). Improvement of the doctor–patient relationship (DiMatteo, 1979; 1982), or nonverbal communication between patient and doctor (Friedman, 1979a; 1982), has potential for maximizing the benefits of suggestion.

Hypnosis

Hypnotic suggestion may be a useful method for helping patients cope with stressful medical exams. Greene and Reyher (1972) compared the effectiveness of two types of suggestion for increasing tolerance to electrical stimulation. The subjects were tested for pain tolerance, hypnotized, and given one of two suggestions: (*a*) to imagine their arms as numb and insensitive; or (*b*) to imagine a pleasant event. A third group was given both suggestions. Those who received the suggestion for analgesia and those who received both suggestions showed a significant increase in pain tolerance, whereas those who imagined pleasant scenes did not. These results contradict previous studies that have found that distraction (imagining pleasant events) is effective in altering tolerance (e.g., Neufeld, 1970). Pleasant imagery may be effective when anxiety is involved.

Chaves and Barber (1974) found that simply suggesting that pain would be reduced led to lowered ratings of discomfort. They instructed subjects to (*a*) imagine a pleasant event; (*b*) imagine their fingers insensitive to the discomfort; or (*c*) expect a reduction in pain (without instructions to engage in any cognitive strategy). The two cognitive strategies involving imagery each significantly reduced self-reports of pain, in comparison with the positive-expectation control. However, a greater reduction was observed for a group led to expect this change than for a no-treatment control group. In a similar experiment, Spanos, Barber, and Lang (1974) found that the most effective among several methods for reducing subjective reports of pain was imagining the effects of anesthesia. Patients were told to ''think of the hand as numb and insensitive, as if it were a piece of rubber.''

Not all people are equally affected by hypnotic and other suggestions. Scales have been developed to measure how susceptible individuals are to hypnotic suggestions (Weitzenhoffer & Hilgard, 1967), and these measures have been quite useful in identifying those who will receive analgesic benefits from hypnotic suggestion (Hilgard, Hilgard, MacDonald, Morgan, & Johnson, 1978). Other studies have also demonstrated that methods such as acupuncture, which gain effectiveness through suggestions, are most effective for those who are hypnotizable (Knox & Shum, 1977).

Relaxation Training

Both experimental studies (Grimm & Kanfer, 1976) and clinical observations (Sternbach, 1968) suggest that people experience more pain when they are anxious. Several studies suggest that the discomfort associated with most types of laboratory-induced pain results more from anxiety than from physical stimulation. For example, Shor (1962) found that subjects show very little physiological response to painful stimulation when they are not anxious. Thus, it is often difficult to determine whether observed reactions are attributable to stress or to pain.

One study attempted to separate reactions to painful stimulation from reactions to stressful stimulation. Subjects were either exposed to painful pressure on the skin or asked to view unpleasant slides of homicide victims. Among many measures, there were very few significant differences between these two groups. Only frontal muscle tension and respiration rate separated pain reactions from stress reactions (Davidson & Neufeld, 1974).

A variety of other experiments demonstrate that muscle relaxation training can help subjects cope with many different types of unpleasant stimulation (Lehrer, 1972; Paul, 1969). However, the effectiveness of relaxation training tends to be most apparent for measures involving physiological arousal. Typically, relaxation is shown to control effectively heart rate (Paul, 1969), skin conductance (McAmmond, Davidson, & Kovitz, 1971), or habituation (Lehrer, 1972).

If reactions to unpleasant stimulation are partly the result of anxiety, methods that control anxiety might decrease this aversive nature of the experience. Clinical psychologists have shown that relaxation training can help control anxiety (Goldfried & Davison, 1976). Relaxation training is a simple behavioral method for training the relaxation of muscle groups through a series of exercises. After a few sessions most individuals can learn to identify muscle tension and to relax. Bobey and Davidson (1970) compared the relative effectiveness of relaxation, cognitive rehearsal of the upcoming procedure, and increased anxiety (produced by listening to a tape recording of women in labor). After experiencing one of these treatments, subjects were exposed to either radiant-heat or intense-pressure stimulation. The relaxation group was best able to tolerate radiant heat, and all three treatment conditions were better able to tolerate the heat than was the control group. Among the three treatment groups, however, only the relaxation group was significantly better able to tolerate pressure than was the control group.

Avoidant Thinking and Attention Diversion

A variety of studies have attempted to determine the effects of different mental strategies upon coping with laboratory pain. Some of these studies test the folklore notion that it is better just to avoid thinking about threatening situations. When giving immunizations, for example, some pediatricians routinely advise children to imagine they are somewhere else. Some studies consider the effects of diverting attention prior to the painful experience (analogous to sitting in the waiting room before a stressful medical procedure), whereas others evaluate the effects of mental strategies during a painful procedure.

More than 30 years ago John Dollard and Neal Miller suggested that *avoidant thinking* was a useful method for coping with stress. People can avoid stress, they suggested, by turning their attention away from the stress-causing situations and by thinking about other things (Dollard & Miller, 1950). More recently, several studies have supported the use of avoidant thinking. In one such demonstration subjects were told that they would receive electric shocks. They were not told, however, when they would receive the shocks or how often they would get them. The subjects' self-reports about coping strategies indicated that the use of avoidant thinking was associated with less psychophysiological activity and distress than was paying attention to the threatening situation (Monat, Averill, & Lazarus, 1972). In other words, the people benefited from turning their attention toward something else.

Not all experiments support the use of avoidant thinking. In one study subjects were informed that they would receive a shock at some time within a 6-min period, but they were not told when within the period they would receive it. As expected, the uncertainty was stress producing. The subjects were then given an opportunity either to engage in an avoidant-thinking activity (listening to music) or to attend to the threat (listening for a tone that was emitted 5 sec before each shock was presented). The results indicated that those who chose to avoid thinking about the shock showed the greatest amount of psychophysiological activity and distress (Averill & Rosenn, 1972).

Since the findings of these experiments had been contradictory, Houston and Holmes (1974) decided to devote more study to the issue. They were aware that the earlier studies had been correlational in nature, with the question of causation remaining largely unanswered. That is, it was not quite clear whether avoidant thinking caused psychophysiological distress or if psychophysiological distress caused avoidant thinking.

In order to clarify the causal relationship, Houston and Holmes began with the hypothesis that avoidant thinking is an effective coping mechanism. Subjects were told that they would either receive or not receive electric shocks at some time during the experiment. For half of the subjects, distraction was created by having them read an interesting story while they were waiting for the experiment to get under way. Reading the stories, it was presumed, would cause avoidant thinking. The other half of the subjects did not read the distracting material. Among the subjects who thought they were to receive the shocks, psychophysiological reactions were highest for those who had read the distracting story. These findings were just the opposite of what was expected. After further analysis Houston and Holmes discovered that those who were not given the distracting reading material used the time to reappraise the seriousness of the threat. Upon reappraisal, their stress level went down. Subjects who had engaged in avoidant thinking did not have the opportunity for reappraisal, and, therefore, their stress level remained high. In any event, it became clear that avoidant thinking seemed to increase, rather than decrease, stress reactions.

Most of the early studies on avoidant thinking evaluated the effects of attention diversion while a subject waits for an unpredictable painful stimulus. Another set of studies considers the effects of diverting a subject's attention *while* the pain stimulus is being presented. These studies may have a quite different impact on the feeling of personal control over the stressor. Unpredictable painful experiences can minimize feelings of personal control, and attention diversion may do little to restore control. On the other hand, attention diversion as an active coping method while the stressor is present may increase perceived personal control. Thus, it is not surprising that attention diversion has been found to be more useful for coping with ongoing painful experiences as opposed to threats of painful stimulation. For example, Kanfer and Goldfoot (1966) found that distracting subjects by showing slides while they held their hands in cold water significantly increased the time they were able to tolerate the water. In comparison to strategies such as expecting severe pain, verbalizing the sensory experiences, or setting goals for cold tolerance, the distraction strategy was the most effective.

Barber and Cooper (1972) compared the effectiveness of three attention-diversion strategies: (a) listening to a taped story; (b) adding aloud; and (c) counting aloud. Each of these strategies was effective for only a short period of time, and it was concluded that with continued stimulation, distraction becomes ineffective. Thus distraction may be useful for helping patients cope with medical exams but may not be effective for managing long-term pain.

Not all attention-diversion approaches are equally effective. Spanos, Horton, and Chaves (1975) asked subjects either to reevaluate the sensory stimulation experienced (immersing a hand in ice-cold water) or to imagine an irrelevant scene. Reevaluation was more effective for increasing tolerance of the cold water. Further, a high involvement in images was found to be associated with greater pain tolerance. In a similar experiment Blitz and Dinnerstein (1971) found that subjects instructed to dissociate the experience of cold and pain and focus on the sensation of cold or to focus on the cold sensation and then interpret it as pleasant were significantly better able to tolerate the cold pressor than were comparable subjects who were not asked to divert their attention.

Accurate Sensory Information

As we have seen, directing attention away from a stressor can be of benefit in coping with an aversive experience. If these methods are effective, it is worth considering the opposite approach. Rather than avoiding information about the stress-producing situation, how about focusing on it and gathering more information? Medical and dental examinations are cases in point. Many times patients report being frightened about upcoming medical examinations. Their fears are not entirely groundless. It is quite possible that in many cases they will be subjected to painful experiences, such as being jabbed by a needle, cut by an instrument, or inspected via a scope. How, then, might patients react if they were told in advance the details of the forthcoming experience? "I don't even want to hear about it" is a common response.

Jean Johnson (1973) probed deeply into mechanisms for coping with pain and distressing experiences. Her belief is that fear comes about as the result of inaccurate expectations about the sensations we experience. In one experiment she exposed two groups of subjects to blood pressure tests. She told one group that the cuff used in the blood pressure tests would cause pressure, tingling of the hand, aching, and blueness—which, in fact, it does. These people were given accurate information. The other group was told how the cuff would be placed on and inflated but was not told exactly what sensations to expect. Those who knew what sensations to expect gave significantly lower ratings when asked to indicate how distressful the situation had been. In a similar experiment it was shown that subjects were less distressed by an electric shock if they had accurate expectations of what the shock would feel like (Staub & Kellett, 1972). These (perhaps counterintuitive) findings suggest that accurate information about the sensations about a physical examination will produce may help patients cope with the unpleasant experience.

Cognitive-Behavior Modification

Cognitive-behavior modification programs teach patients to relax and to develop positive ways to talk to themselves. It is the internal dialogue, or talking to oneself, that determines expectations, evaluations, and the focus of attention. Meichenbaum (1977) believes that coping abilities can be increased by altering what people say to themselves in stressful situations. For example, people who have difficulty coping with medical exams may say to themselves, "This is awful, I can't put up with this." Meichenbaum recommends training them to say positive things to themselves, such as "Take it easy. Good—you're doing fine! Just take a deep breath and relax; it will be over soon." This procedure has been labeled stress-inoculation training. Meichenbaum's procedure applies the technology of behavior therapy to the modification of thoughts or cognitions. The other component is behavioral, which involves training people to relax in specific situations. The Meichenbaum procedure has been shown to be remarkably effective for reducing stress in a wide variety of situations (Meichenbaum, 1977).

Turk (1975) successfully applied cognitive-behavior modification as a preparation for experimentally induced pain. After carefully considering many of the studies cited earlier in this chapter, Turk selected an assortment of cognitive strategies with some documented effectiveness. Trainers described a variety of coping strategies from which subjects could choose to deal with the sensory-discriminative, motivation-affective, and cognitive-evaluative components of pain. Subjects were taught to relax their muscles, divert their attention, or to imagine being in some other situation. In addition, they received instructions for generating positive self-statements to enhance coping with each phase of the pain experience. Measures obtained before and after the procedure included time that the ischemic pain (which is created by tightening a blood pressure cuff) was tolerated as well as verbal report of pain intensity. Results suggested a 15-min increase in tolerance for subjects in the training condition in comparison to a 1-min increase for an attention–placebo control group. This 15-min improvement in tolerance is particularly impressive since Smith, Chaing, and Regina (1974) found that subjects' tolerance for ischemic pain was prolonged by only 5–10 min following the administration of 10 mg of morphine. Since noxious medical exams are of brief duration, cognitive-behavioral interventions may suggest alternatives to the use of drugs with toxic side effects.

Not all individuals respond equally well to cognitive-behavioral interventions, and these differences may be related to the use of self-control strategies in daily life. Rosenbaum (1980) reported that individuals differ in the use of self-control behaviors that are quite similar to those taught in the cognitive-behavioral package. Those who tend to use many self-control strategies in their daily lives are better able to cope with brief-duration pain than are people who use fewer of these strategies. Thus, the cognitive-behavioral package may simply be teaching strategies that individuals who are able to cope well have acquired through other experiences.

Comment on Coping with Brief Aversive Stimulation

Results from research on coping with brief-duration noxious stimulation have been mixed and sometimes contradictory. However, a general pattern of results seems to emerge from the accumulation of data. Thus far, I have avoided providing a definition of pain because, as Melzack (1974, 1980) so convincingly argues, pain is a complex multidimensional set of experiences for which no single definition has proven satisfactory. Melzack has shown that approaches to pain that consider only sensory experience have been inadequate because they ignore the motivational and affective properties.

It is now widely acknowledged that anxiety, fear, and other emotional experiences play an important role in reactions to painful stimulation (Bonica, 1980). Psychologists may be able to do little about the application of various medical instruments that cause undesirable sensations. However, psychological interventions may be very useful for the management of the affective and cognitive components of the pain experience. Thus, it is not surprising that interventions that have been successful for helping patients cope with pain resemble other methods that help people cope with stress.

One of the most consistent findings to emerge from the research on painful stimulation is that patients are better able to cope when they have some feelings of personal control over the situation (Averill, 1973; Orne, 1980; Staub, Tursky, & Schwartz, 1971.) Similarly, belief in control is effective for relief from a variety of other stressful experiences (Rodin & Janis, 1982; Taylor, 1982).

In evaluating why belief in control is helpful, it is necessary to consider the various components of many control manipulations. Giving individuals personal control over a situation may also make the aversive stimulation more predictable. Thus, most experiments confound predictability and control.

Experiments by Johnson (Johnson, 1973, 1977; Johnson, Kirchhoff, & Endress, 1975; Johnson & Leventhal, 1974), which consistently demonstrate that providing accurate sensory information is helpful to patients undergoing stressful stimulation, may be successful because accurate sensory information makes the experience more predictable. Reactions that would ordinarily signal danger are placed in context by accurate sensory information. Instead of panicking when he or she experiences a certain sensation, a patient might realize that the uncomfortable sensations are normal and to be expected. Having information about a forthcoming undesirable event is consistently preferred by subjects over the opportunity to avoid this information (Lanzetta & Driscoll, 1966).

The concept of predictability also helps clarify some of the inconsistent results concerning the effects of avoidant thinking. Studies on avoidant thinking seem to fall into two categories. Some encourage subjects to avoid thinking about an impending shock that may be delivered at some unpredictable time. These studies tend to show that avoidant thinking is not a successful coping strategy.

This strategy allows the subject neither to predict nor to control the sensations. On the other hand, experiments that encourage subjects to divert their attention *while* they are enduring painful stimulation give them some feelings of personal control over the situation. As would be expected by this theory, manipulations that direct attention away from the presentation of the stressful event successfully enhance coping abilities. They gain effectiveness by providing the feeling of control over the aversive stimulation.

Although control and predictability are often confounded in experimental studies, it appears that the two have independent effects. Schulz (1976) carefully designed studies that separated personal control from predictability. He found that both control and predictability had desirable effects upon the well-being of a group of elderly persons. Even though control and predictability have different or independent effects, some evidence suggests that perceived control and predictability of aversive stimulation are functionally equivalent (Burger & Arkin, 1980). Further, physical symptoms that have been found to be associated with the presentation of unpredictable aversive stimulation can be diminished when people exercise more personal control over the situation by attempting to focus their attention on the unpredictable event (Matthews, Scheier, Brunson, & Carducci, 1980).

Manipulations that make the nature of the aversive stimulation more predictable or those that give the patient personal control over the situation should be most useful for helping patients cope with stressful medical experiences.

COPING WITH SPECIFIC MEDICAL PROCEDURES

As I have noted, a growing number of papers have demonstrated that cognitive and behavioral interventions can increase pain tolerance and the perception of laboratory-induced pain (see also Weisenberg, 1977). These experiments typically induce pain by having subjects immerse one hand in cold water (cold pressor task) or by restricting the blood flow in an arm (ischemic pain). Although the results of these studies are frequently generalized to clinical pain, only a few experiments have attempted to assess the interventions in a clinical setting. As Ledwidge (1978) emphasized, research on the effectiveness of cognitive and behavioral interventions will be more convincing if the data are collected in a clinical setting with the same patient population to whom the results are to be generalized. In a clinical setting patients may experience more uncertainty and anxiety than they do in the laboratory. For example, clinically induced pain may be compounded by anxiety. In comparison to the laboratory analogue, clinical patients are less likely to be reassured about potential damage, cause of pathology, or the nature of the procedure (Sternbach, 1968).

Fortunately, evidence is now available that suggests that cognitive and behavioral interventions can be helpful to patients who must undergo a variety of specific medical procedures. These specific procedures include: endoscopy, sigmoidoscopy, electromyography, cardiac catheterization, and dental surgery.

Endoscopy

Endoscopy is a common examination used to diagnose diseases of the gastrointestinal tract. Throughout the 15–20 min examination the patient must endure a series of threatening and uncomfortable steps. During the course of the exam, a small flexible fiber optic tube is inserted in the patient's mouth and passed through in order to inspect visually and photograph the gastrointestinal tract. Prior to the examination, the patient's throat is swabbed with a novocaine-like medicine, and many patients are sedated with a narcotic and/or a tranquilizer (usually Valium). Although the patients are sedated, they cannot have general anesthesia because it is essential for them to be able to follow instructions. If the patient is not able to breathe through the mouth when the throat is swabbed and make swallowing motions when the tube is passed, the exam can be considerably more dangerous and time-consuming. Patients who can control their behavior during the exam will gag less and get through the procedure sooner.

In a study on reactions to endoscopic examinations, Johnson and Leventhal (1974) prepared 48 hospitalized patients for the procedure by giving them either one of two types of preparatory instructions, both types of instructions, or no instructions at all. One type of instruction described the specific set of sensations that would be experienced: what would be seen, heard, felt, and tasted. The other instructions were for "danger control" and told the subjects what they would have to do during the examination: that the chin should be kept down, and that swallowing motions should be made.

The results of the experiment showed that the instructions giving a description of the expected sensations reduced scores on selected measures of emotional stress. The danger-control instructions were only of benefit when they were used in combination with the sensory description instructions. These findings show how simple and accurate information can increase coping with potentially stressful situations.

Another benefit of information has been described by Vernon and Bigelow (1974). These investigators tested the effect of giving accurate information about a hernia-repair operation to 80 men who were about to enter such surgery. They found that those given the information: (a) were more able to concentrate on the specific problems involved in the operation; (b) had greater confidence in the physician; and (c) were less likely to have fits of anger after the operation. However, the instructions did not immunize the men against fear and worry.

Other experiments tend to confirm the importance of accurate expectations for patients undergoing the endoscopic examination. For example, Shipley et al., (1979) prepared a videotape of a patient undergoing the endoscopic examination and showed it to patients either zero, one, or three times. As evaluated by a variety of measures, patients who had viewed the tape three times experienced less distress while they went through the examination than did patients who had seen the film only once or not at all. However, not all patients who had seen the film three times actually experienced less distress.

Shipley and his colleagues divided their patients into two groups according to a well-known psychological dimension known as repression–sensitization. Sensitizers display a coping style that is characterized by seeking information about a stressor as a means of getting ready for the experience. Patients who scored high on sensitization became less distressed as a function of repeated exposure to the film. However, the other group of patients were categorized as repressors—a group usually characterized as avoiders. Repression is a defense mechanism that involves avoiding thoughts about distressing events. For this group, the most arousal occurred upon a single viewing of the tape.

In a later study Shipley and his colleagues replicated this experiment using 36 patients who had previously undergone the endoscopic exam. Since the patients had already gained firsthand experience with the examination, they would be expected to be aware of the sensations it would produce. Averaging all of the subjects, they found that repeated exposure to a videotape of an endoscopic exam had little benefit. However, a finer-grained analysis demonstrated that anxiety and heart rate was much better controlled for sensitizers who had seen the tape three times. The opposite pattern emerged for repressors. For these patients, repeated exposure to the tape actually decreased coping during the exam. These findings suggest that personality variables must be taken into consideration in preparing patients for stressful endoscopic examinations. Patients who are sensitizers or who use information as a method of preparation might become desensitized by repeated exposures to films showing the examination. However, repeated exposures may actually stimulate anxiety among repressors, who prefer to avoid thinking about stressful events (Shipley et al., 1979).

Cardiac Catheterization

Cardiac catheterization is a relatively common medical procedure that is used to diagnose problems of the heart and the major arteries that supply blood to it. During the procedure, a small tubular, flexible surgical instrument is inserted through the vein of either an arm, a leg, or the neck. This instrument, known as a catheter, is passed through the vein and into the heart. It can be used to secure blood samples, determine pressure within the heart, and to inspect for abnormalities of heart muscle and tissue. During the procedure a dye is injected into the heart to provide a contrast medium for X-ray studies. In addition to the anxiety and discomfort the procedure may cause, the injection of the dye can cause some patients to experience a ''hot flash.''

In one study, cognitive-behavioral and patient-education interventions were shown to be effective for helping patients cope with cardiac catheterization. The cognitive-behavioral intervention taught patients to identify their own fears and how to use specific methods to cope with their anxiety during the catheterization. The patient-education intervention provided information about the procedure but did not focus on individual responses to the procedure. The patients were 44 adult males from the Veterans Administration hospital in Palo Alto, California. The cognitive-behavioral and the patient-education intervention were compared with an attention-placebo group in which a therapist actively listened to the patients. An additional no-treatment control group was also included. In this group patients were treated according to the usual hospital policy.

Ratings of the patients by doctors and technicians who were blind to the experimental conditions and patient self-ratings demonstrated that those who had experienced the interventions adjusted to the catheterization significantly better than those who had been randomly assigned to a control group. Further, those exposed to the cognitive-behavioral intervention fared better than those assigned to the patient-education group. These results provide further evidence that a relatively brief (45 min) and inexpensive intervention may aid patients in facing a frightening and painful experience (Kendall *et al.* 1979).

Electromyograph

Electromyography (EMG) is a common neurological procedure that is performed to diagnose neuromuscular disorders and to gain information about the site and nature of the pathology. There are two parts to the examination: (*a*) the electrical stimulation of nerves and muscles by means of applied electrical currents; and (*b*) the recording of action potentials during spontaneous or voluntary activity. During the first portion of the exam a series of electric shocks with durations of .1 to 1 msec and output from 50 MV to 250 MV is applied by means of surface electrodes. The second portion involves the insertion of needle electrodes into the muscles. Most patients experience some discomfort during the procedure, and the anticipation of forthcoming shocks and needle insertions tends to arouse anxiety and tension. Electromyography has been studied as a medical procedure amenable to behavioral preparations because it tends to arouse anxiety and produce considerable discomfort without requiring the administration of any tranquilizers or anesthetics.

One experiment illustrated how cognitive and behavioral interventions can be used to help patients cope with this most unpleasant examination. In this experiment, the cognitive and behavioral components of a cognitive-behavior-modification treatment package were systematically varied. In preparation for the EMG, half of the 40 male patients at the La Jolla Veterans Administration hospital were trained to say positive, coping things to themselves during the examinations. An example of a positive self-statement might be, "Just relax, you're in control; take it easy—it will soon be over."

The other half of the subjects were not given the training. The other manipulation was for relaxation training. Half of the subjects were given breathing exercises and muscle-relaxation training, whereas the other half were not. The resultant treatments were (*a*) cognitive only; (*b*) relaxation only; (*c*) cognitive plus relaxation; and (*d*) neither cognitive nor relaxation (control). The results demonstrated that the cognitive treatment was most successful when assessed by physician rating of distress, whereas the relaxation treatment was most useful for lowering heart rate (Kaplan & Metzger, 1980).

Overall, the results provided the greatest support for the use of the cognitive-behavior modification package. Although the relaxation training did reduce physiological arousal (heart rate), the cognitive-behavioral combination controlled heart rate nearly as well. Further, the relaxation treatment had little effect upon self-report or behavioral ratings. The cognitive intervention lowered self-rated reports of distress and physician distress ratings but had little effect upon physiological or behavioral measures. The combination cognitive-behavioral intervention had the most impact when considering cognitive, behavioral, and arousal measures. Thus, it appears the combination cognitive-behavioral method may be the most useful for helping patients cope with this particularly distressing examination. It is worth noting, however, that there were strong differences between the three treated groups and the control group, but weaker differences among the three experimental interventions.

Sigmoidoscopy

This year 110,000 new cases of cancer of the colon and rectum will be detected in the United States (American Cancer Society Statistics, 1979). This makes rectal and colon malignancies the most common internal cancer among American adults. The key to survival for patients with these maladies is early detection, since only early treatment is associated with lower fatality rates (Gilbertson, 1974; Hertz, Deddish, & Day, 1960; Winawer, Sherlock, Schottenfeld, & Miller, 1976). All men and women over the age of 40 are considered at risk for colon cancer (Copeland, Miller, & Jones, 1968), and annual screening of adults over 40 is now strongly advocated (Winawer *et al.,* 1976). Baseline studies show the detection rates among asymptomatic patients to be 3–6 per 1000 examinations (Strum, Landres, & Berry, 1976).

Sigmoidoscopy is a common medical examination that is performed to examine the mucose of the bowel and to determine whether there are any unusual growths in the last 10 in. of the colon. New evidence supports the increased use of the procedure because it significantly enhances detection of malignancies during routine physical examinations (Winawer *et al.,* 1976).

Although the examination is not believed to be particularly painful or dangerous, it causes mental anguish for significant numbers of patients. Some of this results from the medical procedure itself because the scope causes the bowel to be stretched. Other aspects of the discomfort result from the uncomfortable situation the patient finds himself or herself in. Since the exam requires that a scope be inserted in the anal cavity, the patient, who is nude below the waist, is placed face down in an unfamiliar environment with little personal control over the situation. Because of the unpleasantness of the exam, many patients avoid the situation altogether by refusing the exam or by failing to show up for an appointment. The effectiveness of brief interventions for coping with the exam was investigated by Kaplan, Atkins, and Lenhard (in press).

This study considered two separate factors. One factor was for self-instructional training: Patients were given brief training to focus their attention on either their own control over the situation (internal) or the doctor's control over the situation (external). A third (control) group received attention but did not experience self-instructional training. Half of each of these three groups also received relaxation training, whereas the other half did not. Patients experiencing the internal intervention rated themselves as least anxious during the procedure, followed by the external and attention control groups, respectively. The internal and external groups moved and verbalized less, allowing the doctor to complete the exam in less time than for the control group. Patients experiencing relaxation training tended to overestimate the duration of the exam but had fewer spasms and emitted less verbalizations. Overall, the results encourage the use of a brief psychological intervention prior to this most unpleasant medical experience.

Dental Surgery

Going to the dentist is one of the most common and one of the most disliked health behaviors. Concern over emotional reactions among dental patients has been expressed in the dental literature for more than 45 years (Richardson, 1936). As a result of emotional reactions to the dental experience, many patients avoid regular dental checkups or become behaviorally unmanageable once they see a practitioner (Train, 1969). Because of these problems, helping patients cope with a dental situation may be of benefit to both the patients and the practitioner.

Throughout the last decade dentists have been told by psychologists that a variety of methods are successful for helping their patients cope with the dental experience. These interventions include relaxation, distraction, and personal control. One experiment compared the effectiveness of these three interventions in a dental clinic. Patients scheduled for minor dental surgery were randomly divided into four groups. One group received relaxation training via an audiotape. A second group experienced attention diversion. This was accomplished by having the patients play a video Ping-Pong game before and during the procedure. A third group was given the feeling of personal control over the situation by being better able to communicate with the dentist. The patient was given a button that turned on a light signaling the dentist to stop. The fourth group was a control that received the dental treatment but did not experience a psychological intervention.

Patients who had experienced either relaxation training or distraction were better able to tolerate the procedure as assessed by ratings from both the patients and their dentists. The personal-control intervention group did not differ significantly from the control group. Thus, it appears that either distraction or relaxation may be beneficial for preparing patients for dental surgery. It is worth noting that patients appear to prefer the distraction method over the relaxation technique (Corah, Gale, & Illig, 1979).

Visits to the dentist may be of particular concern to young children. One issue in childhood dentistry is just how much information should be given about the procedure. In an Australian study, 422 children were given one of three types of preparatory information before a dental examination and then again before a restoration. The preparations differed in the amount of information given. Some children simply learned about dental health in the clinic, a second group heard a lecture and was familiarized with the operating room, whereas the third group was given a more detailed explanation of the procedures. There was a tendency for children who had been given a moderate amount of information (familiarization with the operating room) to be the least anxious during the procedure. Too many details may increase rather than decrease anxiety among youngsters (Herbertt & Innes, 1979).

The cognitive-behavioral intervention, which has been effective for adults with several types of medical exams, also has been shown to be useful for children in dental situations. In one study, a brief cognitive-behavior modification intervention was compared with an attention-control and a no-treatment control group as a preparation for a visit to the dentist by 7–12-year-old children. Ratings by an observer revealed that those who had undergone the cognitive-behavioral treatment remained most calm during the dental procedure in comparison to the other two groups. This finding was consistent for children of different ages within the 7–12-year-old range (Nocella & Kaplan, in press). However, younger children in all conditions had more difficulty than the older children. Some studies have shown that the anxiety common to very young children can be eased by the presence of the mother during the procedure. However, for older children, mother presence may actually increase anxiety (Venham, 1979).

Research also suggests that personality characteristics of the patients must also be taken into consideration when designing interventions for use in dental offices. In one study on preparation for tooth extraction, patients were given either general information about the clinic or specific information about the extraction procedure. The responsiveness of patients to these instructions was contingent on their perceived locus of control (Phares, 1976; Rotter, 1966). Patients who were categorized as internal (i.e., believed that rewards and punishments are a function of their own behavior) adjusted better during the surgery if they had been given the specific information. However, the opposite pattern emerged for patients who were classified as external (i.e., believed that rewards and punishments are independent of their behavior). These external patients adapted better during surgery if they had been given general information (Auerbach, Kendall, Cuttler, & Levitt, 1979).

It is worth noting that an enormous number of articles discuss their results as relevant to the dental situation. Nevertheless, relatively few studies have actually been conducted in dental clinics.

CONCLUSIONS

With the increase in medical technology and the access to medical care, we are witnessing a rapid expansion in the use of diagnostic procedures. Many of these procedures are found to be noxious by the millions of patients who experience them each year. Evidence is accumulating of how simple cognitive and behavioral interventions can be used to increase tolerance to noxious laboratory stimulation. Further, a small but growing literature expands upon the laboratory work to demonstrate that similar procedures help patients cope with actual medical examinations. To date, the application of psychological methods to help patients cope with medical examinations has been limited to a small sample of stressful procedures. However, there is reason to believe that the interventions will be effective in other medical situations. Similar methods have also been shown to be effective for preparing patients for other stressful medical experiences such as surgery (Kendall & Watson, 1981).

Studying methods for helping patients cope with stressful examinations provides unique opportunities for both basic and applied research. In the future, the most productive line of research will be experimental trials in which patients are randomly assigned to treatment groups. At least one of the groups should be an "attention-control" group in which the patients receive attention and support but do not experience the treatment that is theoretically linked to benefit. This group is necessary in order to demonstrate that the effectiveness results from the specific intervention and not just attention. The experiments should also include a variety of outcome measures. Some of these measures should be ratings by observers who are unaware of the condition to which the patient had been assigned. Experimentation on preparation for examinations is relevant to not only a personal concern of many patients but also several theoretical positions such as attribution theory, reactance theory, and social learning theory, which can be evaluated using the data.

Because research on coping with stressful medical exams is only now beginning, clinical application of these methods has not been common. However, many physicians are concerned about the unpleasant experiences they subject patients to and are eager to learn about new approaches. Johnson's work (noted earlier) on endoscopy, for example, is now well disseminated, and I am aware of several physicians who apply her suggestions. Thus, research in this area has the potential to be rapidly disseminated and absorbed into practice as well as to be practical and theoretically challenging.

It is worth noting that the effects observed in most studies on interventions for stressful medical exams are not particularly strong. Longer and repeated interventions might be more effective in producing distinctive experimental effects. However, psychological preparations for brief examinations would not be useful in practice if they were time-consuming or required repeated visits. The brief interventions applied in most of the studies could be utilized within the period that patients typically spend in a waiting room and would not require serious constraints on scheduling. The modest experimental effects suggest that the interventions could be useful within the clinical practice of medicine. With a minimal increase in time and effort for medical staff to deliver the preparatory information, patients may be given more control over their own reactions to procedures they find stressful and painful. Patients are likely to be more relaxed and cooperative, to cope more successfully, and to experience minimal discomfort during the medical procedure. Further, the methods may circumvent the need for administering pharmaceuticals.

In our enthusiasm to become more active in health care delivery, health psychologists must be aware of the limitations of their offerings. To date, few psychological procedures have been demonstrated to be effective in clinical settings, and we must continue experimental testing until we are certain that the benefits of these methods offset the added costs and inconvenience they may produce. For example, several authors have suggested that personality test results be evaluated in order to tailor specific interventions for helping patients cope with brief medical exams. However, assessing personality characteristics may not be practical in many applied settings. Indeed, personality assessment may be more time-consuming than the treatments themselves. Further, personality testing requires additional consent, and time must be taken to give patients feedback on their test results. Thus, practical considerations must be exercised in the use of personality assessment as an adjunct to behavioral and cognitive interventions.

In the development of new intervention strategies it will also be important to stick closely to the data. Laboratory studies have provided guidance for those interested in stressful medical exams because the stimuli used in the laboratory are not dissimilar to those used in clinical settings. However, the clinical use of these methods must depend upon their demonstrated effectiveness in clinical settings. It is important to realize that other pain problems, such as chronic back pain, are qualitatively different from either laboratory pain or stressful medical exams. Data summarized in this chapter may not be relevant to more severe and enduring sources of pain. Research in clinical settings, with researcher and clinician working side by side, will eventually produce answers to many important theoretical and practical issues.

IV

PATIENTS' DEMANDS AND
THE HEALTH CARE ENVIRONMENT

Health care is rapidly emerging as one of the most critical political problems facing the United States today. Costs are soaring and significant segments of our society do not have access to adequate health care services. Furthermore, survey results suggest that even with access to care, many consumers are dissatisfied with the way the services are delivered (Kasteler, Kane, Olsen, & Thetford, 1976). Consumers are no longer so tolerant of a system oriented to a physician-dominated ''fixing'' of acute problems, especially considering the high costs involved. Issues of preventive medicine, health maintenance, disclosure of information, cost control, and medical ethics have become social and political problems.

Patients as consumers of health care services are painfully aware that these broader issues are usually not raised by their health professionals. Patients note the lack of completeness and continuity in their care, as well as the impersonality with which care is often delivered by overworked health care providers. Such impersonality and dehumanization may become obstacles to the patient's successful treatment and recovery. For this reason, the health care environment is an important—although often overlooked—area of study.

One cause of patient dissatisfaction involves the widely accepted attitudes held by health professionals concerning what they feel to be the necessary medical environment for patient care. Many health care professionals who function under the pressures of life-and-death situations believe they require total control in order that the environment in which they attempt to save lives be maximally efficient and predictable. Unfortunately, the bureaucratization required to achieve this goal directly conflicts with the patient's psychological needs to be treated as a person and to feel in control of his or her life. This struggle between the patient's demands and the health care environment is the focus of this fourth and final part. Here we see that the struggle is not between the patient's emotional self-fulfillment and his or her physical well-being. Rather, self-fulfillment and physical well-being are highly related and directly affect each other. Thus, the social psychological factors in patient care are part of, not adjunct to, the physical care of the patient. The challenge for social psychologists is to integrate these two seemingly antagonistic dimensions in the health care environment.

Both of the following chapters search for means to inject patient freedom into medical bureaucracies that concentrate on efficient care of human bodies but not of human beings. One promising approach involves modifying the hospital environment to allow the minor exercise of control and to combat depersonalization. Another approach involves the *hospice*—a system of care for the terminally ill that focuses on the patient and family as individuals. Ironically, as we will see in the last chapter, there is a tendency for innovations that provide patient control to themselves become bureaucratized, thereby destroying the autonomy they were designed to create.

11

Shelley E. Taylor

Hospital Patient Behavior: Reactance, Helplessness, or Control?

About 37 million patients will be admitted this year to the more than 7000 hospitals (American Hospital Association, 1977) in the United States. Today people no longer go to hospitals only when they are sick. Hospitalization occurs whenever involved tests are required, when special medical equipment is needed, or when a support system of additional personnel and adjunct services is required. Hospitals are now a common and normal aspect of the management of many different health conditions (Rosen, 1963). However, hospitals are often regarded as unpleasant places to be (Roth, 1972). They are total institutions (Goffman, 1961) that manage all aspects of patient life. Though few people spend more than a few days in the hospital over an entire lifetime, the impact of these few days can be tremendous. Why is this the case?

The hospital is one of the few places where an individual forfeits control over virtually every task he or she customarily performs. This chapter will analyze the implications that loss of control has for hospital patients. We will suggest that loss of control helps depersonalize the patient and that many patients adjust to depersonalization by assuming either ''good patient'' or ''bad patient'' behavior (cf. Lorber, 1975). An analysis of these roles, however, will reveal that many ''good patients'' are actually in a state

Interpersonal Issues in Health Care

of depressed or anxious helplessness, whereas the "bad patient" is exhibiting anger against the arbitrary exercise of control by the hospital (reactance). We will argue that both helplessness and reactance produce physiological, cognitive, behavioral, and affective consequences that can strongly interfere with the course of recovery and that helplessness and reactance in patients evoke reactions in hospital staff that also have undesirable consequences for treatment and recovery. Next, drawing on research results that demonstrate the physical and psychological benefits of control-restoring interventions, we will suggest that feelings of control, the development of appropriate expectations, and the belief that one can affect one's own condition lead to a better physical and psychological state than does the absence of such beliefs. We will argue that use of control-based interventions that encompass a wide range of the hospital patient's activities and draw upon the patient's abilities to manage his or her own care can offset many of the pernicious side effects that the loss of control—reactance—helplessness cycle creates.

ASSUMING THE HOSPITAL PATIENT ROLE

> The patient comes unbidden to a large organization which awes and irritates him, even as it also nurtures and cures. As he strips off his clothing so he strips off, too, his favored costume of social roles, his favored style, his customary identity in the world. He becomes subject to a time schedule and a pattern of activity not of his own making [Wilson, 1963, p. 70].

The patient's reactions to hospitalization have received remarkably little attention from social scientists despite the centrality of the patient to the hospital's functioning and the patient's role in unifying the diverse goals of the hospital. Part of the reason for this lack of attention may be that the hospital-patient population is transitory, so it is impossible to study it longitudinally. A second reason may be that patients are usually sick and often cannot or do not want to respond to researchers' questions. A third reason may be that just as the personnel within the hospital do, the social scientist may come to see patients as "products" of the hospital, recipients of services who, though they are the central focus of the organization, are also passive participants in its activities (Wilson, 1963).

We do know that few people are happy with the prospect of being hospitalized for an illness (see, for example, Tagliacozzo & Mauksch, 1972). Many people, particularly older people, are terrified of hospitals either because they associate them with pain and death or because the hospital atmosphere is frightening and disorienting. Other people become upset in hospitals because they are restricted and infantilized by the system.

And still others become quite dependent and helpless, unable to make the smallest effort to help in their own treatment. Hospitals are so commonly regarded as unpleasant places to be that psychiatrists are inclined to study those who want to stay in the hospital rather than those who want to leave as quickly as possible (Roth, 1963).

When patients arrive at the hospital, they may already be feeling a loss of control. Illness, particularly serious illness, leads to a sense of alienation from one's body, in that one is usually able to count on good health and no longer can (see Leventhal, 1975). Patients usually also experience literal loss of control in that they no longer can manage their daily activities and roles. The hospital regimen exacerbates these already-existent feelings. Activities are mobilized around patient care, but not necessarily around the patient as a person. The patient is the body upon which the ministrations and talents of the staff are exerted, but the patient is not expected to take on an active role in his or here own care. She or he is expected to be cooperative, pleasant, and quiet. Indeed, as Goffman (1961) has suggested, it would be much easier for the staff overall if the patient were not a person but, rather, a noninteracting object. In an effort to approximate this unattainable state, medical staff subtly communicate to each new patient the critical components of the hospital patient role.

From this point of view, the ideal hospital patient role would be an inanimate state (see, for example, Cartwright, 1964; Coser, 1962; Goffman, 1961; Lorber, 1975). Hospital staff, at least partially, accomplish this state by depersonalizing the patient. Depersonalizing of the patient in the hospital occurs through several means: by routinization of treatment procedures, by the obfuscation of bureaucratic procedures, by nonperson treatment by medical staff, and by not providing information to the patient regarding the state of his or her health or the nature of his or her treatment (cf. Goffman, 1961). Each of these means deserves some elaboration. Before doing so, however, it is important to distinguish between values or intentions of medical personnel and their actual behavior. In the following discussion of depersonalization, we will be concerned with the effects of staff behavior on patients; we do not wish to imply that patient depersonalization reflects a value or intention on the part of staff. Indeed, the opposite is the case. It is clear that hospital staff are strongly committed to the concept of personalized patient care (see, for example, Skipper & Leonard, 1965). However, for reasons that will become clear in the following sections, medical staff are often unable to act upon this value and instead fall back on depersonalizing treatments for reasons of efficiency and self-protection. With this caveat in mind, we can now turn to a discussion of patient depersonalization.

The routinization of procedures facilitates the patient's loss of identity within the hospital by substituting formulas for personalized care. Patients first arrive at the hospital with anxiety from the illness itself, from the prospect of hospitalization, and from all the role obligations they must leave behind unfulfilled. The hospital intake procedure does little, if anything, to calm anxiety, and in some cases it exacerbates it. The admission is often conducted by an impersonal clerk who asks about scheduling, insurance, and money. The patient is then ushered to a strange room, given new clothes, provided with an unfamiliar roommate, and subjected to confusing tests. The patient must entrust his or her body completely to strangers, in a peculiar, uncertain, unfamiliar environment in which many procedures are new (Kornfeld, 1972; Wilson, 1963). He or she is expected to be cooperative, dependent, and helpful without demanding too much attention. The patient learns quickly that in many respects the hospital is organized for the convenience of staff, rather than for patients. Thus, joining the ranks of the sick by seeking formal treatment means moving into a category in which one's individuating characteristics—job, relationships, clothing, hobbies—are irrelevant as a basis for identity, because it is precisely these characteristics that must be temporarily suspended. The patient becomes part of the staff's schedule, appearing on a number of different lists as the recipient of a number of different services (Roth, 1963; Tagliacozzo & Mauksch, 1972).

The hospital bureaucracy depersonalizes the patient by placing him or her in a complex organization that cannot be controlled by the patient to his or her own advantage. The patient is in an institution whose structure she or he does not understand and is subject to the directives of several different lines of authority with several different levels within each line. As a result, the patient may receive contradictory instructions from different people and have no means of determining which are correct. Each hospital staff member can put off the patient's questions by referring them to another level of authority. Orderlies often tell the patient to ask the nurse; the nurse tells the patient to ask the doctor; and when the doctor drops in unexpectedly for a visit, the patient may be taken so by surprise that he or she fails to ask questions at all (Kornfeld, 1972; Roth, 1963). As a result of these different loci of authority, care is fragmented. As many as 30 different staff persons may pass through a patient's room each day, conducting tests, taking blood, bringing food, or cleaning. Even the nursing staff, which theoretically provides some continuity in care, shifts three times a day (Brown, 1963).

When staff members interact in proximity to the patients, the interaction often depersonalizes the patient still further. It is marked by what Goffman (1961) calls "the wonderful brand of 'non-person treatment' . . . whereby the patient is greeted with what passes as civility, and said farewell to in the same fashion, with everything in between going on as if the patient weren't there as a social person at all, but only as a possession someone has left behind [pp. 341-342]." Nonperson treatment results in part from simple lack of courtesy. Cartwright (1964) found that medical staff often forget the most basic civilities in their interactions with patients. Patients are often referred to (and thought of) in terms of their symptoms, disease, or condition. ''People get in and they become arms or legs or kidneys, or bladders or something besides Joe Smith the human being [Scanlan, in Terkel, 1972, p. 494].'' Commenting on depersonalization in the hospital, Kaufman (1970) noted that when medical staff make rounds, they often use either highly technical terms or euphemistic terms when discussing a case with colleagues. These terms often alarm or confuse the nonparticipating but physically present patient, an effect to which physicians are often oblivious.

A fourth source of depersonalizing experiences for patients involves being kept in a state of low information. There are many reasons why hospital staff may not want to communicate full information to patients about their illness. One reason is lack of time; staff may feel they are unable to spend time explaining details of condition or care to one patient when they could instead be spending time on the physical care of other patients. Alternatively, information may be deliberately withheld because it is feared that it will alarm the patient or that he or she will misinterpret it. In other cases, however, withholding information from patients fits the needs of the staff more than it does the needs of the patients. Skipper, Tagliacozzo, and Mauksch (1964) summarize:

> Giving information to patients about their illness may be seen as something which patients do not need to know, would probably not understand anyway, might cause an emotional reaction which would interfere with their instrumental care and cure, and at the very least takes the time of the nurses and physicians away from more important tasks [pp. 35–36].

In addition, the withholding of information from patients prevents their asking further questions (see Duff & Hollingshead, 1968).

Depersonalizing treatment, coupled with any disorientation produced by illness itself, renders patients vulnerable to social influence from the staff, and in this case, staff pressures all work in the same direction, pushing the patient into assuming the good patient role. As Tagliacozzo and Mauksch (1972) observed, the patient becomes concerned with doing precisely as he or she is told and following all instructions literally in an effort to increase his or her chances of recovering. Patients feel they must accommodate all instructions of the staff. Physicians are regarded by patients as expecting cooperation, trust, and confidence, and nurses are seen as expecting undemanding, respectful, and considerate behavior. Thus, the hospitalized patient regards pleasing the doctor and nurse by behaving properly as a chief role obligation. For the patient, ''behaving properly'' means doing what one is told and not making trouble. Tagliacozzo and Mauksch (1972) summarize:

> The obligation to be a "cooperative" patient is learned early in life, and as has been indicated, is apparently taken quite seriously by most patients. More aggressive interpretations of the patient role are not easily verbalized and, apparently not often realistic alternatives for the patient. Prevalent images of the hospital as a crisis institution, the conception that rights and demands should be governed by the seriousness of the illness, and consideration for other, possibly sicker patients, make it extremely difficult to play the "consumer role" openly and without fear of criticism [p. 171].

The observations of Tagliacozzo and Mauksch (1972) and others (e.g., Katz, Weiner, Gallagher, & Hellman, 1970; Lorber, 1975) make it clear that most patients try to adopt the good patient role. Some are more successful than others. According to Lorber's (1975) classifications, about 25% of all patients cause the staff almost no problems, either because their illnesses are easy to manage, or because they try especially hard to be cooperative, or both. Another 50% cause minor problems for staff because their medical problems require more care, and although they are generally cooperative, they have some legitimate complaints due to the pain or discomfort of their conditions. A third group, comprising about 25%, is more problematic still (e.g., Katz et al., 1970; Lorber, 1975). Although some of these patients take up staff time because they are seriously ill and require extensive care, others are just "bad patients." The bad patient is one who is not seriously ill but who complains and demands attention anyway (Lorber, 1975). This patient often plays a consumer role, insisting on his or her rights as a patient, especially the "right to know." Coser (1962), making a similar distinction, refers to good patients as "primary" patients and to bad patients as "instrumental," a reference to their insistence on their autonomy, their right to criticize, their right to be well informed (see also Shiloh, 1965). These patients are suspicious of their treatment, and they react negatively to most efforts to mollify them. Though a minority, their numbers are substantial enought to constitute a major medical problem.[1,2]

Why do some hospitalized patients become angry? One reason may be that many freedoms are withheld from medical patients when they enter the hospital. Some of these restrictions are medically based, such as requiring a patient with a broken leg to refrain from standing on it, or requiring a patient receiving intravenous feeding to stay in bed. Other restrictions are imposed to protect the freedoms of other patients, the abilities of the staff to go about their work, and the ability of the hospital bureaucracy to function. For example, visitors are restricted to particular times of the day; patients are allowed to walk about only at certain times and in certain places; drink-

---

[1] Obviously, patient behavior runs the gamut from very cooperative or "good" to very uncooperative or "bad." Whether one divides this continuum into two groups (e.g., Coser, 1962; Duff & Hollingshead, 1968), three groups (e.g., Lorber, 1975), or more is entirely arbitrary.

[2] The good patient–bad patient distinction comes from terminology often used by hospital staff to refer to these two types of patients.

ing, smoking, and eating of certain foods are in many cases discouraged; and lights and televisions are turned off by particular times at night. Many of these restrictions on freedom may have an unclear rationale for the patient who is bored, thirsty, hungry, and generally restless. This threat to freedom may not be particularly distressing in itself, but when combined with distress resulting from being ill, it can create a "bad patient." The patient is already feeling put upon by illness. She or he has had to suspend normal activities, ones that she or he may have preferred not to give up, in order to get treatment. If hospitalization requires further restriction upon freedoms, it can increase the patient's irascibility and inclination to lash out against authority. There may be pressures on the patient to accomplish things at work. She or he may have planned for a vacation that has now become impossible. As one lies in bed, it is easy to dwell on all the things one would like to do and cannot. Immobility, then, is a continual source of frustration because one is not only kept from doing the things one planned but also left with all the time in the world to dwell upon that very fact. The resulting angry reactions against the abrupt and seemingly arbitrary withdrawal of freedom has been termed reactance (Brehm, 1966).

INDIVIDUAL DIFFERENCES IN ASSUMING THE PATIENT ROLE

Many patients, then, respond to pressures to assume the patient role with one of two reactions: good patient behavior (compliance) or bad patient behavior (resistance). Is there any basis for predicting who will show which reaction to hospitalization? Thus far, little research has addressed this issue, but some speculations are possible. Since the result of patient depersonalization is increasing loss of control, the manner in which an individual reacts to loss of control in general might well predict reactions to hospitalization. For example, in a different but related context, Kubler-Ross (1969) has suggested that among terminally ill patients, those who have lived active, controlling, high-pressured lives have more difficulty adjusting to the prospect of death than do more simple, passive, reactive people. (One can think of the prospect of death as the ultimate loss of control.) In addition, research on coronary-prone behavior patterns has led to the identification of a Type A syndrome, which is marked by a high need to control and succeed (Friedman & Rosenman, 1974; Jenkins, 1971). Type A individuals have a sense of time urgency; they work harder than others; and they tend to become hostile when thwarted. Type B individuals, in contrast, manifest the absence of these same characteristics (Glass, 1977b; Jenkins, 1971). These kinds of data lead one to predict that people who are accustomed to controlling and managing the environment (such as Type A individuals) would be more likely to react to hospitalization with resistive behavior than would Type B individuals, who are more accustomed to being dependent, reactive, or passive in their environment. Consistent with these predictions are Lorber's (1975) findings that younger, well-educated patients (who may be highly motivated to control) most often turned up as problem patients and DeWolfe's, Barrell's and Cummings's (1966) findings that older people and those who prefer an authoritarian hospital environment showed the best adjustment to hospitalization.

Expectations about the hospital experience and perceptions of the rationale for loss of control might also predict who reacts to hospitalization with good or with bad patient behavior. Individuals who expect to make an active contribution to their care, those who anticipate considerable personal attention in the hospital, and those who expect to be able to manage their personal affairs within only limited hospital constraints would presumably be most surprised and upset by the rigidly controlling hospital regimen. This reaction might well be exacerbated if the patient is unaware of the rationale for these constraints on behavior. Research shows that when the withdrawal of freedom is perceived as arbitrary, reactance ensues, and the individual attempts to restore the lost freedoms (Brehm, 1966). These efforts may be behavioral, such as when the patient decides to engage in some forbidden activity despite hospital rules. Or these efforts may be psychological, such as when the patient comes to value the forbidden activity even more than he or she did before and responds to its loss with anger. One would predict, then, that patients who anticipate loss of freedom, either because they have been prepared for it or because they have been hospitalized before, and patients who appreciate the rationale for restrictions on their freedoms and mobility would be more likely to react to the hospitalization experience with good patient behavior. Similarly, people who are generally sensitive to and responsive to social norms might be expected to show good patient behavior since all socialization pressures that the patient receives from hospital staff are toward adopting the normative good patient role. Patients who are responsive to such pressures, such as those with high need for approval or high sensitivity to social desirability, should adopt the desired behavior patterns somewhat faster than those who are less aware of social norms.

Thus far, predictions about patients' reactions to hospitalization have been drawn from assumptions about personality variables, prior experiences, and expectations. There may also be a temporal pattern of reactions to hospitalization whereby an individual's initial reaction to restrictions on freedom is resistance that, in time, gives way to compliant behavior. This prediction derives from Wortman's and Brehm's (1975) analysis of reactions to loss of freedom in which they attempt to reconcile research on helplessness with research on reactance. The research literature on responses to loss of freedom has shown two distinct patterns. One pattern, that of reactance, involves efforts to restore the freedom, and, as noted earlier, these behaviors often make the patient angry and resentful. The second behavior pattern, compliance, involves giving in and accepting the loss of freedom and failing to make any effort to change the environment. In effect, the patient becomes helpless. Assuming that the reactance pattern fits the ''bad patient'' profile, whereas the compliance–helplessness pattern fits the ''good patient'' profile, several predictions can be made. An analysis of the extant data suggests, first, that when people are exposed to short-term and/or mild levels of threat to freedom, they are more likely to respond with reactance, whereas long-term or severe loss of control promotes compliance and helplessness. Thus, among patients who expect control, the initial reaction to loss of freedom might be expected to be reactance. However, if the loss of freedom is extended, one would predict that the patient would eventually become helpless and compliant. Accordingly, patients with short hospitalizations and few restrictions on freedom might show reactance, whereas patients with long hospitalizations and/or extensive restrictions on freedom might be more likely to show helplessness. Furthermore, the patient who initially shows reactance may eventually give up and become compliant if repeated efforts to gain information and control over the environment fail to produce results. These predictions rest on the assumption that compliance in the good patient role is actually helplessness and that the anger of the bad patient is a manifestation of reactance. Evidence for these assumptions will now be presented.

PHYSICAL AND PSYCHOLOGICAL CONCOMITANTS OF LOSS OF CONTROL, THE GOOD PATIENT ROLE, AND THE BAD PATIENT ROLE

Whether ''good patient'' or ''bad patient'' behavior is better from the standpoint of the patient's physical and psychological health is a question of considerable importance. That is, whereas functional analyses of the hospital make it clear that the good patient role is desirable from the perspective of hospital and staff functioning (see, for example, Coser's 1962 discussion), it may not be the case that such a role is desirable from the patient's perspective. It may be true, for example, that fighting depersonalization with anger is a psychologically healthier response than passively accepting it. It is important, then, to examine the cognitive, affective, behavioral, and physiological concomitants of loss of control and of good and bad patient behavior, in order to assess the implications they have for the patient's physical and psychological health.

Reactions to Lack of Control

Research on the effects of lack of control (without controlling for the idividual's response to that lack of control) has yielded many findings that are of possible importance to understanding the situation of the medical patient. Much of this research involves experimental laboratory studies of healthy college students; thus, extrapolating to the hospital setting has certain risks. Nonetheless, this research quite consistently demonstrates that when individuals have no information regarding the onset, timing, and severity of noxious stimuli (such as shock), they find the sensations more painful, show greater physiological reactivity, and show greater impairment in the performance of various tasks than do people who do have such information (see Averill, 1973; Bowers, 1968; Corah & Boffa, 1970; Geer, Davidson, & Gatchel, 1970; Holmes & Houston, 1974; Kanfer & Seider, 1973; Staub & Kellet, 1972; Staub, Tursky & Schwartz, 1971). Generalizing to the situation of the hospital patient, one would predict that if patients have little information regarding the onset, nature, and timing of their symptoms or any noxious medical procedures that they will be undergoing, they should experience discomfort more intensely, manifest a heightened physiological response to that discomfort, and show reduced powers of concentration for other kinds of tasks. In fact, research in hospital settings supports these predictions for both symptoms (Janis, 1958) and medical procedures (e.g., Johnson & Leventhal, 1974). Janis, for example, found that surgery patients who were ill-prepared for postsurgery side effects reacted more strongly to them, required more medications, complained to staff more, and were generally less cooperative with regard to medical treatments than were patients who had received fuller information about the aftereffects of surgery. In a series of intriguing experiments, Pennebaker and his colleagues (e.g., Pennebaker, Burnam, Schaeffer, & Harper, 1977) have found that when people are exposed to aversive stimulation over which they have no control, they report more symptoms than when they feel they do have control. Loss of control engendered by the hospital environment, then, may actually increase the experience of aversive symptoms. There is also evidence that patients who are provided with information regarding the sensations induced by noxious medical procedures, and who are instructed in how to respond to those procedures, are able to withstand them more easily (see, e.g., Johnson & Leventhal, 1974; Johnson, Rice, Fuller, & Endress, 1977). Since studies of hospital settings suggest that absence of information regarding symptoms and treatment is the rule, both the physical and emotional status of the patient may be adversely affected.

A second concomitant of lack of information is nondiscriminating information seeking. Because participation in the management of care is not part of the hospital patient role, patients receive little but cursory information about their medical condition or management. However, as the social psychological research on attribution reveals, people are motivated to maintain some semblance of control over their lives in order to predict and anticipate events (e.g., White, 1959). People gather information, make causal inferences, and strive to control and manipulate the environment.

The tendency to seek information and to draw causal inferences is especially notable during periods of uncertainty (Kelley, 1967). Patients often go to great lengths to gain information about their illnesses and care. Frequently, however, their attempts fail, as their questions go unanswered. The lack of communication between staff and patients is one of the "most universal complaints of hospitalized patients in western society [Skipper *et al.*, 1964, p. 38]." As one patient put it: "My physician has upset me. It drives me nuts. What's up? I don't know what's up. It's driving me crazy. . . . I have to have an explanation. I just could not live with it any other way. I can live with anything I can understand [p. 38]." One result of this serious lack of communication is that patients often go to non-discriminating, devious, or extreme measures to gain information about their illnesses (Peck, 1977; Roth, 1963; Seeman & Evans, 1962; Skipper & Leonard, 1965; Suchman, 1972), often initiating frantic searches for clues. Patients may compare their cases with what they believe (often erroneously) are similar cases. They seek out information from people such as friends and relatives, and the result is often an odd assortment of misconceptions and contradictory information (Klagsbrun, 1971; McIntosh, 1974). Some patients then use this information as a basis for refusing treatments, discharging themselves from the hospital, or supplementing treatment with remedies of their own. Thus, the experience of loss of control can itself lead to adverse effects on health status. How the individual reacts to that loss of control may also have implications for health status, an issue to which we will now turn.

Good Patient Behavior

> To be a "patient" is a unique status because one thinks it means that one has relinquished the right to ask questions, although one must accept the obligation of answering questions and permitting one's self to be examined. Asking questions seems to be the right of everyone else—especially physicians, strangers, and others who can deny emotional ties to the patient. Thoroughly exposed, the patient is expected patiently to submit to all manner of indignities [Cooper, 1976, p. 43].

What are the behavioral, cognitive, affective, and physiological concomitants of the good patient role that might influence the health status, both physical and psychological, of the hospital patient? The "good patient" is highly regarded by the staff because he or she is compliant, noncomplaining, nondemanding, and generally passive. However, the good patient may also be helpless and anxious. Tagliacozzo and Mauksch's studies of hospital patients (1972) point out that the "good patient," rather than being the calm, accepting, content person the hospital staff believes him or her to be, is often torn between the desire for attention and information and the need to be well behaved. The result can be helplessness. Behaviorally, helplessness is manifested as extreme passivity and the inability to take steps to change one's condition. The outcome of this state is not only the patient's inability to do anything to improve his or her own health status but also a tendency to refrain from disclosing information that would help staff members manage him or her more effectively (see also Lederer, 1952; Roth, 1963; Seligman, 1975).

> Many patients prefer not to risk appearing too demanding or too dependent. They accept what appears to them to be deviations from the physician's orders, and even violate what they believe is expected of them by the physician. They anxiously watch a medication being late, rather than object to the delay, and they watch the specimen get cold rather than point this out to a nurse [Tagliacozzo & Mauksch, 1972, p. 164].

As the following quotation demonstrates, patients may also keep to themselves information that could help hospital staff manage other patients: "I could have told him [the physician] everything she did before she went into a coma, but why should I say anything when he doesn't even bother to ask me? Every time you try to tell these people anything around here they act as if you're trying to run their business. I've learned to keep my mouth shut [Roth, 1963]." Thus, the compliant patient who withholds information may actually negatively affect his or her own or another's health.

The helpless patient may fail not only to give out information, but also to take in information, at least on certain topics. Tagliacozzo and Mauksch (1972) have suggested that one such topic is patients' rights: "Patients who were asked directly what they 'considered their rights' had some difficulties responding. One-fourth of the respondents admitted they did not know what their rights were; some patients stated outright that they had no rights [p. 167]." Another such area may be in making decisions regarding care. The good patient role, marked as it is by helplessness, is not conducive to effective decision making. Thus, patients who are forced to make decisions regarding their care may have trouble doing so. Rather than considering information objectively, the good patient may ignore information that contradicts some initial inclination and accept information that supports it (Janis & Mann, 1977).

Another potential outcome of loss of control is *learned helplessness* (Seligman, 1975). Research has shown that when an individual's efforts to control an environment are repeatedly thwarted, not only does the individual cease responding in that environment, but he or she may also fail to respond in some new environment where possibilities for control do exist. People, then, can *learn* to be helpless and generalize that learning. Under some circumstances, they can become unable to emit appropriate controlling responses to any environment.

How might learned helplessness affect the hospital patient? First, if the hospital patient has learned that his or her comments or questions continually remain substantially unanswered, he or she is unlikely to contribute to the staff information that is highly valuable. Second, the hospital patient may find extremely difficult the eventual transition back to private person. This is likely to be especially problematic for patients who suffer from chronic disease, since after their discharge from a hospital, they will be expected to assume the responsibility of self-management. The patient who is accustomed to having every aspect of care and treatment monitored and administered by others may have considerable difficulty assuming these tasks. Consistent with this point is Coser's (1962) observation that a significant problem encountered by staff was the reluctance of "good patients" to leave the hospital. Although learned helplessness as engendered by the hospital environment is likely to be short term, its timing is especially problematic. Just at the point when the individual must learn to self-manage a treatment regimen (i.e., discharge), learned helplessness, to the extent it exists, will be maximal.

What is the cognitive and affective situation of the "good patient"? Tagliacozzo and Mauksch (1972) and Coser (1962) suggest that cognitions of at least some "good patients" center around feelings of helplessness and that the good patient's mood may alternate between anxiety and depression. Anxious patients are caught in the bind of desiring information about their care but fearing the consequences of asking for this information. Two-thirds of the patients in the Tagliacozzo and Mauksch (1972) study indicated needs and criticisms of the hospital system but reported that they had not felt free to express them.

> Being on good terms was seen by these patients not only as convenient, but as an essential factor for their welfare. They directly expressed their awareness of their inability to control those who were in charge of their care. Patients felt that they were subject to arbitrary rewards and punishment and that essential services could be withheld unless they made themselves acceptable [p. 166].

Depressed patients have given up entirely. "Feelings of helplessness were directly expressed in observations that 'one is at their mercy,' that 'trying to change things is futile,' and 'won't get you anywhere' and that patients feel 'helpless' [p. 166]." As one patient put it:

> When you are really sick, you are at the mercy of the hospital staff. In my opinion, you've got to have luck on your side. You've got to be lucky enough to get key people in the hospital who are really alert and who wish to do a job; and have someone on the shift at the time you need them who wants to give the service or you are just out of luck. I think you could die in one of these hospitals of a heart attack before anybody came to help you [p. 169].

These reactions of hospital patients fit the observations of researchers in other contexts who have also found that helplessness can eventually lead to depression (Seligman, 1975).

> In severe cases, there often is complete paralysis of the will. The patient has no
> desire to do anything, even those things which are essential to life. Conse-
> quently, he may be relatively immobile unless prodded or pushed into activity by
> others. It is sometimes necessary to pull the patient out of bed, wash, dress and
> feed him. In extreme cases, even communication may be blocked by the patient's
> inertia [Beck, quoted in Seligman, 1975, p. 83].

Interview studies of patients awaiting surgery, cancer diagnosis, or other serious procedures or outcomes (e.g., Katz *et al.*, 1970; Renneker & Cutler, 1952; Sutherland & Orbach, 1953) reveal that good patient behavior may be a mask for regressive, often maladaptive psychological withdrawal. Some patients practice denial, maintaining a rigidly pleasant facade and behaving as if there were no threat when, in fact, the threat may be substantial. Although in the short run, denial may not be a psychological problem, it is regarded as a primitive, unsuccessful defense that leaves the individual immobilized by anxiety when defenses break down. Furthermore, patients exhibiting denial may be unable to process information about their care, or to make appropriate decisions when required to do so. Good patient behavior may also be a mask for fatalism—the belief that it is "one's turn" and that nothing can be done to change what is inevitable. The resources of these patients, too, cannot be mobilized in services of their own care.

In summary, the so-called good patient is often actually in a state of helplessness, to which he or she reacts initially with anxiety and later with denial or depression. This emotional state scarcely seems conducive to a speedy recovery. In fact, there are important implications of helplessness and depression for the patient's physical state. The most consistent finding is that adrenalin depletion accompanies depression (see Seligman, 1975), helplessness, and, at extreme levels of aversive stimulation, loss of control (e.g., Weiss, Stone, & Harrell, 1970). The individual's physiological reserves, which customarily mobilize the organism against threat, may become depleted, and the individual may be unresponsive to stimuli as a consequence. Feelings of helplessness have also been associated with poor or deteriorating physical health in studies of sudden death (Engel, 1968; Schmale, 1971), in investigations of the health status of the elderly (Langer & Rodin, 1976; Schulz, 1976), and in research on the onset of other physical disabilities, such as heart conditions and possible cancer (Schmale & Iker, 1971). Thus, although there is no direct evidence that helplessness, induced by adopting the good patient role, actually worsens the patient's physical state, the data that bear on such a relationship suggest that if there is an effect, it is negative.

What behaviors are helpless patients likely to evoke in staff? On the one hand, because patients are docile and noncomplaining, staff are inclined to treat them well, albeit routinely. Were helpless patients to voice complaints, the staff would probably pay this unusual behavior more attention. During the normal course of events, however, it is likely that staff would refrain from soliciting information from good patients, and, over time, these patients would learn not to volunteer it. Thus, although in an emergency good patients may fare well, in the normal course of events good patient behavior tends to reduce communication between patient and staff—communication that might lead to improved treatment.

Obviously, not all good patients are helpless and depressed. However, the available evidence strongly suggests that enough so-called good patients *are* helpless and depressed, so that the potential debilitating effects of their concomitant mood, beliefs, physiological changes, and treatment by staff merit study and intervention.

Bad Patient Behavior

In refusing to become helpless, the "bad patient" exhibits continuous efforts to obtain attention and information. Is this fighting role a more constructive mode of responding to depersonalization, or does it, too, produce behaviors, emotions, physiological reactions, and staff behaviors that undermine the patient's physical and psychological health?

First, what are the behavioral concomitants of reactance? Brehm (1966) has suggested that reactance leads to efforts to restore lost freedoms. In hospital patients, reactance is manifested behaviorally as petty acts of mutiny, such as making passes at nurses, drinking in one's room, smoking against medical advice, and wandering up and down the halls. Such minor incidents tend to irritate nursing and custodial staff but rarely do any damage. However, petty acts of mutiny can turn into self-sabotage, such as failing to take medications that are essential to recovery, or engaging in acts that have potentially fatal consequences. Coupled with these mutinous acts against the hospital routine and treatment regimen are frequent demands upon the staff for attention, treatment, and medication and frequent complaints regarding the quality of same (Katz *et al.,* 1970; Lorber, 1975). Behaviorally, then, the patient who experiences reactance creates potential health risks.

What are the emotional and cognitive concomitants of reactance? The patient is likely to believe that he or she is being ignored and that not as much is being done for him or her as could be. The patient may be suspicious to the point of paranoia that the staff are providing medication merely to placate and that staff members are deliberately withholding information (Katz *et al.,* 1970); some of these beliefs are occasionally correct (Lorber, 1975). Many angry patients insist that they have the right to information about their treatment and feel that the hospital has an obligation to treat them as consumers of health care (see, e.g., Coser, 1962).

What is the physiological state of the angry patient? Research from many sources indicates that the usual physiological reaction to anger is heightened catecholamine secretion (adrenalin and noradrenalin). Studies of angry hospital patients have also found high levels of hydrocortisone, an indicator of stress (Katz *et al.,* 1970). Still other studies (see Glass, 1977b) demonstrate that the physiological reaction to loss of control is heightened adrenalin secretion, in that individuals become frustrated when their efforts to control are thwarted. In sum, the physiological state of the angry patient is likely to be one of arousal. This arousal may have any of several effects, depending upon other aspects of the patient's physical condition. Heightened arousal can lead to or aggravate high blood pressure, hypertension, tachycardia, or angina pectoris. It can eventually lead to adrenalin depletion, in which case the individual's capacity to respond to the environment is sapped. Available studies, then, concur that unrelieved anger in a medical patient is likely to have negative effects on health.

How does the hospital staff react to the angry patient? Because a relatively small number of patients reacts to hospitalization with anger, medical staff are inclined to dismiss these individuals as unusual cases ("Some people are just like that"), in other words, to regard the problem as due to a quirk of personality. At its most benign, the staff treats the irascible patient with good-humored condescension, the proverbial "good boy" or "good girl" baby-talk approach. Somewhat more problematic, medically, is the tendency of staff to ignore the angry patient and avoid listening to his or her complaints. Certain patients are labeled "difficult" early in treatment; staff come to regard their complaints less seriously than they might the complaints of more complacent patients (e.g., Katz *et al.,* 1970; Lorber, 1975). If the angry patient does have a complaint that has medical significance, the staff may overlook it by ignoring it or prematurely medicating it.

In some cases, complaining patients are referred to psychiatrists (Katz *et al.,* 1970; Lorber, 1975). Psychiatrists often term angry patients "projective paranoics." Anger at medical personnel, according to this psychiatric view, can be traced to the anger that the patient feels toward himself or herself for being ill. Being temperamentally disinclined toward blaming themselves or turning their anger inward, as some people do, angry patients direct anger about their fates outward against the staff. It is believed, then, that the projective paranoic would find something wrong with hospital treatment, even if everything were perfect, simply because this is how she or he is constructed psychologically. There may well be such patients, and certainly some individuals are more inclined toward blaming others for their problems than they are toward blaming themselves. However, interpreting all complaining behavior as paranoid projection raises the possibility of ignoring objective privations patients experience, stresses they feel, or new or worsening symptoms.

Even more serious consequences of "bad patient behavior" are suggested by Lorber's (1975) study of surgical patients. She found some evidence that bad patients were medicated, especially tranquilized, so that they would be easier to manage. Under the guise of treating symptoms, hospital staff, in fact, ''treated'' the complaint. In one or two cases, these patients were even discharged prematurely. It may be that patients who are angry appear less sick to staff than do patients who are compliant, or it may be simply that staff distort perceptions of the patient's progress toward recovery so as to be rid of them. In sum, there is evidence that ''bad patients'' who react to their situation with anger and irritation, rather than with good patient behavior, actually run health risks at the hands of the staff who care for them.

The possible behavioral, cognitive, affective, and physiological concomitants of both loss of control and the two patient roles, as well as the behaviors they elicit from staff, are summarized in Table 11.1. Clearly, neither good patient behavior nor bad patient behavior is conducive to good physical and psychological health. The good patient may be resigned to helplessness, whereas the bad patient is often angry and complaining. Is there not some third patient role that could avoid the problems of the roles that currently exist? This possibility deserves exploration.

A NEW ROLE FOR HOSPITAL PATIENTS?

Both good patient behavior and bad patient behavior are predicated on the loss of control that the patient experiences, in part, as a result of depersonalization in the hospital. Thus, both reactions can be viewed as efforts to cope with the loss of control. But, as Table 11.1 indicates, loss of control itself produces negative behaviors that may interfere with treatment efforts. Thus, to develop a hospital patient role that avoids the pitfalls of the existing roles, the solution must hinge on removing the problem of loss of control itself, rather than on leading patients to cope with loss of control differently. The significance of this point can be illustrated by proposing a hypothetical intervention and examining its probable results. Suppose a reduction in the incidence of bad patient behavior is initiated by drawing on the prediction (offered in the first section of this chapter) that inappropriate expectations regarding the rationale for hospital restrictions lead to bad patient behavior. Accordingly, a prehospitalization intake program could be developed in which patients are carefully prepared for these restrictions, so as to facilitate adjustment. However, according to the model developed in this chapter, no advantages, save a bureaucratic one, will have been achieved. That is, with this intervention, prospective ''bad patients'' become ''good patients,'' who are now compliant and well behaved. But good patient behavior, like bad patient behavior, can produce physical and psychological effects that may adversely affect health status. Thus, it is evident that a purely psychological intervention that fails to take into account

TABLE 11.1

The **Possible Consequences of Loss of Control, Good Patient Behavior, and Bad Patient Behavior in Hospital Patients**

State	Behaviors	Cognitions	Affect	Physical state	Response from staff
Loss of control (depersonalization)	Nondiscriminant information seeking and use; complaints to staff	Inadequate expectations; confusion	Anxiety	Heightened physical reactions to symptoms and noxious medical procedures; possible increased need for medication, lengthened hospital stay	Nonperson treatment
Good patient behavior (helplessness)	Compliance; passivity; learned helplessness; inability to take in information; failure to provide condition-relevant information	Feelings of helplessness, powerlessness; possible denial or fatalism	Anxiety and depression	Possible norepinephrine depletion; helplessness also related to sudden death and gradual erosion of health	Responsiveness to emergencies but routine failure to solicit information from patient
Bad patient behavior (reactance)	Complaints to staff; demands for attention; mutinous behavior; possible self-sabotage	Commitment to a right to know; suspicion (or paranoia) regarding condition, treatment and staff behavior	Anger	Heightened catecholamine secretion and hydrocortisone production; possible aggravation of blood pressure, hypertension, tachycardia, angina; eventual adrenalin depletion	Condescension; ignoring patients' complaints; medication to placate; psychiatric referrals; possible premature discharge.

the structural and functional conditions that give rise to good and bad patient behavior is unlikely to improve significantly patient health.

If the concept of patient control were applied to the hospital-patient population, what form might it take? The major problem created by loss of control is that in responding with either helplessness or reactance, the patient has directed his or her behavioral and cognitive resources against his or her own care rather than in the service of it. Methods for rechanneling the focus of these resources need to be found. Control-based interventions provide an appropriate model and have in the past consisted of two types: those that involve providing control in limited treatment settings, and those that involve system-wide changes.

Specific Procedure or Disease-Related Interventions

A number of studies exist that have examined the effects of providing control to hospital patients in constrained and limited contexts. One such group of studies, which examined the effects of preparation for surgery, owe their genesis to the groundbreaking observations of Janis (1958). Janis observed that patients who adjusted well to surgery were those who had learned and understood information about the side effects of surgery. Drawing on these observations, a number of researchers designed interventions to help surgical patients adjust to surgery more favorably. Egbert and his colleagues (Egbert, Battit, Welch, & Bartlett, 1964), for example, found that intraabdominal surgery patients who had been informed about the normality, duration, and severity of postoperative pain, and who had been instructed in exercises that would reduce the pain, coped better than did patients who received no instructions. They required fewer narcotics and were able to leave the hospital earlier than the patients who were not prepared for the surgical pain (see also Egbert, Battit, Tundorf, & Beecher, 1963). Langer, Janis, and Wolfer (1975) varied whether or not surgical patients received preparatory information and whether they received instruction in a cognitive-reappraisal coping device. This coping device consisted of teaching patients how they could reappraise their own symptoms and distract themselves by thinking about other things. The authors found that, by itself, preparatory information did not affect adjustment. However, when information was combined with the coping device, patients left the hospital somewhat earlier and required somewhat fewer pain killers than did patients who received no instructions or only preparatory information. Similar effects have been used with cholecystectomy (gallbladder surgery) patients: Receiving behavioral instruction in deep-breathing and leg exercises reduced to some degree the amount of analgesics required by these patients, increased their ambulation, and reduced fear and anger among those who had been fearful prior to surgery. Being informed of specific sensations to be expected reduced both postoperative anger and length of hospitalization (Johnson *et al.*, 1977).

To date, most of the evaluative criteria for these interventions have been physical, including such measures as number of analgesics needed and length of hospitalization. One reason for this emphasis has been that differences in physical-treatment variables make these interventions "marketable" to skeptical physicians and hospital administrators. However, as the value of these programs has come to be established on physical grounds, psychological criteria, such as the patient's satisfaction with care and level of anger, have come to be more closely monitored. From this monitoring emerges evidence that the patient's mood, satisfaction with care, and compliance, as well as physical recovery, are improved by these preparatory interventions (Wolfer, 1973; see also DiMatteo, 1979).

Since a patient's postsurgical recovery can be facilitated by interventions that emphasize preparatory information and instructions in coping, it is worth considering how these concepts might be applied more generally to the improvement of the patient's hospital environment. How might one eliminate depersonalization and avoid the patient anger and helplessness that lead not only to a poor psychological environment but also to interference with treatment? On what issues can the patient be informed? What services and information can be provided to reduce helplessness? How can one draw upon the patient's own resources to work in favor of care, rather than against it?

Although most of the control-based research has been done with surgical patients, it is certainly the case that a similar intervention format is applicable to nonsurgical hospitalized groups. In one study (Putt, 1970), 36 peptic ulcer patients were divided into three groups. One group received standard nursing care. The second group was given "psychological care," in which the nurses spent several minutes a day listening to the patient's problems and helping him or her explore feelings. The third group of patients was given information about and instruction in their own care, including how the stomach works, how ulcers develop, and how treatment goals are accomplished. Both of the experimental groups had shorter hospitalization compared with that of controls, and they reported less pain for less time. Of the two experimental groups, the one receiving instructions left the hospital first.

Other noxious procedures can also draw on the presurgical-preparation model to enhance feelings of control. For example, Johnson and Leventhal (1974) gave patients awaiting an endoscopic examination specific instructions as to the sensations they could expect to experience and behaviors they could engage in to make easier the passage of the tube they had to swallow. Sensory information by itself and in combination with the behavioral manipulation reduced emotional distress, and the effects were particularly pronounced among over-55 patients, an at-risk group. There is evidence that preparing children in advance for bone marrow transplants reduces some anxiety during the procedure itself (McCue, 1980).

Preparation need not be confined to treatment alone. Similar use of informational material to improve understanding of one's illness can also reduce anxiety and enhance feelings of control. Some health maintenance organizations have begun to use standardized presentations of etiology, symptoms, and treatments for common disorders, which can be viewed on film or slides by patients at their leisure while they are waiting to see the physician.

In short, providing information or specific behaviors that an individual can engage in to contribute to his or her care can reduce patient anxiety, and in some cases reduce operating costs.

System-Wide Control-Based Interventions

Several studies provide a basis for designing and predicting the impact of an environment-wide control-based intervention. Perhaps the most dramatic work in this area involved providing control to the institutionalized elderly. In a study by Langer and Rodin (1976), patients on one floor of a nursing home were given a small plant to care for and were allowed to make decisions about when to see a movie and when to participate in other available activities. The patients on the comparison floor were likewise given plants, but staff cared for them, and these patients were assigned to particular times when they had to go to activities, rather than being able to choose those times. The effects on individuals provided with small amounts of control were dramatic. Staff reported that the patients who were given control had improved mood and health, and a year later they tended to show a mortality rate lower than that of patients on the comparison floor. That such findings should be produced by such small amounts of control is surprising. Consider, however, that the institutional environment for the elderly is impoverished. There is very little to do, activities are highly standardized, and individuals have very few choices. When choice is provided against such an impoverished background, its effects are likely to be dramatic (see also Schulz, 1976). Given similar conditions of environmental impoverishment in the hospital, one might expect similar small-scale interventions to have a large impact in the hospital as well.

A model of a somewhat more elaborate system-wide intervention is provided by experimental self-help units for alert, ambulatory, usually chronic patients (Hoge, 1964) that make use of patients' energies. In these units patients often run their own errands, make their own beds, and provide other aspects of their own custodial care. Patients even perform these chores for other patients who are too sick to care for themselves. Several hospitals have developed occupational therapy programs for long-term patients or for patients who do not feel ill in order to break up the monotony of hospitalization and to keep them out of the way of the staff (Elman, 1950). Other changes designed to make use of ambulatory patients' abilities, to meet social needs, and to reduce boredom have included the extension of visiting hours, the provision of small dining and lounging facilities for noncontagious ambulatory patients, and the provision of facilities such as games and movies (Brown, 1963). The coupling of small responsibilities with expanded social facilities has greatly improved morale among patients (Kornfeld, 1972). Other programs have gone so far as to involve patients in their own treatment. Some patients on self-help wards administer their own medications, take their own temperatures, and monitor their own conditions. They are given phones so that they can page their doctor if necessary (Klagsbrun, 1971; Kornfeld, 1972; Roth, 1963). Most such programs, however, currently exist on a demonstration basis only, and whether this is a practical model for a system-wide intervention remains to be seen.

We are sometimes more generous to our children than we are to ourselves, and the history of hospitalization with children may provide a model for intervention with adults. As recently as the 1950s, children were placed on drab wards with little to occupy their attention, little preparation for specific procedures they would undergo, and little contact with others, whether family members or other children. As this author well remembers from her own childhood hospitalization, hospitals were boring and frightening places to be. Because of high rates of adverse reactions in children (between one-third and one-half in pre-1960 studies; see Gofman, Buckman, & Schade, 1957), a concerted effort was undertaken to change this situation. We now know that children can profit greatly from: prehospitalization preparation that informs them about what they can expect during admission (Gofman et al., 1957); the presence of a warm, colorful environment with toys and volunteer playmates (Bronstetler, 1969; Gellert, 1958; Prugh, Staub, Sands, Kirschbaum, & Lenihan, 1953); specific preparation for any unusual or uncomfortable medical procedure, which outlines exactly what will occur and how it will feel (Gofman et al., 1957); and facilities that make it possible for a family member to stay with the child (Bronstetler, 1969). These changes in the child's hospitalization are believed to have reduced the rate of adverse reactions in children (Gofman et al., 1957), and as a consequence, the World Health Organization formalized many of these recommendations into its report on hospitalized children (Bulletin of the World Health Organization, 1955). That we are so quick to intervene to provide feelings of control, adequate preparation, and a good social environment in a population whose needs for control may actually be less than is the case for adults is striking. If we were as conscientious about adult needs, the current rate of adverse effects of hospitalization with adults might also be reduced.

In summary, the problems associated with little information, loss of identity, and inadequate preparation for the hospital setting have not gone completely unnoticed. For some patient groups, such as children, surgical patients, and some chronically ill ambulatory patients, interventions have been developed to offset the negative effects of loss of control in the hospital environment. However, these steps have yet to be extended to other patient groups in the hospital population. Although the goal of this chapter is not to provide the details of an informed and participant patient role, some general guidelines can be outlined. One requirement would be an individual assessment of the patient's ability to understand and make a contribution to his or her care. Another would involve providing detailed information both about ongoing care and about any specific treatments that would be required, such as surgery. Third, training in any kind of self-help activities that the patient is capable of discharging would be needed. Conceivably, staff at all levels could be involved in this educational process, though clearly nursing staff would be most directly affected. Indeed, experimental nursing programs have already begun to train nurses in precisely these kinds of educational activities (Skipper & Leonard, 1965).

CONCLUSIONS

Researchers have been aware for some time that so-called bad patients encounter health risks and that good patients, rather than being content, compliant individuals, may be helpless, anxious, and desperate for information that is not forthcoming. What has been lacking in this area is a theoretical model in which to cast these observations, and the need for it is great. Sociological models that analyze good and bad patient behavior from the standpoint of hospital structure and functioning underscore the adaptiveness of good patient behavior for the hospital's smooth regulation. These models, however, overlook or minimize many of the psychological liabilities of good patient behavior. The control–helplessness–reactance literature thus provides a badly needed perspective that underscores, as previous work has not, the extent of these liabilities. This perspective also provides a basis not only for predicting who will engage in which kind of patient behavior but also for specifying the causes, consequences, and alternatives to those behaviors. In concrete terms, the theory argues that both good and bad patient behavior may result from the experience of loss of control, specifically, the absence of information regarding one's condition and treatment and the inability to take steps or make a contribution in one's own behalf. This psychological model in turn leads to a structural solution; that is, what the helplessness–reactance–control literature clearly points to is the difficulty of individual coping efforts to be successful within a structure that promotes depersonalization and loss of control. What is implied as a solution to this problem is an informed-participant role for the patient (Taylor & Levin, 1976). Research examining such a role in the limited contexts of preparation for surgery and self-help units for chronic patients clearly points to its benefits. Giving the patient control over those aspects of care that he or she can assume and giving the patient a participant role in those aspects of care that he or she cannot manage alone acknowledge the patient's mature status and can prevent the patient's reduction to total helplessness and dependence. Both psychological and physical adjustment appear to be improved by interventions that draw on the patient-participation approach. In many cases, symptom incidence and complaints are reduced, morale is higher, there is a reduced need for medication, and patients often leave the hospital sooner.

Is an expanded role based on informed participation cost-effective? Cost-effectiveness is, of course, a necessary condition for the expanded patient role to gain acceptance in hospital settings. There are many reasons to expect it might be. Whereas patient participation involves a larger initial output of time and resources, this outlay may be more than offset by a diminution in the hidden costs of the current system. Whereas staff time would be required to inform patients about their treatment, time taken up by complaints and bids for attention would be reduced. Whereas staff would be needed to teach patients various aspects of self-management, once patients assumed these tasks on their own, staff resources would be saved. Furthermore, some such training can be done in groups. Shorter hospitalizations and reduced need for medication have direct impact on resource outlay. Medical error rates may even be reduced (see Roth, 1972). Finally one of the hidden costs of depersonalization, namely, discretionary malpractice litigation, might be reduced. Increasingly, malpractice suit initiation has been tied to feelings of helplessness, lack of responsiveness from the physician, and failure to provide information (see, for example, Blum, 1957; Halberstam, 1971). Given the enormous increase in the costs of malpractice insurance and suits, the savings in malpractice fees alone could conceivably offset the costs of an expanded patient role.

The problems of the hospital patient are not simple. It is one thing for a researcher to say, "Give the patient control," and quite another to implement that idea in a manner that maintains a high level of physical care and allows the hospital bureaucracy to continue to function. Changes proceed gradually only after careful planning. Nonetheless, the currently available evidence provides a basis for cautious optimism that just as the hospital's prior association with death has begun to fade so may its current association with depersonalization.

ACKNOWLEDGMENTS

The author is grateful for the helpful comments of M. Robin DiMatteo, John Eckenrode, Steve Edelman, Howard S. Friedman, David Glass, Irving Janis, Smadar Levin, Tom Pettigrew, Paul Pilkonis, Susan Radius, John Stoeckle, Charles Taylor, Jennifer Walters, Janet Weiss, and Susanne Whitehead.

12

Robert Kastenbaum

Dying is Healthy and Death a Bureaucrat: Our Fantasy Machine is Alive and Well

Death has stimulated humankind's fantasy and imagination from the most ancient days. Examine the history of arts and sciences, and we find centuries of effort to comprehend or transcend mortality, strivings to maintain contact with loved ones over the abyss of death, magical devices and biomedical innovations. The imaginative response to death has contributed much to our general cultural heritage. I might like to believe I am seeing life and death through my own eyes, but in truth I am following biases and instructions that have settled upon me—and upon you—from an immense accumulation of prior thought and experience.

Does this mean that we are merely the passive recipients of deathways from the past? Not at all. Fresh ideas continue to emerge, in particular that dying is healthy and death a bureaucrat. I make two qualifications first:

1. None of the current phenomena and concepts are totally new; they represent instead novel configurations of material from the past and present.
2. Fantasy and reality do not come to us with clear labels; we have to work out way through quite a bit of mispackaging.

233

Two qualifications were promised. Here is one more as a bonus: It is unlikely that any two observers would come to precisely the same conclusion about so vast and complex a topic. This writer is himself two observers. There is the person who examined the scene and introduced the concept of ''healthy dying'' not very long ago, and there is the person who has since been exposed to additional phenomena and has had the opportunity to reconsider this controversial view. Continued developments, particularly in the widening arena of the hospice movement, have suggested that this is not the time to repent and disavow. Instead, it appears increasingly pertinent to address another facet of our contemporary fantasy machine. The bureaucratization of death is proceeding rapidly.[1] Death itself has moved up the promotional ladder within the bureaucracy. The tension between these two rather different fantasies—healthy dying and death as bureaucrat—and the relationship of both to reality demand examination. This chapter is intended not to persuade but to invite attention to developments that concern us all.

THE QUEST FOR "HEALTHY DYING" IN HISTORICAL CONTEXT

The quest for healthy dying has become more conspicuous in the past few years. It might be spoken of almost as a ''consumer demand.'' In establishing the historical context of this phenomenon it might be useful to focus first on the experience of one individual.

The place: one of the world's great cities. The time: our own century. A young man burning with fever has been admitted to the hospital after an intake procedure almost lethal in its bureaucracy. He awakens in the stuffy, crowded ward to see

> old Numero 57 lying crumpled up on his side, his face sticking out over the side of the bed, and towards me. He had died some time during the night, nobody knew when. When the nurses came they received the news of his death indifferently and went about their work. After a long time, an hour or more, two other nurses marched in abreast like soldiers, with a great clumping of sabots, and knotted the corpse up in the sheets, but it was not removed till some time later. Meanwhile, in the better light, I had had time for a good look at Numero 57. Indeed I lay on my side to look at him. Curiously enough he was the first dead European I had seen. I had seen dead men before, but always Asiatics and usually people who had died violent deaths. Numero 57's eyes were still open, his mouth also open, his small face contorted into an expression of agony.

---

[1] Ugly word that it is, *bureaucratization* is apt in this context. Dying is now a topic for consideration by the health care bureaucracy.

The young man's psychological response was fully in keeping with the fixed image that met his eyes:

> As I gazed at the tiny screwed-up face it struck me that this disgusting piece of refuse, waiting to be carted away and dumped on a slab in the dissecting room, was an example of ''natural'' death, one of the things you pray for in the Litany. There you are, then, I thought, that's what is waiting for you, twenty, thirty, forty years hence: that is how the lucky ones die, the ones who live to be old. One wants to live, of course, indeed one only stays alive by virtue of the fear of death, but I think now, as I thought then, that it's better to die violently and not too old. People talk about the horrors of war, but what weapons has man invented that even approaches in cruelty some of the commoner diseases?

The next statement is perhaps even more repugnant: '' 'Natural' death, almost by definition, means something slow, smelly, and painful.''

This characterization of ''natural'' death affronts our sensibilities today perhaps even more than it did when the experience occurred in the Paris of 1929. Public and professional awareness of the dying person's situation has increased dramatically throughout the past decade. ''Death with dignity'' has become a rallying cry. Many deplore what is seen as misguided technology in the terminal care situation. Rather than to prolong relentlessly enfeebled life, health care providers are being pressured to facilitate ''natural death''—the same expression from which George Orwell's mind recoiled in horror when he described ''How the Poor Die'' (Orwell, 1975, p. 36). The impressions formed during his hospital stay contributed to the bleak, arresting vision of *1984*. This masterwork has in turn alerted millions of readers to the possibility of a dehumanized future.

Orwell's blunt and unflattering depiction of ''natural'' death appears out of keeping with the humanism and hopefulness of the current death-awareness movement. It is for this very reason that this view has been selected as our starting point. Numero 57 and his impact on Orwell represent the kind of phenomena that public and health care professionals alike are now trying to prevent. Blatant negative instances are easy to identify. But how *should* people die? What is desirable? And what is realistic? The relationship between facts and values is less clear in this realm, a situation that can contribute to expectations so outsized that they might justly be called fantasies.

I will be suggesting that Americans are now more prepared to integrate dying and death into our general view of life—but with the proviso that the terminal condition achieves standards of psychosocial health that are seldom encountered in ordinary life. Attention must be given to our assumptions and expectations as well as to the concrete reality of the terminal situation.

The quest for healthy dying has certain distinguishing features that should now be spelled out more specifically:

1. Criticism of the way in which biomedical technology is applied to the terminally ill person. According to this view, too much is done, too long, and too expensively—all to the detriment of the individual's human sensitivities. The aggressive, all-out application of technology has come to be seen often as enemy rather than as friend. Family and other loved ones are seen as covictims. Rampant technology and professional management are experienced as alienating factors, interfering with intimacy and leave-takings and intensifying the survivors' grief.

2. Criticism of the general attitudinal climate and interpersonal network that closes in around the terminally ill person. This includes the development of "mutual pretense" communication patterns in which both the dying person and the caregiver act as though the other individual does not know the truth (Glaser & Strauss, 1965). Physicians, with their power and prestige, have become especially popular targets of criticism. A typical criticism, for example, is that physicians are attracted to their occupation by their own need to master high death anxiety. This is said to lead them into a peculiar pattern of obsessive cure-oriented actions that give way to abrupt withdrawal—emotional and physical—when it is apparent that they will be defeated by death. The actual situation is more complicated than this, as continuing research and clinical experience indicates. Nevertheless, it is clear enough that once a person is defined as terminally ill, he or she tends to become property of a health care network and is threatened by possible loss of autonomy and personhood. It is as though the following dialogue ensues: "Mend my body or at least relieve my pain." "Of course. Now, put your soul on this tray."

3. Reaction against the "lingering" course of terminal illness. Our society in general appears to favor a quick transition between life and death (Kastenbaum, 1976). This is the attitude of most people who are themselves in good health, including physicians and nurses as well as the lay public. But this orientation that "the less dying, the better" has come up against an altered biosocial reality. People are now approaching death more often through a "lingering trajectory" (Glaser & Strauss, 1968). This is related both to the heightened association betwen aging, chronic disease, and death and to medical techniques for prolonging life.

4. Fear of being held captive in a state between life and death. This is not a totally new theme. (More than a century ago there was a nearly parallel dread of being buried alive; Kastenbaum & Aisenberg, 1972). However, to the dysphoric prospects of a lingering terminal course has been added the image of indefinite suspension on life-support machines when one scarcely exists any longer as a person.

5. Reaction against the physical distress and loss of control associated with terminal illness. On the face of it, this is a peculiar statement to make about any given time in human history. When have most people *ever* favored

conditions of pain and dependency? However, our *expectations* for suffering have changed. We seek relief for relatively minor symptoms throughout our lives. Pharmaceutical houses prosper on our expectation that we should be without pain and discomfort in the ordinary course of life. A visit to the dentist often is dreaded even though sophisticated equipment, techniques, and pain-controlling substances will be employed. As a generation that has high expectations for symptom control and low expectations for suffering, we are likely to regard the prospect of dying with a degree of apprehension that was less common to those who came before us.

6. An image, if vague, of the "good," "acceptable," or "self-actualized" death. The preceding points centered around what most of us do *not* want to befall us. Gradually, however, a set of positive images has been emerging. Kubler-Ross (1969) influenced many with her notion of the "stage of acceptance" that a person can achieve at the very end of life. Weisman (1972) offers the concept of an "appropriate death," meaning by this the particular form of exit that a person would select to be consistent with his or her total lifestyle if given the opportunity to do so. The new freedom to depict dying in the media has reacquainted us with a variety of other orientations from which to choose: the romantic death, the brave death, the death that integrates and confirms the individual's distinctive identity. It is not enough, then, just to be reasonably free of pain and distress. Increasingly, the person with a life-threatening illness has some kind of positive conception of the death to be achieved. This is a distinct departure from the interpersonal climate that existed only a few years ago when death was not considered a fit topic of contemplation for either patient or caregiver.

7. The growth of "consumerism" in general is making its mark on the health care establishment. The "Patient's Bill of Rights" has become commonplace and, under some jurisdictions, mandated by law. There is more public expectation and demand for informed consent, access to clinical records, more detailed and justified invoices, and so on. As we consumers become increasingly "pushy" across the board, it is also increasingly natural to demand that our health service vendors provide us with the type of care we desire in all situations, not least of all, life-threatening illness.

8. Holistic medicine is another broad trend that has specific applications to our expectations for terminal care. In some instances the public seems to be ahead of the general health care establishment in its demand that treatment encompass the "whole person" and his or her interconnectedness with society and that the modes of treatment themselves draw upon our total social and spiritual as well as technical resources. Certain clusters of health care professionals are more than receptive to this approach, but others retain a more narrow model. Rising general expectations for holistic medicine thus are virtually guaranteed to find some happy matches and

some painful mismatches with the particular services they happen to encounter. The concept of "healthy dying" has some contexts in which it appears more reasonable than others.

CONFLICT AND TENSION

It is evident that there are multiple conflicts in this new orientation and that these generate tension. More and more people are including the prospect of death—their own and their loved ones'—in their overall life perspective. Yet the existing health care system as often as not appears to be unresponsive, even at times antagonistic, to the emerging values that people hope to actualize. Perhaps this tension can be relieved or at least placed into better perspective by further attention to the history of dying and death.

Return first to George Orwell's depiction of his experiences in a large urban hospital half a century ago. What he witnessed and went through himself was not fully representative of medical facilities at that time. Nevertheless, his observations offer a stark reminder that over the centuries the terminal phase of life often has been far from "healthy." "Good deaths" were achieved by some individuals in a variety of times and places. However, many people suffered to an extent that would be completely unacceptable today. Their distress often was intensified by medical practice every bit as "aggressive" as today's—but woefully lacking in knowledge. "The doctor is worse than the disease" was a common sentiment, and hospitals a place to avoid at all costs. As we read accounts of how kings and queens as well as commoners met their death, it is difficult to reconcile the facts of history with today's nostalgic sentiment that "they really knew how to die back then." Sunlight, fresh air, and nourishing food often were withheld from the critically ill person as if these would do harm, while debilitating and painful procedures were carried out that served only to increase misery. It has taken physicians, nurses, and hospitals many years to earn their generally favorable reputations of today. The "saw-bones," the plague nurse, and the "pest-house" bore little resemblance to the present medical care establishment. Criticism of the impersonal and overly technological aspects of medical care today, then, has been floating on an idealized image of how people died in earlier times. The past has been made the stuff of fantasy or, at best, of highly selective memory. (A similar case could be made for the familiar and sweeping criticisms of the services that modern morticians perform: Few of us would be pleased with sanitation and burial conditions of the past!)

Many of us rebel against the bureaucratic, professional, highly regulated medical and nursing practice that we encounter today. And yet this practice is itself an achievement, and the outcome of a previous revolution! The community is outraged when it comes across isolated examples of truly slipshod or wrongheaded care that once would have been unremarkable.

This perspective does not oblige us to accept the problems of today without complaint. But it does suggest a different approach to their solution. Look at the situation from the standpoint of, say, a physician or nurse who has been around long enough to see marked strides made in knowledge and technology. This person probably realizes that chaos is still not very far away. Even with the best of contemporary measures, it is still possible for "all hell to break loose." Errors can be made in treatment. Infections can be generated in the hospital situation itself. An apparently well-managed situation can give way to emergency. There is still a felt need, in other words, for the exercise of control, for adhering closely to regulations and procedures that appear so restrictive and rigid from an outsider's standpoint. It might not be advantageous to relinquish what has been laboriously achieved over the years in health care management. It is more a question of balance and timing.

How much can modern medical technology afford to "let go" in the interest of the human values that the technology was created to serve in the first place? Instead of regarding the existing technology as the sworn enemy of humane care, then, we might search for ways to use it more appropriately. "You can relax a little, now," one might in effect say to the physician and nurse. "You have come a long way in controlling physical distress and supporting life—it is time to sit down with the patient again and see what both of you really want."

Another dimension of change in our "death system" (Kastenbaum, 1977a) should also be considered here. In comparison with the past, we are considerably more adept both at curing and killing. Since the mushroom cloud over Hiroshima we have lived in a world in which "megadeath"—extending perhaps to the complete destruction of life on earth—is a possibility quite within human means. At the same time, an increasing number of life-threatening conditions have yielded to public health and medical advances.

The emphasis on killing and curing has led to a relative neglect of other functions served by our death system. Rituals of mourning and social consolidation after death have been on the retreat in recent years. There appears to be less tolerance for the survivor's grief; he or she is expected to "snap right back" after a short while (Fulton, 1976). The expectation—at times, the demand—that a bereaved person bury the sorrow and return quickly to normal life runs counter to what clinicians and behavioral scientists have learned about the nature of grief (e.g., Glick, Weiss, & Parkes, 1974; Parkes, 1973). It ignores the fact that the bereaved person is exceptionally vulnerable to accidents, psychophysiological reactions, disease, and disturbances throughout the entire range of action and relationships (e.g., Frederick, 1976; Parkes, 1975a). The bereaved person is a kind of casualty, but our cultural milieu does not consistently recognize this situation.

Comfort care for the person approaching death also was neglected until recently. A major thrust of the death awareness movement has been to bring appropriate measures to the individual who might otherwise be abandoned because "cure" is beyond medicine's reach. Our society has also been relatively stagnant in its response to the "why" questions. In the past, religious and philosophical traditions were on steady call. There was not much curing and not enough comforting available from the health care providers. Under such circumstances it was especially important to have a "reason" for death and a rationale for dying. What could not be altered much in physical reality could be invested with meaning.

The *ars moriendi* tradition gained prominence early in the fifteenth century and achieved perhaps its most compelling expression in Jeremy Taylor's *The Rule and Exercise of Holy Dying* (1977 reprint) of 1665, a work that stayed in print for another 2 centuries. Illness and death might be regarded as tests of faith, trials of the soul. The way in which a person confronted death could be seen as of supreme importance, and a confrontation to be practiced in days of health as well as the final night of passage. This attitude stands in obvious contrast to the twentieth-century orientation, in which the dying person tends to be seen as a useless or failed machine. The current death-awareness movement, then, has about it something of a revival of the significance of the dying person as a person—but without yet a clear framework of values and principles from which the significance might be derived.

The death-awareness movement itself became visible, if dimly, in the 1950s. Isolated clinicians, educators, and researchers had explored the psychology of death, but their contributions seldom registered on either colleagues or the public. Psychologist Herman Feifel encountered strong resistance from the health care establishment when he attempted to study the terminally ill. He persevered, however, and his edited volume *The Meaning of Death* (1959) heralded the development of a field of inquiry that is sometimes known as *thanatology* (a term introduced by Elie Metchnikoff in 1908). The first struggle was to break down the barriers to discussing death. Feifel characterized the treatment of death in America at that time as a *taboo* topic. We would have to overcome our inhibitions about bringing this topic into the open before anything could be accomplished.

Although many people still find it difficult to shatter the taboo, the momentum of the field has since moved well past this point. The next "discovery" was of the dying person himself or herself. Elisabeth Kubler-Ross emerged as an exceptional communicator. In her book *On Death and Dying* (1969) and her charismatic lectures, Kubler-Ross brought some of the emotional needs of the dying person to general attention. Her specific orientation and conclusions were accepted rather hastily by people who had no previous framework for understanding the dying process. Critical examination of her methods and conclusions (e.g., Kastenbaum & Costa, 1977) does not detract from her arousal of widespread concern and compassion for the terminally ill. By the early 1970s, people were talking about death, and the dying person was no longer quite so hidden from sight.

The death-awareness movement has continued to gain momentum. Death-education courses have appeared from high school through graduate and professional training. Two journals (*Omega, Journal of Death and Dying,* and *Death Education*) have become well established, and the nearly 4000 references listed by Fulton (1977) will be joined by thousands more in a second volume in press. Changes have taken place within both the community and the mental health establishment. A notable example of the former is the group known as Make Today Count (Kelly, 1978). Orville Eugene Kelly was dismissed from a hospital with the knowledge that he had cancer. Like many other individuals in similar circumstances, he had to work his own way through and learn not to become victim of a self-imposed taboo. Kelly wrote a newspaper article describing his first experiences as a terminal cancer patient, suggesting that an organization be created to discuss the emotional problems of people such as himself. There are now more than 80 chapters of this organization functioning in 30 states. This is one example of the ways in which the voices of terminally ill persons have gradually come to be heard.

The changes that have been taking place within the health care network are not easily summarized. In all the helping professions there have been some people who have tried to behave sensitively and flexibly despite the system's taboos and rigidity. These individuals now have a more encouraging attitudinal climate in which to work. Nurses have led the way in expressing concern for the terminally ill and now are more likely to find a receptive attitude on the part of physicians.

Other health personnel, however, seem to be experiencing the death-awareness movement more as pressure than opportunity. People who were never comfortable in their interactions with the terminally ill person and his or her family are in a more exposed position than they were previously. Patients and family alike are more apt to be explicit and persistent in their demands. Their questions must be answered carefully and thoroughly. The physician's "disappearance act" is resented and called to his or her attention. Additionally, legal and ethical dimensions of terminal care have also come to the fore. Who is entitled to make significant treatment decisions? Are physicians free to follow their own traditional guidelines, or must they now check with the courts? Has the most recent judge's ruling upset the hospital's policy with respect to resuscitation, "heroic measures," and life-support procedures? And if it has, then should the hospital scrupulously obey the new rulings—or subvert them by effective if informal maneuvers? The individual with a keen interest in the interface between medical ethics, the law, and human values has much to contemplate these days (e.g., Horan & Mall, 1977; Veatch, 1976). But the practicing physician and the medical administrator often experience this aspect of the death-awareness movement as a hassle, a threat, a source of unwelcome pressure in an already-difficult situation.

At the least, it is clear that the set patterns of relating to terminally ill people and their families are now being reexamined. Some health personnel regard this as opportunity, others as threat. This means that at times we see tension, conflict, and defensiveness more openly than before. At other times, we see innovations that improve the care of the terminally ill person and provide useful training experiences for the next generation of physicians, nurses, social workers, and other care givers.

ENTER: THE HOSPICE

The major development of practical consequence centers around the *hospice* concept. It represents the application of skill and compassion in the care of the terminally ill person rather than simply talking about dying and death. There is still more talk than action, but the ratio is starting to close. The establishment of a hospice system is a challenge that requires the talents and energies of many different kinds of people, ranging from fundraisers and legal experts to designers, health care planners, and the entire spectrum of care providers. Furthermore, the hospice requires an unusual level of participation by the community as well. Both the expressed enthusiasm for and the criticism of the hospice movement in the United States might lead one to believe that such services are already in place and numerous. This is not yet the case, although hospice organizations are developing rapidly and have their own coordinating structure (the National Hospice Organization, along with a number of local coordinating groups).

Roots of the Hospice Movement

A sense of journey, of passage, has been central to the hospice concept from the very beginning. The term itself was known as early as the twelfth century. The Knights Hospitallers of the Order of Saint John of Jerusalem decreed that the sick pilgrim should be carried to bed, refreshed charitably with food, and cared for tenderly. The sick should be served cheerfully, without grumbling or complaining. Strangers were to perform these acts of kindness for people journeying to and from sacred places. Life itself could be conceived as a journey from earthly existence to a more blessed state.

Hospices of this type became fairly common, especially along the route of the Crusades. Terminal care was not the hospices' original or distinctive function, but the dying person was not turned away. Long before this time, hospitals in something approaching the modern sense had existed (among the Greeks and Romans, for example). However, the hopelessly wounded or ill person was not especially welcome in such facilities, especially those that had cultivated reputations as centers of curing and rehabilitation (Stoddard, 1978). What was to become of the dying person who had no shelter, nobody to look after him or her? During the Middle Ages many people came to such a crisis because of famine, epidemic, and the warfare that tore apart families and social structure. The hospice orientation opened the door for some of these sufferers. Debilitated people literally were carried in from the side of the road and given food, shelter, and whatever other comforts were available. Religious faith was a vital dimension of these early hospices. The dying person often was placed so that he or she could gaze upon religious symbols and icons until the very end.

Even in the past, then, one did not expect to find compassionate care for the terminally ill within the confines of the conventional medical situation but had to create another approach that had its own people, places, and philosophy.

The Contemporary Hospice

A hospice today is a system or network of care for people with limited life expectancies. It is sometimes thought to be simply a place. This is a mistaken impression; as a matter of fact, most of the hospice organizations operating in the United States together consist of a coordinated network of services without a specially constructed facility for inpatient care. It is the purpose of the hospice orientation to maintain continuity of care for the individual regardless of his or her location at the moment. Fledgling hospice organizations typically emphasize services for patients at their own homes, and some hospices intend to concentrate on this approach on a permanent basis, staying clear of constructing and operating an inpatient facility. Some hospices are freestanding organizations; others have developed within an existing hospital as a specialized form of home care. The term *palliative care unit* is often applied to hospice-type services within a larger hospital context. Without underestimating the value of a specially designed physical facility, those intimately involved in the hospice movement generally emphasize principles and attitudes that transcend any particular environment. The multidisciplinary hospice team is central, whether its services are limited to the home, or whether it also has either a separate facility or a palliative care unit within an established hospital.

St. Christopher's Hospice (Sydenham, England) is without doubt the most influential hospice of our time, a beacon and model for many that are still coming into existence. The opening of St. Christopher's in 1967 was preceded by almost 2 decades of preparation led by Dr. Cicely Saunders. She is widely regarded as the key person in the international hospice movement and has served as St. Christopher's medical director since its inception. It is a relatively small facility: 54 beds. Yet in a year's time St. Christopher's serves about 500 people directly and provides information and other services to another thousand. Although there is a strong sense of religious presence in the design and staffing of the facility, St. Christopher's serves people of all socioeconomic strata and various religious persuasions, including the agnostic and atheist. It is funded in part by Great Britain's National Health Service system and in part by private contributions. Patients are not billed, although families often make small donations.

The aims and many of the techniques pioneered by St. Christopher's have been adopted subsequently by hospices throughout Europe, the United States, and Canada. Control of pain and other symptoms receives high priority. Severe pain—or fear of severe pain—has been a common problem for those seeking admission to a hospice. Following St. Christopher's model, hospices typically attempt to relieve not only the physical distress as such but also the accompanying tension, fatigue, and dread. The hospice approach to pain control is interpersonal and environmental as well as medical. Frequently it is careful management of the person's total condition, the time given directly to the patient by attentive staff, and the general atmosphere of serenity and confidence that seems to have the most efficacy in restoring a sense of well-being. Expert use of medication (e.g., various versions of the celebrated "Brompton Cocktail") is important but does not have to carry the entire burden of pain relief. The use of all available options to prevent both pain and the expectation of pain from ruling a patient's life has come to be one of the hallmarks of the hospice (Saunders, 1978).

The philosophy emphasizes "comfort care." Staff do not come running from all sides for frantic exercises in medical "heroics." However, comfort care is interpreted as requiring careful assessment of the person's total condition and the continuation of those measures that might prolong useful or desirable life.

The relatively small size of St. Christopher's furthers its purposes. There is more opportunity for staff, volunteers, patients, and family to interact on an individual basis and also to feel themselves to be part of a community. Previous experience in England (e.g., Hinton, 1963) and elsewhere had indicated that the terminally ill person has a more difficult time in a large facility.

Emphasis on services to the patient and family at home, backed by a small, specially designed residential facility, has made it possible for existing hospitals to develop hospice-like programs. One recent and particularly successful example is the palliative care service of the Royal Victoria Hospital in Montreal (Wilson, Ajemian, & Mount, 1978). It is also an example of establishing a hospice in a cultural context rather different from the original model. The origins and early operation of this unit are instructive to review.

The hospital staff had become increasingly aware of the needs of terminally ill patients and their families through death-education programs. However, their aims remained the traditional ones of diagnosis and remission, rather than centering on the quality of life remaining to the patients. Observations suggested that the terminally ill were not receiving the desired level of care in the hospital as then constituted. Economic analysis indicated that it would be more feasible to establish a palliative care service in the existing hospital rather than to set up an independent facility. This would also enable the hospital to provide continuity of care for people who had been patients in other phases of their lives. Advocates of the palliative care service devoted more than a year to building political and economic support for their project. (Other hospice-oriented organizations have had to work even harder and longer to develop a climate of acceptance.)

The interpersonal activity stirred up by the planning process itself was rather impressive. Large public meetings were held, presentations were made through the media, a core group of representatives from six different fields met regularly, prospective staff members went to St. Christopher's for experience, and a team of 50 volunteers was developed after careful screening and training. Furthermore, a physicians' advisory committee was set up with consultants from various medical specialties. The main task of this committee was to make sure that no conflicts of interest would arise between the palliative service and other physicians in decisions to suspend "active treatment." Failure in interpersonal communication and rapport could have aborted the hospice-oriented effort before it became firmly established. Interpersonal problems among the various groups of people involved in hospice planning and function have indeed led to their own casualties in various settings.

The Palliative Care Unit itself admits only patients for whom it has been determined that cure and life prolongation are no longer appropriate goals. Priority is given to those in the home-care programs who now require additional services and those in other areas of the hospital whose physical or psychosocial situations cannot be managed well in their present location. The philosophy of this unit, typical of the hospice orientation in general, can be read in statements such as the following:

Use of personal name cards, greetings by name, and bedside flowers are part of the unit's style of operation. Both patient and family are familiarized with ward routines and the family is reassured that they can continue to be involved in the patient's care to whatever degree they feel comfortable. There are no "visiting hour" restrictions and no age minimum for visitors. A family may stay overnight if need arises. A pet may visit if it is important to the patient. The family is encouraged to bring in the patient's favorite foods—there's a microwave oven, refrigerator, etc., for preparing meals and snacks [Wilson *et al.*, 1978, p. 9].

The patient–family unit is considered the focus of care. Staff include physicians, nurses, nurse's aides, social workers, ward clerk, dietician, physiotherapist, chaplains, recreational therapist, music therapist, and volunteers. (Hospice-type operations in all settings require an ample supply of competent volunteers.) A patient may return home if symptoms come under sufficient control and the family feels able to cope with the situation. When death is near, the emphasis is on comfort and reassurance to the patient–family unit rather than on strenuous efforts to prolong life.

The home-care program is staffed by nurses and a physician on a 7-day, 24-hour basis, with additional support by volunteers, a physiotherapist, and social workers. The goals are not only pain control but also resolution of difficulties in the emotional, interpersonal, and financial spheres. Families and patients know that they can call on somebody for help at any time, or gain admission to the residential unit if necessary. People still undergoing active treatment for possible cure or life prolongation are also accepted for this program if patient load permits.

Another program centers around a consulting team. This team, consisting chiefly of the Palliative Care Unit medical director and nurses, makes itself available to terminally ill patients throughout the hospital on request of their physicians. In-hospital teaching is another important function of the consulting team.

The Royal Victoria Hospital service, like other hospice-oriented operations, continues its interest in the family after the patient's death. The bereavement follow-up service in a sense begins while the patient is still living. Family members who are especially close to the patient are evaluated for the health and psychosocial risks they might encounter after the loss of their loved one. Telephone and in-person contacts are maintained with the closest survivors, making use of those staff–family relationships that had already developed in a particular constellation. The multidisciplinary staff meets regularly to assess the situation of bereaved family members and to make recommendations.

Another typical feature of this service is its reliance upon active participation of patient and family throughout the entire process. Treatment plans are developed with patient and family as part of the team. By including patient and family as care givers as well as receivers, it is hoped "to counter the institutional depersonalization many of these patients have experienced. It also assists the key persons in their anticipatory grief [Wilson *et al.*, 1978, p. 12]."

A decade ago the hospice was a symbol, an attitude, and a hope, with but a few actual systems in place. Now there are approximately 300 hospices in 35 states, many of these quite young, with an unknown number still in the process of formation. Some hospices have only one paid staff member, and some have no paid staff at all, although there are hospices with more than 20 paid employees. Volunteers are important in all types of ongoing hospices and generally outnumber paid staff. Hospice organizations, like other health-delivery systems in the United States, must find dependable and sufficient funds to perform their services. As a relatively new type of service and one that focuses on a highly sensitive and long-neglected problem area, the hospice faces some distinctive challenges as well. Engage the director of an American hospice in conversation, and one is perhaps more likely to learn of problems, anxieties, and frustrations in securing financial support than of any other matter, including the actual process of comforting the terminally ill. This does not—yet—represent an erosion of hospice principles. What it does represent is the painful bump of idealism against (current) reality. People motivated by the desire to be helpful are becoming forced either to flee in the face of bureaucracy or to undergo a bureaucratic transformation themselves. This situation leads us to undertake a brief critical review of the hospice in contemporary American life and to identify more clearly the second of the problems suggested earlier—the bureaucratization of death.

CRITICISMS, RESERVATIONS, AND TRANSFORMATIONS

There are physicians who believe that traditional hospital care of the terminally ill is basically sound and adequate. The establishment of a separate system for the dying patient is regarded as unnecessary and, perhaps, as insulting. Others have privately expressed concern about the encouragement of a new ''death doctor'' specialty. Still others fear that the hospice concept will serve as a disguise for expensive but shoddy custodial operations. Questions could be raised about the suitability of the model hospice program (St. Christopher's type) in cultural contexts that differ appreciably from the original. Would it be effective, for example, in a situation where religious systems and sentiments are weak?

Hospice services have come to be identified largely with the management of intractable cancer. Has this focus resulted, as some think, in a false sense of general accomplishment, while people with other forms of life-threatening illness remain relatively neglected? Would concepts and techniques developed chiefly in this context prove as effective with people whose terminal illness does not involve cancer?

The bureaucratization of death involves an ill-defined mix of fantasy and reality. The well-informed person will certainly want to know what diseases are ''reimbursable'' today. It would be unwise to perish with a condition that is not on the list for hospice services. The services themselves may or may not be reimbursable. A skillful bed bath from a visiting nurse is likely to be reimbursable, as well as "meals on wheels," for example. But—as I heard one hospice pioneer report recently—"bereavement is not reimbursable." Take just this latter example for a moment. It is part of virtually everybody's hospice philosophy to provide follow-up services to survivors as needed. This is a straightforward, core service for St. Christopher's and other hospices where financial arrangements are solid and relatively hassle free. In the United States, however, if services are to be offered to the bereaved, these generally must be provided on a volunteer basis. This means that one of the most emotionally sensitive and responsible tasks in the entire hospice operation is placed in the hands of people who are outside the "professional orbit." This is not as unfortunate as it may seem. A hospice that is living up to its own standards will be very careful in its selection and training of volunteers. Their services often may prove quite comforting to bereaved family members. Nevertheless, the division of labor in this instance has been sanctioned not by clinical judgment but by an essentially arbitrary "cost-effective" bureaucratic decision made outside of the hospice. The volunteer enters a very sensitive emotional arena in which, despite the best of intentions, people can hurt one another. "Is this best for the patient and family?" is a question the regulatory bureaucracy asks less often than it asks, "How much will it cost?"

Death was an outsider not so long ago. Death's work was done after hours, when our backs were turned, in specialized places. Numero 57 and his successors were not to die "on my shift." Few perished in the operating room, but many failed to make it in the "recovery room," thereby cooperating with statistical and psychological fantasies of The Establishment. Commonplace evasions of the physical evidences of death (e.g., false-bottomed stretchers to transport corpses invisibly) were but the overt expression of covert psychological boundaries. Death did not belong.

Today Death sits around the conference table. He[2] is part of the management team. His advice and consent is politely solicited as regulations are promulgated, special interests accommodated, and finances scrutinized. Once represented by artists as a skeletonal figure adorned with a regal crown, Death is now one of us, part of the bureaucratic process. He points his finger, and another cul-de-sac is added to the labyrinth of regulations. He demands to "get his" in one situation but is willing to let other interests prevail in another. The health care bureaucracy has started to accept Death. In return, Death must play the bureaucratic game. It is just now being realized—if dimly—that Death brings astounding new resources to The Establishment. Those who can add Death to their team gain the potential for enhanced power: the millions who will be taken by Death! their needs and anxieties, transformed into allegiances and money! the well-

[2] Death has most often been personified as a male, although female personifications are not unknown.

intentioned but politically somewhat naive "natural leaders" who have brought the hospice movement up to this point!—what a gift to The Establishment!

To put it bluntly, The Establishment is in the process of discovering that it can "use" Death (and not simply the health care establishment but the larger political–economic system as well). Death was ignored as inimical to the self-image and other interests of The Establishment. The hospice movement was also ignored to some extent, but it did not go away. I do not think it is going too far to say that Death has been admitted to the conference room in order to be transformed into one more tool of power. This is not a novel role for Death, as a glance at human history—virtually any time, any place—will verify.

And yet, The Establishment is not really comfortable with its new acquisition. Most of the people who have learned to live with Death remain outside the corridors of power. Those who are in positions of legitimated authority are apt to protect their own sensitivities by entangling Death in more subtle webbings. Death is on his way to being standardized, neutralized, trivialized, one more item along with the others, a trend whose danger has previously been pointed out in the realm of death education (Kastenbaum, 1977b).

The humanitarian impulse behind the hospice movement is endangered by its growing association with and dependency on the established bureaucracy. The sensitivities and energies that have brought the movement this far may not suffice. The price for success, in other words, could be a crippling transformation. The Establishment's fantasy once was that Death could be ignored. The operative fantasy today is that Death can be accommodated without really examining—let alone, revising—the principles and process of The Establishment itself. In the name of "due process" and "cost-efficiency" we might see the ruination of the hospice movement in its most pure and distinctive forms.

The conclusion need not be this unfortunate. Encouragement may be taken, for example, in the fact that hospice-type attitudes have been dormant in a number of conventional health care settings and are now starting to flourish. At the same time that the hospice "invasion" may be threatened by deleterious modification, there is a kindred approach developing within The Establishment itself.

"HEALTHY DYING"

Belief that Death can be safely bureaucratized is a major fantasy of The Establishment. It is time to return to a major fantasy of the public at large.

Our rising expectations for comfort and autonomy have already been touched upon. At the moment, many people are (rightfully, I think) impressed by the achievements of hospices and palliative care units as well as by such community-initiated efforts as Make Today Count. However, this level of improvement may not satisfy us for long. Already there are indications that we expect the terminal phase of life to be more than merely pain-free, dignified, and comfortable. It should also be "special," exalted, fulfilling—something well beyond the ordinary dimensions of daily experience.

Part of this orientation derives from our generally rising expectations for quality of life and freedom from distress or even inconvenience. Another source may be our reaction against the mass and technological aspects of our society in general, as well as their specific intrusions into the health care situation. The more bland and aloof the face that health care delivery turns toward us, the more we conjure a vision of warmth and fulfillment.

Still a third source of idealization of the dying–death experience must be acknowledged. In recent years there has been a strong revival of interest in dying as a spiritual or transcendental experience. Raymond Moody's *Life after Life* (1975) and the public statements of Kubler-Ross have been central to this phenomenon. (For a research approach to these phenomena, however, see Kastenbaum, 1979; Osis & Haraldsson, 1977; Ring, 1980).

Moody's (1975) major contribution was the collection and interpretation of experiences from people who have returned after a close encounter with death. The typical experience in his collection has a quality of free-floating pleasure and liberation. Whatever the experiences might "mean," it is evident that they do not resemble stereotypes of dying as an agonized and fearful condition. I see no reason to doubt the honesty and accuracy of most of these reports. Some people do have such experiences when in the borderlands between life and death (although not necessarily *only* in that circumstance), and there is a core of common elements among many of the reports.

Kubler-Ross and some others go beyond these reports to the conclusion that death as such does not exist. Dying is the pleasurable transition to a higher or more exalted form of existence. On the surface of it, there is nothing new in this latter contention. But what is relatively new is its claim to be associated with "scientific data" of the type already described, and, perhaps, even more significantly, with the prestige of a famous authority on dying and death. If the best-known psychiatrist in this area declares that she has *certain* knowledge that dying and death are extraordinarily satisfying conditions, then who dares or cares to raise a voice in protest?

The point we can deal with here, unfortunately, is *not* whether this optimistic view of dying and death is justified by "reality." I do not know how to formulate and answer this question as a behavioral scientist. But we can be aware of the influence this view has within the social climate. Here is an opportunity for any of us to project and displace onto the dying–death situation all of our frustrated longings. Disappointments throughout life, the blows of faith, our own limitations, the senselessness of accidents and disasters and bureaucracies—all that has buffeted our hopes—perhaps can be conquered by the sweetness of dying and the fulfillment of death.

The general dynamics are familiar enough: Take me to the promised land, set me free from suffering and degradation! But now this orientation is not limited to a particular segment of the populations that has suffered systematic discrimination and exploitation. Any of us might keep our hopes and values insulated from the inhospitality of daily reality because dying and death will somehow cure our ills, free our spirits.

I am not presenting this view in an ironic or parodistic vein. Values are too precious, suffering is too real, and the realities we denote by ''dying'' and ''death'' are too unfathomed for glib dismissal of the present swelling of ideals and fantasies. The point is that we may be expecting too much of the health care establishment, both present and future. It is still an achievement to help a person maintain self-integrity during the terminal phase of life. A positive quality of life is a reasonable expectation, given basic resources within the individual himself or herself and those dedicated to his or her care and comfort.

But perhaps we should start to examine our underlying fantasies about what we expect. The dying–death situation is still not intimately known to many people. It is, therefore, a tempting screen on which to project aspirations and fantasies that have no other place to be displayed. At the extreme, it can lead to the assumption that a glorious death will compensate for a disappointing life—or that one need not bother too much with laborious, routine care for the terminally ill person with his or her family.

References

Abrams, R. D. The patient with cancer: His changing pattern of communication. *New England Journal of Medicine,* 1966, *244*(6), 317–322.

Abrams, R. D., & Finesinger, J. Guilt reactions in patients with cancer. *Cancer,* 1953, *6,* 474–482.

Achte, K. A., & Vauhkonen, M. L. Cancer and the psyche. *Omega,* 1971, *2,* 46–56.

Adams, J. Mutual-help groups: Enhancing the coping ability of oncology clients. *Cancer Nursing,* 1979, *2*(2), 95–98.

Adler, N. E. Emotional responses of women following therapeutic abortion. *American Journal of Orthopsychiatry,* 1975, *45,* 446–454.

Adler, N. E. Abortion: A social-psychological perspective. *Journal of Social Issues,* 1979, *35*(1), 100–119.

Adler, N. E., & Stone, G. C. Social science perspectives on the health system. In G. C. Stone, F. Cohen, & N. E. Adler (Eds.), *Health psychology.* San Francisco: Jossey-Bass, 1979. Chapter 2.

Aitken-Swan, J. Nursing the late cancer patient at home. *Practitioner,* 1959, *183,* 64–69.

Ajzen, I., & Fishbein, M. Attitudinal and normative variables as predictors of specific behaviors. *Journal of Personality and Social Psychology,* 1973, *27,* 41–57.

Allport, G. W. *The nature of prejudice.* Garden City, N.Y.: Addison-Wesley, 1954.

Alpert, J. J. Broken appointments. *Pediatrics,* 1964, *34,* 127–132.

Altman, I. The communication of interpersonal attitudes: An ecological approach. In T. L. Huston (Ed.), *Foundations of interpersonal attraction.* New York: Academic Press, 1974.

American Board of Internal Medicine. Clinical competence in internal medicine. *Annals of Internal Medicine,* 1979, *90,* 402–411.

American Cancer Society. *1978 facts and figures.* New York, 1978.

American Cancer Society Statistics, 1979, 1980.

American Hospital Association. *Hospital statistics.* Chicago: American Hospital Association, 1977.

Andreason, N.J.C., & Norris, A. S. Long-term adjustment and adaptation mechanisms in severely burned adults. *Journal of Nervous and Mental Disorders,* 1972, *154*(5), 352–362.

Antonovsky, A. *Health, stress and coping.* San Francisco: Jossey-Bass, 1979.

Appelbaum, S. A. The refusal to take one's medicine. *Bulletin of the Menninger Clinic,* 1977, *41,* 511–521.

Appley, M. H., & Trumbull, R. (Eds.). *Psychological stress: Issues in research.* New York: Appleton-Century-Crofts, 1967.

Argyle, M. *Bodily communication.* London: Methuen, 1975.

Arney, W. R., & Trescher, W. H. Trends in attitudes toward abortion, 1972–1975. *Family Planning Perspective,* 1976, *8,* 117–124.

Artiss, K. L., & Levine, A. S. Doctor–patient relations in severe illness. *New England Journal of Medicine,* 1973, *288*(23), 1210–1214.

Athanasiou, R., Oppel, W., Michelson, L., Unger, T., & Yager, M. Psychiatric sequelae to term birth and induced early and late abortion: A longitudinal study. *Family Planning Perspectives,* 1973, *5*(4), 227–231.

Atthowe, J. M. Token economies come of age. *Behavior Therapy,* 1973, *4,* 646–654.

Auerbach, S. M., Kendall, P. C., Cuttler, H. F., & Levitt, N. R. Anxiety, locus of control, type of preparatory information, and adjustment to dental surgery. *Journal of Consulting and Clinical Psychology,* 1979, *44,* 809–818.

Averill, J. R. Personal control over aversive stimuli and its relationship to stress. *Psychological Bulletin,* 1973, *80,* 286–303.

Averill, J. R., & Rosenn, M. Vigilant and nonvigilant coping strategies and psychological stress reactions during the anticipation of electric shocks. *Journal of Personality and Social Psychology,* 1972, *23,* 128–141.

Bakan, D. *Disease, pain, and sacrifice: Toward a psychology of suffering.* Chicago: University of Illinois Press, 1968.

Bakker, C. G., & Dightman, C. R. Psychological factors in fertility control. *Fertility and Sterility,* 1964, *15,* 559–567.

Baldwin, B. A. Problem pregnancy counseling: General principles. In R. R. Wilson (Ed.), *Problem pregnancy and abortion counseling.* North Carolina: Family Life Publications, 1973.

Balint, E., & Norell, J. Six minutes for the patient. In *Interactions in general practice consultation.* London: Tavistock, 1973.

Balint, M. *The doctor, his patient, and the illness* (2nd ed.). London: Pitman, 1964.

Bandura, A. Self-efficacy: Toward a unifying theory of behavioral change. *Psychological Review,* 1977, *84,* 191–215.

Bandura, A., Adams, N. E., & Beyer, J. Cognitive processes mediating behavioral change. *Journal of Personality and Social Psychology,* 1977, *35,* 125–139.

Banks, F. R., & Keller, M. D. Symptom experience and health action. *Medical Care,* 1971, *9,* 498–502.

Barber, T., & Cooper, B. Effects on pain of experimentally induced and spontaneous distraction. *Psychology Reports,* 1972, *31,* 647–651.

Bard, M. The sequence of emotional reactions in radical mastectomy patients. *Public Health Reports,* 1952, *67,* 1144–1148.

Bard, M., & Waxenberg, S. E. Relationship of Cornell Medical Index responses to postsurgical invalidism. *Journal of Clinical Psychology,* 1957, *13,* 151–153.

Barnlund, D. C. The mystification of meaning: Doctor–patient encounters. *Journal of Medical Education,* 1976, *51,* 716–725.

Bart, P. B. Social structure and vocabularies of discomfort: What happened to female hysteria? *Journal of Health and Social Behavior,* 1968, *9,* 188–193.

Basbaum, A. *Physiology and anatomy of pain.* Paper presented at the Management of Pain Conference, San Francisco, 1978.

Bean, G., Cooper, S., Alpert, R., & Kipnis, D. Coping mechanisms of cancer patients: A study of 33 patients receiving chemotherapy. *Ca—A Cancer Journal for Clinicians,* 1980, *30*(5), 256-259.

Beck, A. T. *Depression: Clinical, experimental and theoretical aspects.* New York: Harper, 1967.

Beck, N. C., Geden, E. A., & Brouder, G. T. Preparation for labor: A historical perspective. *Psychosomatic Medicine,* 1979, *41,* 243-258.

Becker, M. H. (Ed). The health belief model. *Health Education Monographs,* 1974, *2*(Whole No. 4).

Becker, M. H., Drachman, R. H., & Kirscht, J. P. Predicting mothers' compliance with pediatric medical regimens. *Journal of Pediatrics,* 1972, *81,* 843-854.

Becker, M. H., & Maiman, L. A. Sociobehavioral determinants of compliance with health and medical care recommendations. *Medical Care,* 1975, *13,* 10-24.

Becker, M. H., & Maiman L. A. Strategies for enhancing patient compliance. *Journal of Community Health,* 1980, *6*(2), 113-135.

Beecher, H. K. Relationship of significance of wound to the pain experience. *Journal of the American Medical Association,* 1956, *161,* 1609-1613.

Beecher, H. K. *Measurement of subjective responses: Quantitative effects of drugs.* New York: Oxford University Press, 1959.

Beecher, H. K. The placebo effect as a non-specific force surrounding disease and the treatment of disease. In R. Janzen, W. D. Keidel, A. Herg, C. Steichele, J. P. Payne, & R.A.P. Burt (Eds.), *Pain: Basic principles, pharmacology, therapy.* Stuttgart, West Germany: Geaze Thieme, 1972.

Beecher, H. K., Keats, A. S., Mosteller, F., & Lasagna, L. The effectiveness of oral analgesics (morphine, codeine, acetylsalicylic acid) and the problem of placebo "reactors" and "nonreactors." *Journal of Pharmacology and Experimental Therapeutics,* 1953, *109,* 393-400.

Bennett, A. E. *Communication between doctors and patients.* Oxford: Oxford University Press, 1976.

Bennis, W. G., Berlew, D. E., Schein, E. H., & Steele, F. I. Some interpersonal aspects of self-confirmation. In W. G. Bennis *et al.* (Eds.), *Interpersonal dynamics* (3rd ed.). Homewood, Ill.: Dorsey, 1973.

Ben-Sira, Z. The function of the professional's affective behavior in client satisfaction: A revised approach to social interaction theory. *Journal of Health and Social Behavior,* 1976, *17,* 3-11.

Ben-Sira, Z. Affective and instrumental components in the physician–patient relationship: an additional dimension of interaction theory. *Journal of Health and Social Behavior,* 1980, *21,* 170-180.

Benson, H., & Epstein, M. The placebo effect: A neglected asset in the care of patients. *Journal of the American Medical Association,* 1975, *232*(12), 1225-1226.

Benson, H., & McCallie, D. P., Jr. Angina pectoris and the placebo effect. *New England Journal of Medicine,* 1979, *300,* 1424-1429.

Bergman, A. B., & Werner, R. J. Failure of children to receive penicillin by mouth. *New England Journal of Medicine,* 1963, *268,* 1334-1338.

Bernstein, L., & Bernstein, R. S. *Interviewing: A guide for health professionals* (3rd ed.). New York: Appleton-Century-Crofts, 1980.

Berscheid, E., & Walster, E. H. *Interpersonal attraction.* Reading, Mass.: Addison-Wesley, 1969.

Bertakis, K. D. The communication of information from physician to patient: A method for increasing patient retention and satisfaction. *Journal of Family Practice,* 1977, *5,* 217-222.

Bille, D. A. Patients' knowledge and compliance with post-hospitalization prescriptions as related to body image and teaching format. (Doctoral dissertation, University of Wisconsin, Madison, 1975). *Dissertation Abstracts International,* 1976, *36,* 6070B-6071B. (University Microfilms No. 76-6068, 205).

Binger, C. M., Ablin, A. R., Feuerstein, R. C., Kushner, J. H., Zoger, S., & Mikkelson, C. Childhood leukemia: Emotional impact on patient and family. *New England Journal of Medicine,* 1969, *280*(8), 414–418.

Bird, B. *Talking with patients.* Philadelphia: J. B. Lippincott, 1973.

Black, R. G. The chronic pain syndrome. *Surgical Clinics of North America,* 1975, *55,* 999–1011.

Blackman, S. *The effects of nonverbal expression and cognition on the perception of pain.* Unpublished doctoral dissertation, University of California, Riverside, 1980.

Blackman, S. L. *Toward an individual case study approach to pain.* Paper presented at the Western Psychological Convention, Los Angeles, 1981.

Blackwell, B. The drug defaulter. *Clinical Pharmacology Therapy,* 1972, *13,* 841.

Blackwell, B. Drug therapy: Patient compliance. *New England Journal of Medicine,* 1973, *289,* 249–253.

Blackwell, B. Treatment adherence. *British Journal of Psychiatry,* 1976, *129,* 513–531.

Blackwell, B., Bloomfield, S. S., & Buncher, C. R. Demonstration to medical students of placebo responses and non-drug factors. *Lancet,* 1972, *1,* 1279–1282.

Blair, C., & Mahoukis, C. Comparing notes: The nurse as patient/The nurse as labor coach. *Maternal–Child Nursing,* 1980, *5,* 102–106.

Blauner, R. Death and social structure. *Psychiatry,* 1966, *29,* 378–394.

Blitz, B., & Dinnerstein, A. J. Role of attentional focus in pain perception: Manipulation of response to noxious stimulation by instructions. *Journal of Abnormal Psychology,* 1971, *77,* 42–45.

Bloch, M. *The royal touch* (F. E. Anderson Trans.). Montreal: McGill-Queen's University Press, 1973. (Orginally published, 1961.)

Blondis, M. N., & Jackson, B. E. *Nonverbal communication with patients.* New York: John Wiley & Sons, 1977.

Bloom, J. R., Ross, R. D., & Burnell, G. The effect of social support on patient adjustment after breast surgery. *Patient Counseling and Health Education.* 1978, *1*(2), 50–59.

Bloom, S. W. *The doctor and his patient: A sociological interpretation.* New York: Russell-Sage Foundation, 1963.

Blum, L. S. *The psychology of mastectomy: Time to move on.* Paper presented at the 88th Annual Convention of the American Psychological Association, Montreal, September, 1980.

Blum, R. H. *The psychology of malpractice suits.* San Francisco: California Medical Association, 1957.

Blum, R. H. *The management of the doctor–patient relationship.* New York: McGraw-Hill, 1960.

Blumberg, B. D., Golbus, M. S., & Hanson, K. H. The psychological sequelae of abortion performed for a genetic indication. *American Journal of Obstetrics and Gynecology,* 1975, *122,* 799–808.

Bobey, M. J., & Davidson, P. O. Psychological factors affecting pain tolerance. *Journal of Psychosomatic Research,* 1970, *14,* 371–376.

Boeck, M., & Leventhal, B. The adolescent cancer patient: Social function and mood. *Proceedings of the 70th Annual Meeting of the American Association for Cancer Research,* 1979, *20,* 430.

Bolter, S. The psychiatrist's role in therapeutic abortion: The unwitting accomplice. *American Journal of Psychiatry,* 1962, *119,* 312–316.

Bond, M. R. The relation of pain to the Eysenck Personality Inventory, Cornell Medical Index, and Whitely Index of Hypochondriasis. *British Journal of Psychiatry,* 1971, *119,* 671–678.

Bond, M. R. Personality studies in patients with pain secondary to organic disease. *Journal of Psychosomatic Research,* 1973, *17,* 257–263.

Bond, M. R., & Pearson, I. B. Psychological aspects of pain in women with advanced cancer of the cervix. *Journal of Psychosomatic Research,* 1969, *13,* 13–19.

Bond, M. R., & Pilowsky, I. Subjective assessment of pain and its relationship to the administration of analgesics in patients with advanced cancer. *Journal of Psychosomatic Research,* 1966, *10,* 203–208.

Bonica, J. J. Organization and function of a pain clinic. In J. J. Bonica (Ed.), *Advances in neurology* (Vol. 4). New York: Raven Press, 1974.

Bonica, J. J. *Pain: Research publications of the association for research in nervous and mental diseases.* New York: Raven Press, 1980.

Boring, E. G. *History, psychology, and science* (R. I. Watson & D. T. Campbell, Eds.). New York: Wiley, 1963.

Bowers, K. Pain, anxiety and perceived control. *Journal of Clinical and Consulting Psychology,* 1968, *32,* 596–602.

Boyd, J. R., Covington, T. R., Stanaszek, W. F., & Coussons, R. T. Drug-defaulting. II: Analysis of noncompliance patterns. *American Journal of Hospital Pharmacy,* 1974, *31,* 485–491.

Boyle, E. Biological patterns in hypertension by race, sex, body weight, and skin color. *Journal of the American Medical Association,* 1970, *213,* 1637–1643.

Bozeman, M. F., Orbach, C. E., & Sutherland, A. M. Psychological impact of cancer and its treatment. III: The adaptation of mothers to threatened loss of their children through leukemia. Part I. *Cancer,* 1955, *8,* 1–19.

Brackbill, Y. Obstetrical medication and infant behavior. In J. D. Osofsky (Ed.), *Handbook of infant development.* New York: Wiley, 1979.

Bracken, M. B. Psychosomatic aspects of abortion: Implications for counseling. *Journal of Reproductive Medicine,* 1977, *10,* 265–272.

Bracken, M. B. A causal model of psychosomatic reactions to vacuum aspiration abortion. *Social Psychiatry,* 1978, *13,* 135–145.

Bracken, M. B., Grossman, G., Hachamovitch, M., Sussman, D., & Schrier, D. Abortion counseling: An experimental study of three techniques. *American Journal of Obstetrics and Gynecology,* 1973, *117,* 10–19.

Bracken, M. B., Hachamovitch, M., & Grossman, G. The decision to abort and psychological sequelae. *Journal of Nervous and Mental Disease,* 1974, *158,* 154–162.

Bracken, M. B., & Kasl, S. V. Delay in seeking induced abortion. *American Journal of Obstetrics and Gynecology,* 1975, *121,* 1008–1019.

Bracken, M. B., & Kasl, S. V. Psychosocial correlates of delayed decisions to abort. *Health Education Monographs,* 1976, *4,* 6–44.

Bracken M. B., Klerman, L. V., & Bracken, M. Coping with pregnancy resolution among never-married women. *American Journal of Orthopsychiatry,* 1978, *48,* 320–333.

Breath and body odors may be diagnostic tools. *UPI* (Chicago), December 3, 1978.

Brehm, J. W. *A theory of psychological reactance.* New York: Academic Press, 1966.

Brehm, S. *The application of social psychology to clinical practice.* Washington D.C.: Hemisphere, 1976.

Brener, J. Visceral perception. In J. Beatty & H. Legewie (Eds.), *Biofeedback and behavior.* New York: Plenum, 1977.

Brickman, P., & Bulman, R. J. Pleasure and pain in social comparison. In J. M. Suls & R. L. Miller (Eds.), *Social comparison processes.* Washington, D.C.: Hemisphere, 1977.

Brim, O. G. (Ed.). *The dying patient.* New York: Russell-Sage Foundation, 1975.

Brody, H., Meikle, S., & Gerritse, R. Therapeutic abortion: A prospective study. *American Journal of Obstetrics and Gynecology,* 1971, *109,* 347–352.

Bronstetler, E. The young child's response to hospitalization: Separation anxiety or lack of mothering care? *American Journal of Public Health,* 1969, *59,* 92–97.

Brown, E. Meeting patients' psychosocial needs in the general hospital. *Annals of the American Academy of Political and Social Science,* 1963, *346,* 117–122.

Brown, E. R. *Rockefeller medicine men: Medicine and capitalism in America.* Berkeley, Calif.: University of California Press, 1979.

Brown, W. A. *Psychological care during pregnancy and the postpartum period.* New York: Raven Press, 1979.

Brownell, L. D., Heckerman, C. L., Westlake, R. J., Hayes, S. C., & Monte, P. M. *The effect of couples' training and partner cooperativeness in the behavioral treatment of obesity.* Paper presented at the annual meeting of the Association for the Advancement of Behavior Therapy, Atlanta, 1977.

Buehler, J. A. What contributes to hope in the cancer patient? *American Journal of Nursing,* 1975, *75,*(8), 1353–1356.

Bulletin of the World Health Organization, 1955, *12,* 427–468.

Burger, J. M., & Arkin, R. M. Prediction, control, and learned helplessness. *Journal of Personality and Social Psychology,* 1980, *38,* 482–491.

Burnum, J. F. Outlook for treating patients with self-destructive habits. *Annals of Internal Medicine,* 1974, *81,* 387–393.

Buss, A., & Portnoy, N. Pain tolerance and group identification. *Journal of Personality and Social Psychology,* 1967, *6,* 106–108.

Byrne, D. *The attraction paradigm.* New York: Academic Press, 1971.

Caines, D., Thomas, L., Mooney, V., & Pace, B. A comprehensive treatment approach to chronic low back pain. *Pain,* 1976, *2,* 301–308.

Caldwell, D., & Mishara, B. L. Research on attitudes of medical doctors toward the dying patient. *Omega,* 1972, *3,* 341–346.

Campbell, D. T., & Fiske, D. W. Convergent and discriminant validation by the multitrait-multimethod matrix. *Psychological Bulletin,* 1959, *56,* 81–105.

Cancer: More than a disease, for many a silent stigma. *New York Times,* May 4, 1977. p. 1.

Caplan, E. K., & Sussman, M. B. Rank-order of important variables for patient and staff satisfaction. *Journal of Health and Human Behavior,* 1966, *7,* 133–138.

Caplan, G. Emotional implications of pregnancy and influence on family relationships. In H. Stuart & D. Preigh (Eds.), *The healthy child.* Cambridge, Mass.: Harvard University Press, 1964.

Caplan, G. Psychological aspects of pregnancy. In N. I. Lief (Ed.), *The psychological basis of medical practice.* New York: Harper & Row, 1973.

Caplan, N., & Nelson, S. D. On being useful: The nature and consequences of psychological research on social problems. *American Psychologist,* 1973, *28,* 199–211.

Caplan, R. Social support, person–environment fit, and coping. In L. Furman & J. Gordis (Eds.), *Mental health and the economy.* Kalamazoo, MI: Upjohn Institution, 1979.

Caplan, R. D. Patient, provider, and organization: Hypothesized determinants of adherence. In S. J. Cohen (Ed.), *New directions in patient compliance.* Lexington, Mass.: D. C. Heath, 1979. Pp. 75–110.

Caplan, R. D., Robinson, E.A.R., French, J.R.P., Jr., Caldell, J. R., & Shinn, M. Adhering to medical regimens: Pilot experiments in patient education and social support. Ann Arbor, Mich.: Research Center for Group Dynamics, Institute for Social Research, University of Michigan, 1976.

Caporael, L. R. Ergotism: The satan loosed in Salem? *Science,* 1976, *192,* 21–26.

Caporael, L. R. The paralanguage of caregiving: Baby talk to the institutionalized aged. *Journal of Personality and Social Psychology,* 1981, *40,* 876–884.

Carey, R. C. Emotional adjustment in terminal patients: A quantitative approach. *Journal of Counseling Psychology,* 1974, *21,* 433–439.

Carlson, B., & Sumner, P. E. Hospital "At home" delivery: A celebration. *JOGN Nursing,* 1976, *5,* 21–27.

Cartwright, A. *Human relations and hospital care.* London: Routledge & Kegan Paul, 1964.

Cartwright, L. Sources and effects of stress in health careers. In G. C. Stone, F. Cohen, & N. E. Adler (Eds.), *Health psychology.* San Francisco: Jossey-Bass, 1979.

Casey, P. H., & Whitt, J. K. *Effect of pediatric well child care on the mother–infant relationship and infant cognitive development.* Paper presented at the biennial meeting of the Society for Research in Child Development, San Francisco, 1979.

Cassileth, B. R., Zupkis, R. V., Sutton-Smith, K., & March, V. Information and participation preferences among cancer patients. *Annals of Internal Medicine,* 1980, *92,* 832–836.

Center for Disease Control. *Abortion Surveillance 1976.* Atlanta, Ga.: Center for Disease Control, U.S. Department of Health, Education, and Welfare, 1978.

Chafetz, M. E. No patient deserves to be patronized. *Medical Insight,* 1970, *2,* 68–75.

Chang, P. *The effects of quality of self-disclosure on reactions to interviewer feedback.* Unpublished doctoral dissertation, University of Southern California, 1977.

Chapman, C., Sola, A., & Bonica, J. Illness behavior and depression compared in pain center and private practice patients. *Pain,* 1979, *6,* 1–7.

Char, W. F., & McDermott, J. F. Abortions and acute identity crisis in nurses. *American Journal of Psychiatry,* 1972, *128,* 952–957.

Charles, A. G., Norr, K. L., Block, C. R., Meyering, S., & Meyers, E. Obstetric and psychological effects of psychoprophylactic preparation for childbirth. *American Journal of Obstetrics and Gynecology,* 1978, *131,* 44–52.

Charney, E. Patient–doctor communication: Implications for the clinician. *Pediatric Clinics of North America,* 1972, *19,* 263–279.

Charney, E., Bynum, R., Eldredge, D., *et al.* How well do patients take oral penicillin? A collaborative study in private practice. *Pediatrics,* 1967, *40,* 188–195.

Chaves, J. F., & Barber, T. X. Cognitive strategies, experimenter modeling and expectation in attenuation of pain. *Journal of Abnormal Psychology,* 1974, *83,* 356–363.

Chertok, L. Psychosomatic methods of preparation for childbirth. *American Journal of Obstetrics and Gynecology,* 1967, *98,* 698–707.

Chesser, E. S., & Anderson, J. L. Psychological considerations in cancer of the breast. *Proceedings of the Royal Society of Medicine,* 1975, *68,* 793–795.

Christopher, B. & Pfeiffer, C. Varying the timing of information to alter preoperative anxiety and postoperative recovery in cardiac surgery patients. *Heart and Lung,* 1980, *9,* 854–861.

Clark, C., & Hunt, H. Pain. In J. Downey & R. Darling (Eds.), *Physiological basis of rehabilitative medicine.* Philadelphia: W. B. Saunders, 1971. Pp. 373–401.

Clausen, J. P., Flook, M. H., & Ford, B. *Maternity nursing today.* New York: McGraw-Hill, 1977.

Cleghorn, J. M., & Streiner, B. J. Prediction of symptoms and illness behavior from measures of life change and verbalized depressive themes. *Journal of Human Stress,* 1979, *5,* 16–23.

Coates, D., & Wortman, C. B. Depression maintenance and interpersonal control. In A. Baum and J. E. Singer (Eds.), *Advances in environmental psychology, Volume 2: Applications of personal control.* Hillsdale, N.J.: Lawrence Erlbaum Associates, 1980.

Coates, D., & Wortman, C. B. Control, social interaction, and depression maintenance. In A. Baum, J. Singer, & Y. Epstein (Eds.), *Advances in environmental psychology* (Vol. 2). Hillsdale, N.J.: Lawrence Erlbaum Associates, 1980.

Coates, D., Wortman, C. B., & Abbey, A. Reactions to victimization: A social psychological analysis. In I. Frieze, D. Bar-Tel, & J. Carroll (Eds.), *Applications of attribution theory.* San Francisco: Jossey-Bass, 1979.

Cobb, B. Why do people detour to quacks? *The Psychiatric Bulletin,* 1954, *3,* 66–69.

Cobb, B. Nurse–patient relationships. *Journal of the American Geriatric Society,* 1956, *4,* 690–698.

Cobb, S. Social support as a moderator of life stress. *Psychosomatic Medicine,* 1976, *38,* 300–314.

Cobb, S. Social support and health through the life course. In M. W. Riley (Ed.), *Aging from birth to death: Interdisciplinary perspectives.* Boulder, Colo. Westview Press, 1979.

Cobb, S., & Erbe, C. Social support for the cancer patient. *Forum on Medicine,* 1978, *1*(8), 24–29.

Cobb, S., & Rose, R. M. Hypertension, peptic ulcer, and diabetes in air traffic controllers. *Journal of the American Medical Association,* 1973, *224,* 489–492.

Cobliner, W. G. Psychosocial factors in gynecological or breast malignancies. *Hospital Physician,* 1977, *13*(1), 38–40.

Cohen, F. Personality, stress, and the development of physical illness. In G. C. Stone, F. Cohen, & N. E. Adler (Eds.), *Health psychology: A handbook.* San Francisco: Jossey-Bass, 1979.

Cohen, M., Goldenberg, I., & Goldenberg, H. Treating families of bone marrow recipients and donors. *Journal of Marriage and Family Counseling,* 1977, *3,* 45–51.

Cohen, P., Dizenhuz, I. M., & Winget, C. Family adaptation to terminal illness and death of a parent. *Social Casework,* 1977, *58*(4), 223–228.

Cohen, R. L. Some maladaptive syndromes of pregnancy and the puerperium. *Obstetrics and Gynecology,* 1966, *27,* 562–570.

Cohen, S., & McKay, G. Social support, stress and the buffering hypothesis: A review of naturalistic studies. In A. Baum, J. E. Singer, & S. E. Taylor (Eds.), *Handbook of psychology and health* (Volume 4). Hillsdale, New Jersey: Erlbaum, in press.

Cole, S. A., O'Connor, S., & Bennett, L. Self-help groups for clinic patients with chronic illness. *Primary Care,* 1979, *6*(2), 325–340.

Coley, S. B., & James, B. E. Delivery: A trauma for fathers? *Family Coordinator,* 1976, *25,* 359–363.

Collins, B. E., & Hoyt, M. F. Personal responsibility for consequences: An integration and extension of the forced compliance literature. *Journal of Experimental Social Psychology,* 1972, *8,* 558–593.

Colman, A. D. Psychological state during first pregnancy. *American Journal of Orthopsychiatry,* 1969, *39,* 788–797.

Colten, M. E., & Janis, I. L. Effects of self-disclosure and the decisional balance-sheet procedure in a weight reduction clinic. In I. L. Janis (Ed.), *Counseling on personal decisions: Theory and field research on short-term helping relationships.* New Haven, Conn.: Yale University Press, in press.

Conolley, E., Janis, I. L., & Dowds, M. Effects of variations in type of feedback from the counselor. In I. L. Janis (Ed.), *Counseling on personal decisions: Theory and research on short-term helping relationships.* New Haven, Conn.: Yale University Press, in press.

Cooper, B. A child with cancer: How three families cope with life, not death. *Chicago Magazine,* April 1980, pp. 174–179, 224, 228.

Cooper, I. S. *Living with chronic neurologic disease.* New York: Norton, 1976.

Copeland, E., Miller, L., & Jones, R. Prognostic factors in carcinoma of the colon and rectum. *American Journal of Surgery,* 1968, *116,* 875–881.

Corah, N. L., & Boffa, J. Perceived control, self-observation, and response to aversive stimulation. *Journal of Personality and Social Psychology,* 1970, *16,* 1–4.

Corah, N. L., Gale, E. N., & Illig, S. J. Psychological stress reduction during dental procedures. *Journal of Dental Research,* 1979, *58,* 1347–1351.

Coser, R. L. *Life in the ward.* East Lansing, Mich.: Michigan State University Press, 1962.

Cousins, N. *Anatomy of an illness as perceived by the patient.* New York: W. W. Norton, 1979.

Coyne, J. C. Depression and the response of others. *Journal of Abnormal Psychology,* 1976, *85*(2), 186–193. (a)

Coyne, J. C. Toward an interactional description of depression. *Psychiatry,* 1976, *39,* 28–39. (b)

Craig, K. D. Social Modeling determinants of pain processes. *Pain,* 1975, *1,* 375–378.

Craig, T. J., & Abeloff, M. D. Psychiatric symptomology among hospitalized cancer patients. *American Journal of Psychiatry,* 1974, *131*(12), 1323–1327.

Crano, W., & Brewer, M. *Principles of research in social psychology.* New York: McGraw-Hill, 1973.

Cronbach, L. J., & Snow, R. E. *Aptitudes and instructional methods: A handbook for research on interactions.* New York: Irvington, 1977.

Cronenwett, L. R. Elements and outcomes of a postpartum support group program. *Research in Nursing and Health,* 1980, *3,* 33–41.

Crown, S., & Crown, J. Personality in early rheumatoid disease. *Journal of Psychosomatic Research,* 1973, *17,* 189–196.

Dailey, C. A. The effects of premature conclusions upon the acquisition of understanding of a person. *Journal of Psychology,* 1952, *33,* 133–152.

D'Andrade, R. G. Memory and the assessment of behavior. In H. M. Blalock (Ed.), *Measurement in the social sciences. Theories and strategies.* Chicago: Aldine, 1974.

Danziger, S. K. Treatment of women in childbirth: Implications for family beginnings. *American Journal of Public Health,* 1979, *69,* 895–901.

Dattore, P. J., Shontz, F. D., & Coyne, L. Premorbid personality differentiation of cancer and noncancer groups: A test of the hypothesis of cancer proneness. *Journal of Consulting and Clinical Psychology,* 1980, *48*(3), 388–394.

Daubenmire, M. J. Nurse–patient–physician communicative interaction process. In H. Werley, A. Zuzich, M. Zajkowski, & A. Zngornik (Eds.), *Health research: The systems approach.* New York: Springer, 1976.

Dauber, B. Profile of an abortion counselor. *Family Planning Perspectives,* 1974, *6,* 185–187.

Dauber, B., Zalar, M., & Goldstein, P. J. Abortion counseling and behavioral change. *Family Planning Perspectives,* 1972, *4,* 23–27.

Davidson, P., & Bobey, M. Repressor–sensitizer differences: A repeated exposure to pain. *Perceptual and Motor Skills,* 1970, *31,* 711–714.

Davidson, P., & Neufeld, R. Response to pain and stress: A multivariate analysis. *Journal of Psychosomatic Research,* 1974, *18,* 25–32.

Davies, R. K., Quinlan, D. M., McKegney, F. P., & Kimball, C. P. Organic factors and psychological adjustment in advanced cancer patients. *Psychosomatic Medicine,* 1973, *35*(6), 464–471.

Davis, M. S. Variations in patients' compliance with doctors' orders: Analyses of congruence between survey responses and results of empirical investigations. *Journal of Medical Education,* 1966, *41,* 1037–1048.

Davis, M. S. Physiologic, psychological, and demographic factors in patient compliance with doctors' orders. *Medical Care* 1968, *6,* 115–122. (a)

Davis, M. S. Variations in patients' compliance with doctors' advice: An empirical analysis of patterns of communication. *American Journal of Public Health,* 1968, *58,* 274–288. (b)

Davis, M. S. Variations in patients' compliance with doctors' orders: Medical practice and doctor–patient interaction. *Psychiatry in Medicine,* 1971, *2,* 31–54.

Davitz, J. R. *The communication of emotional meaning.* New York: McGraw-Hill, 1964.

Deci, E. *Intrinsic motivation.* New York: Plenum, 1975.

Degenaar, J. J. Some philosophical considerations on pain. *Pain,* 1979, *7,* 281–304.

Delaphaine, R., Ifabumuji, O., Mersky, H., & Zarfas, T. Significance of pain in psychiatric hospital patients. *Pain,* 1978, *4,* 361–366.

DelliQuadri, L., & Breckenridge, K. *Mother care: Helping yourself through the emotional and physical transitions of a new motherhood.* Los Angeles: J. P. Tarcher, 1978.

Denenberg, V. H. Stimulation in infancy, emotional reactivity, and exploratory behavior. In D. C. Glass (Ed.), *Neurophysiology and emotion.* New York: Rockefeller University Press, 1967.

Derogatis, L. R., Abeloff, M. D., & Melisaratos, N. Psychological coping mechanisms and survival time in metastatic breast cancer. *Journal of the American Medical Association,* 1979, *242*(14), 1504–1508.

DeWolfe, A. S., Barrell, R. P., & Cummings, J. W. Patient variables in emotional response to hospitalization for physical illness. *Journal of Consulting Psychology,* 1966, *30,* 68–72.

DiCicco, L., & Apple, D. Health needs and opinions of older adults. In D. Apple (Ed.), *Sociological studies of health and sickness.* New York: McGraw-Hill, 1960.

DiMatteo, M. R. A social-psychological analysis of physician-patient rapport: Toward a science of the art of medicine. *Journal of Social Issues,* 1979, *35*(1), 12–33.

DiMatteo, M. R., & DiNicola, D. D. Social science and the art of medicine: From Hippocrates to holism. In H. S. Friedman & M. R. DiMatteo (Eds.), *Interpersonal issues in health care.* New York: Academic Press, 1982.

DiMatteo, M. R., & DiNicola, D. D. Sources of assessment of physician performance: A study of comparative reliability and patterns of interrelatedness. *Medical Care,* 1981, *19,* 829–842.

DiMatteo, M. R., & Friedman, H. S. *Social psychology and medicine.* Cambridge, Mass.: Oelgeschlager, Gunn & Hain, 1982.

DiMatteo, M. R., Friedman, H. S., & Taranta, A. Sensitivity to bodily nonverbal communication as a factor in practitioner–patient rapport. *Journal of Nonverbal Behavior,* 1979, *4,*(1), 18–26.

DiMatteo, M. R., & Hall, J. A. Nonverbal decoding skill and attention to nonverbal cues: A research note. *Environmental Psychology and Nonverbal Behavior,* 1979, *3,* 188–192.

DiMatteo, M. R., & Hays, R. The significance of patients' perceptions of physician conduct: A study of patient satisfaction in a family practice center. *Journal of Community Health,* 1980, *6*(1), 18–34.

DiMatteo, M. R., & Hays, R. Social support and serious illness. In B. Gottlieb (Ed.), *Social networks and social support.* Beverly Hills, Calif.: Sage Publications, 1981.

DiMatteo, M. R., Prince, L. M., & Taranta, A. Patients' perceptions of physicians' behavior: Determinants of patient commitment to the therapeutic relationship. *Journal of Community Health,* 1979,*4,* 280–290.

DiMatteo, M. R., Taranta, A., Friedman, H. S., & Prince, L. M. Predicting patient satisfaction from physicians' nonverbal communication skills. *Medical Care,* 1980, *18,* 376–387.

DiNicola, D. D., & DiMatteo, M. R. Communication, interpersonal influence, and resistance to medical treatment. In T. A. Wills (Ed.), *Basic processes in helping relationships.* New York: Academic Press, 1982.

Dohrenwend, B. S., & Dohrenwend, B. P. (Eds.). *Stressful life events: Their nature and effects.* New York: Wiley, 1974.

Dollard, J., & Miller, N. E. *Personality and psychotherapy.* New York: McGraw-Hill, 1950.

Donovan, W. L., & Leavitt, L. A. Early cognitive development and its relation to maternal physiological and behavioral responsiveness. *Child Development,* 1978, *49,* 1251–1254.

Dowds, M., Janis, I. L., & Conolley, E. Effects of acceptance by the counselor. In I. L. Janis (Ed.), *Counseling on personal decisions: Theory and research on short-term helping relationships.* New Haven, Conn.: Yale University Press, in press.

Doyle, B. J., & Ware, J. E. Physician conduct and other factors that affect consumer satisfaction with medical care. *Journal of Medical Education,* 1977, *52,* 793–801.

Drury, V.W.M., Wade, O. L., & Woolf, E. Following advice in general practice. *Journal of the Royal College of General Practitioners,* 1976, *26,* 712–718.

Dubos, R. *Mirage of health: Utopias, progress, and biological change.* New York: Harper & Row, 1959.

Dubos, R. *Man adapting.* New Haven, Conn.: Yale University Press, 1965.

Dubos, R. The diseases of civilization: Achievements and illusions. In L. King (Ed.), *Mainstreams of medicine.* Austin, Tex.: University of Texas Press, 1971.

Dubos, R., & Dubos, J. *The white plague.* Boston: Little, Brown, 1952.

Duff, R. S., & Hollingshead, A. B. *Sickness and society.* New York: Harper & Row, 1968.

Duffy, D., Hamerman, D., & Cohen, M. Communication skills of house officers. *Annals of Internal Medicine,* 1980, *93,* 354–357.

Duncan, D. S., Jr., & Rosenthal, R. Vocal emphasis in experimenters' introduction reading as unintended determinant of subjects' responses. *Language and Speech,* 1968, *11,* 20–26.

Dunkel-Schetter, C., & Wortman, C. B. Dilemmas of social support: Parallels between victimization and aging. In Kiesler, S. B., Morgan, J. N., & Oppenheimer, V. K. (Eds.), *Aging: Social change.* New York: Academic Press, 1981.

Dyk, R. B., & Sutherland, A. M. Adaptation of the spouse and other family members to the colostomy patient. *Cancer,* 1956, *9,* 123–138.

Ebaugh, F., & Heuser, K. Psychiatric aspects of therapeutic abortion. *Postgraduate Medicine,* 1947, *2,* 325–332.

Ebert, R. H. Medical education in the United States. *Daedalus,* 1977, *106*(1), 171–184.

Edelwich, J., & Brodsky, A. *Burnout: Stages of Disillusionment in the Helping Profession.* New York: Human Sciences Press, 1981.

Egbert, L. D., Battit, G. E., Tundorf, C. E., & Beecher, H. K. The value of the preoperative visit by an anesthetist. *Journal of the American Medical Association,* 1963, *185,* 553–555.

Egbert, L. D., Battit, G. E., Welch, C. E., & Bartlett, M. K. Reduction of postoperative pain by encouragement and instruction of patients: A study of doctor–patient rapport. *New England Journal of Medicine,* 1964, *270,* 825–827.

Eichna, L. W. Medical school education, 1975–1979: A student's perspective. *New England Journal of Medicine,* 1980, *303,* 727–734.

Eisenberg, L. Disease and illness: Distinctions between professional and popular ideas. *Culture, medicine, and psychiatry,* 1977, 9–23. (a)

Eisenberg, L. The search for care. *Daedalus,* 1977, *106,* 235–246. (b)

Ekblad, M. Induced abortion on psychiatric grounds: A follow-up study of 479 women. *Acta Psychiatrica et Neurologia Scandinavica,* 1955, Supplementum 99, 3–238.

Ekman, P., & Friesen, W. V. Nonverbal leakage and clues to deception. *Psychiatry,* 1969, *32,* 88–106.

Ekman, P., & Friesen, W. V. Detecting deception from the body or face. *Journal of Personality and Social Psychology,* 1974, *29,* 288–298.

Ekman, P., & Friesen, W. V. *Unmasking the face.* Englewood Cliffs, N.J.: Prentice-Hall, 1975.

Ekman, P., Friesen, W. V., & Ellsworth, P. *Emotion in the human face.* New York: Pergamon Press, 1972.

Elling, R., Whittemore, R., & Green, M. Patient participation in a pediatric program. *Journal of Health & Human Behavior,* 1960, *1,* 183–191.

Ellsworth, P. Direct gaze as a social stimulus: The example of aggression. In P. Pliner, L. Krames, & T. Alloway (Eds.), *Nonverbal communication of aggression.* New York: Plenum Publishing, 1975.

Ellsworth, P., Friedman, H., Perlick, D., & Hoyt, M. Some effects of gaze on subjects motivated to seek or to avoid social comparison. *Journal of Experimental Social Psychology,* 1978, *14,* 69–87.

Elman, R. Psychogenic factors in surgery. *The Surgical Clinics of North America,* 1950, *30,* 1391–1409.

Elstein, A. S. Clinical judgment: Psychological research and medical practice. *Science,* 1976, *194,* 696–700.

Elstein, A. S., Schulman, L. S., & Sprafka, S. A. *Medical problem solving: An analysis of clinical reasoning.* Cambridge, Mass.: Harvard University Press, 1978.

Engel, G. A life setting conducive to illness: The giving-up–given-up complex. *Annals of Internal Medicine,* 1968, *69,* 293–300.

Engel, G. L. The need for a new medical model: A challenge for biomedicine. *Science,* 1977, *196,* 129–136. (a)

Engel, G. L. The care of the patient: Art or science? *Johns Hopkins Medical Journal,* 1977, *140,* 222–232. (b)

Engel, G. L. A unified concept of health and disease. In T. Millon (Ed.), *Medical behavioral science.* Philadelphia: W. B. Saunders, 1975.

Enkin, M. W., Smith, S. L., Dermer, S. W., & Emmett, J. O. An adequately controlled study of effectiveness of PPM training. In N. Morris (Ed.), *Psychosomatic medicine in obstetrics and gynecology.* Basel: S. Karger, A. G., 1972.

Epstein, A. S. *Pregnant teenagers' knowledge of infant development.* Paper presented at the biennial meeting of the Society for Research in Child Development, San Francisco, March, 1979.

Epstein, L. H., & Masek, B. J. Behavioral control of medical compliance. *Journal of Applied Behavior Analysis,* 1978, *11,* 1–9.

Evans, D. A., & Gusdon, J. P. Postabortion attitudes. *North Carolina Medical Journal,* 1973, *34,* 271–273.

Evans, F. J. The placebo response in pain reduction. In J. Bonica (Ed.), *Advances in neurology* (Vol. 4). New York: Raven Press, 1974.

Ewing, J. A., & Rouse, B. A. Therapeutic abortion and a prior psychiatric history. *American Journal of Psychiatry,* 1973, *130,* 37–40.

Exline, R. V. Visual interaction: The glance of power and preference. In J. Cole (Ed.), *Nebraska Symposium on Motivation, 1971.* Lincoln, Nebr.: Univeristy of Nebraska Press, 1972.

Farina, A., Holland, C. J., & Ring, K. Role of stigma and set in interpersonal interaction. *Journal of Abnormal Psychology,* 1966, *71*(6), 421–428.

Faxel, A.M.H. The birthing room concept at Phoenix Memorial Hospital. Part I: Development and 18 months statistics. *JOGN Nursing,* 1980, *9,* 151–159.

Feifel, H. (Ed.). *The meaning of death.* New York: McGraw-Hill, 1959.

Feifel, H. (Ed.). *New meanings of death.* New York: McGraw-Hill, 1977.

Fein, R. A. Men's entrance to parenthood. *Family Coordinator,* 1976, *25,* 341–348.

Ferlic, M., Goldman, A., & Kennedy, B. J. Group counseling in adult patients with advanced cancer. *Cancer,* 1979, *43,* 760–766.

Ferreira, A. J. Emotional factors in prenatal environment: A review. *Journal of Nervous and Mental Disorders,* 1965, *141,* 108–118.

Festinger, L. A theory of social comparison processes. *Human Relations,* 1954, *7,* 117–140.

Finnerty, F. A., Jr., Mattie, E. C., & Finnerty, F. A., III. Hypertension in the inner city. 1: Analysis of the clinic dropouts. *Circulation,* 1973, *47,* 73–75.

Fleck, S. Some psychiatric aspects of abortion. *Journal of Nervous and Mental Disease,* 1970, *151,* 42–50.

Flexner, A. *Medical education in the United States and Canada* (Bulletin No. 4). New York: Carnegie Foundation for the Advancement of Teaching, 1910.

Flexner, J. Dying, death and the "front-line" physician. In D. Barton (Ed.), *Dying and death.* Baltimore: Williams & Wilkins, 1977.

Flom, P. K. Performance in the medical internship. (Doctoral dissertation, University of California, Berkeley, 1970) *Dissertation Abstracts International,* 1971, *32*(2–B), 1188.

Ford, A. B., Liske, R. E., Ort, R. S., & Denton, J. C. *The doctor's perspective: Physicians view their patients and practice.* Cleveland, Ohio: Case Western Reserve University Press, 1967.

Ford, C., Castelnuovo-Tedesco, P., & Long, K. Abortion: Is it a therapeutic procedure in psychiatry? *Journal of the American Medical Association,* 1971, *218,* 1173–1178.

Fordyce, W. E. Pain viewed as learned behavior. *Advances in neurology* (Vol. 4). New York: Raven Press, 1974. Pp. 415–422.

Fordyce, W. E. Behavioral concepts in chronic pain and illness. In P. O. Davidson (Ed.), *The behavioral management of anxiety, depression, and pain.* New York: Brunner/Mazel, 1976. (a)

Fordyce, W. E. *Behavioral methods for chronic pain and illness.* St. Louis: C. V. Mosby, 1976. (b)

Fordyce, W., Fowler, R., Lehamann, J., De Lateur, B., Sand, P., & Treischmann, R. Operant conditioning in the treatment of chronic pain. *Archives of Physical Medicine and Rehabilitation,* 1973, *54,* 399–408.

Forester, B. M., Kornfeld, D. S., & Fleiss, J. Psychiatric aspects of radiotherapy. *American Journal of Psychiatry,* 1978, *135*(8), 960–963.

Foreyt, J. P. (Ed.). *Behavioral treatments of obesity.* New York: Pergamon, 1977.

Forrest, J. D., Sullivan, E., & Tietze, C. Abortion in the United States, 1977–1978. *Family Planning Perspectives,* 1979, *11,* 329–341.

Forrest, J. D., Tietze, C., & Sullivan, E. Abortion in the United States, 1976–1977. *Family Planning Perspectives,* 1978, *10,* 271–279.

Fosson, S. E. House staff attitudes toward cancer. *Proceedings of 14th Annual meeting of the American Association of Cancer Education* (Vol. 1). September, 1980.

Foster, Z., & Mendel, S. Mutual-help group for patients: Taking steps toward change. *Health and Social Work,* 1979, *4(3),* 82–98.

Fox, R. Ethical and existential developments in contemporaneous American medicine: The implications for culture and society. *Milbank Memorial Fund Quarterly,* 1974, *52,* 445–483.

Fox, R. C. *Experiment perilous: Physicians and patients facing the unknown.* Glencoe, Ill.: The Free Press, 1959.

Francis, V., Korsch, B. M., & Morris, M. J. Gaps in doctor–patient communications: Patients' response to medical advice. *New England Journal of Medicine,* 1969, *280,* 535–540.

Frank, J. D. The medical power of faith. *Human Nature,* 1978, *1,* 40–47.

Frederick, J. F. Grief as a disease process. *Omega,* 1976, *7,* 297–306.

Freeman, G. Gaps in doctor–patient communication: Doctor–patient interaction analysis. *Pediatric Research,* 1971, *5,* 298–311.

Freeman, M. H. Giving family life a good start in the hospital. *American Journal of Maternal–Child Nursing,* 1979, *4,* 51–54.

Freidson, E. *Patients' views of medical practice.* New York: Russell-Sage Foundation, 1961.

French, J.R.P., Jr., & Raven, B. H. The bases of social power. In Dorwin Cartwright (Ed.), *Studies in social power.* Ann Arbor, Mich.: Insititute for Social Research, University of Michigan, 1959. Pp. 150–167.

Freudenberger, H., & Richelson, G. *Burnout: The High Cost of High Achievement.* Garden City: Anchor Press/Doubleday, 1980.

Friedman, H. S. Nonverbal communication between patients and medical practitioners. *The Journal of Social Issues,* 1979, *35,* 82–99.(a)

Friedman, H. S. The interactive effects of facial expressions of emotion and verbal messages on perceptions of affective meaning. *Journal of Experimental Social Psychology,* 1979, *15,* 453–469. (b)

Friedman, H. S. Nonverbal communication in medical interaction. In H. S. Friedman & M. R. DiMatteo (Eds.), *Interpersonal issues in health care.* New York: Academic Press, 1982.

Friedman, H. S., DiMatteo, M. R., & Taranta, A. A study of the relationship between individual differences in nonverbal expressiveness and factors of personality and social interaction. *Journal of Research in Personality,* 1980, *14,* 351–364.

Friedman, H. S., Prince, L., Riggio, R., & DiMatteo, M. Understanding and assessing nonverbal expressiveness: The Affective Communication Test. *Journal of Personality and Social Psychology,* 1980, *39,* 333–351.

Friedman, M., & Rosenman, R. H. *Type A behavior and your heart.* New York: Knopf, 1974.

Fuchs, V. R. *Who shall live?* New York: Basic Books, 1974.

Fulton, R. (Ed.). *Death and identity* (2nd ed.) New York: Wiley, 1976.

Fulton, R. *Death, grief and bereavement. A bibliography: 1845–1975.* New York: Arno Press, 1977.

Gal, R., & Lazarus, R. S. The role of activity in anticipating and confronting stressful situations. *Journal of Human Stress,* 1975, *1,* 4–20.

Gallup, G. "Seventy-five percent back abortions but most say only in certain circumstances." *The Gallup Poll,* news release, Princeton, N.J., January 22, 1978.

Garfield, C. Impact of death on the health care professional. In H. Feifel (Ed.), *New meanings of death.* New York: McGraw-Hill, 1977.

Garfield, C. A. (Ed.). *Psychosocial care of the dying patient.* New York: McGraw-Hill, 1978.

Garner, H. H. *Psychosomatic management of the patient with malignancy.* Springfield, Ill.: Charles C. Thomas, 1966.

Garrity, T. F., Marx, M. B., & Somes, G. W. The relationship of recent life change to seriousness of later illness. *Journal of Psychosomatic Research,* 1978, *22,* 7–12.

Geer, J., Davison, G., & Gatchel, R. Reduction of stress in humans through non-veridical perceived control of aversive stimulation. *Journal of Personality and Social Psychology*, 1970, *16*, 731–738.

Geersten, H. R., Gray, R. M., & Ward, J. R. Patient non-compliance within the context of seeking medical care for arthritis. *Journal of Chronic Disease*, 1973, *26*, 689–698.

Gellert, E. Reducing the emotional stresses of hospitalization for children. *The American Journal of Occupational Therapy*, 1958, *12*, 125–129.

Gelles, R. J. Violence and pregnancy: A note on the extent of the problem and needed services. *The Family Coordinator*, 1975, *24*, 81–86.

Gerle, B., Lundin, G., & Sandblom, P. The patient with inoperable cancer from the psychiatric and social standpoint. *Cancer*, 1960, *13*, 1206–1217.

Giacquinta, B. Helping families face the crisis of cancer. *American Journal of Nursing*, 1977, *77*(10), 1585–1588.

Gilbertson, V. Proctosigmoidoscopy and polypectomy in reducing the incidence of rectal cancer. *Cancer*, 1974, *34*, 936–939.

Gillium, R. F., & Barsky, A. J. Diagnosis and management of patient noncompliance. Journal of the American Medical Association, 1974, *228*, 1563–1567.

Glaser, B. G., & Strauss, A. L. *Awareness of dying*. Chicago: Aldine, 1965.

Glaser, B. G., & Strauss, A. L. *Time for dying*. Chicago: Aldine, 1968.

Glass, D. *Behavioral antecedents of coronary heart disease*. Hillsdale N.J.: Erlbaum, 1977. (a)

Glass, D. *Behavior patterns, stress, and coronary disease*. Hillsdale, N.J.: Erlbaum, 1977. (b)

Glick, I. O., Weiss, R. S., & Parkes, C. M. *The first years of bereavement*. New York: Wiley, 1974.

Goffman, E. *Asylums*. Garden City, N.Y.: Doubleday, 1961.

Goffman, E. *Stigma: Notes on the management of spoiled identity*. Englewood Cliffs, N.J.: Prentice-Hall, 1963.

Gofman, E., Buckman, W., & Schade, G. The child's emotional response to hospitalization. *American Journal of Diseases of Children*, 1957, *93*, 157–164.

Goldenberg, I., & Goldenberg, H. *Family therapy: An overview*. Monterey, Calif.: Brooks-Cole, 1980.

Goldfried, M. R., & Davidson, G. *Clinical behavior therapy*. New York: Holt, Rinehart and Winston, 1976.

Goldsmith, S., Potts, L., Green, L., & Miller, R. Couseling and referral for legal abortion in California's Bay Area. *Family Planning Perspectives*, 1970, *2*, 14–19.

Goodman, R., & Gorlin, R. *The face in genetic disorders*. St. Louis: C. V. Mosby, 1970.

Gordis, L. Methodologic issues in the measurement of patient compliance. In D. L. Sackett & R. B. Haynes (Eds.), *Compliance with therapeutic regimens*. Baltimore: Johns Hopkins University Press, 1976.

Gordon, B. The vulnerable mother and her child. In S. Kitzinger & J. A. Davis (Eds.), *The place of birth*. Oxford: Oxford University Press, 1978.

Gordon, W., Freidenberg, I., Diller, L., Rothman, L., Wolf, C., Ruckdeschel-Hibbard, M., Ezrachi, O., & Gerstman, L. *The psychosocial problems of cancer patients: A retrospective study*. Paper presented at the meeting of the American Psychological Association, San Francisco, September, 1977.

Gorer, G. *Death, grief and mourning*. New York: Arno Press, 1977.

Gough, H. G., Hall, W. B., & Harris, R. E. Admissions procedures as forecasters of performance in medical training. *Journal of Medical Education*, 1963, *38*, 983–998.

Gough, H. G., Hall, W. B., & Harris, R. E. Evaluation of performance in medical training. *Journal of Medical Education*, 1964, *39*, 679–692.

Gray, P. G., & Cartwright, A. Choosing and changing doctors. *Lancet*, Dec. 19, 1953, p. 1308.

Greenberg, M. S. *Patient reported disturbances in the hospital treatment of cancer patients as elicited by the critical incident technique*. Unpublished masters thesis, University of Houston, 1961.

Greenberg, N., & Morris, N. Engrossment: Newborn's impact on the father. *American Journal of Orthopsychiatry,* 1974, *44,* 520–531.

Greene, L. Effects of the counselor's verbal feedback, interpersonal distance and clients' field dependence. In I. L. Janis (Ed.), *Counseling on personal decisions: Theory and research on short-term helping relationships.* New Haven, Conn.: Yale University Press, in press.

Greene, R., & Reyher, J. Pain tolerance in hypnotic analgesic and imagination states. *Journal of Abnormal Psychology,* 1972, *79,* 29–38.

Greenleigh & Associates. Report on the Social, Economic, and Psychological Needs of Cancer Patients in California. California Division, American Society, San Francisco, May 1979.

Grimm, L., & Kanfer, F. H. Tolerance of aversive stimulation. *Behavior Therapy,* 1976, *7,* 216–225.

Grollman, E. (Ed.). *Explaining death to children.* Boston: Beacon Press, 1967.

Gross, M. L. *The doctors.* New York: Random House, 1966.

Gustafson, J., & Whitman, H. Toward a balanced social environment on the oncology service: The cancer patients' group. *Social Psychiatry,* 1978, *13,* 147–152.

Haase, R. F., & Tepper, D. T. Nonverbal components of empathic communication. *Journal of Counseling Psychology,* 1972, *19,* 417–424.

Hackett, T. P., & Cassem, N. H. Psychological management of the myocardial infarction patient. *Journal of Human Stress,* 1975, *1,* 25–38.

Hackett, T. P., & Weisman, A. D. Denial as a factor in patients with heart disease and cancer. *Annals of the New York Academy of Science,* 1969, *164,* 802–817.

Hahn, S. R., & Paige, R. E. American birth practices: A critical review. In J. E. Parsons (Ed.). *The psychobiology of sex differences and sex roles.* New York: McGraw-Hill, 1980.

Halberstam, M. J. The doctor's new dilemma: Will I be sued? *New York Times Magazine,* February 14, 1971.

Hall, E. T. *The hidden dimension.* Garden City, N.Y.: Doubleday, 1966.

Hall, J. A., Roter, D., & Rand, C. Communication of affect between patient and physician. *Journal of Health and Social Behavior,* 1981, *22,* 18–30.

Hamburg, D. A., & Brown, S. S. The science base and social context of health maintenance: An overview. *Science,* 1978, *200,* 847–849.

Harker, B. L. Cancer and communication problems: A personal experience. *Psychiatry in Medicine,* 1972, *3,* 163–171.

Harkins, S., & Chapman, R. Detection and decision factors in pain perception in young and elderly men. *Pain,* 1976, *2,* 253–264.

Harlow, H. F., & Zimmerman, R. R. Affectional responses in the infant monkey. *Science,* 1959, *130,* 421–432.

Harper, R., Wiens, A., & Matarazzo, J. *Nonverbal communication: The state of the art.* New York: John Wiley, 1978.

Harris, J. (Ed.). The great Boston fire, 1872. *Boston Globe,* November 12, 1972, special publication.

Harris, M. *Cows, pigs, wars, and witches.* New York: Random House, 1974.

Harshbarger, D., & Moran, G. A selective bibliography on disaster and human ecology. *Omega,* 1974, *5,* 89–95.

Hatcher, S. Understanding adolescent pregnancy and abortion. *Primary Care,* 1976, *3,* 407–425.

Haverkamp, A. D., Thompson, H. E., McFee, J. G., & Cetrulo, C. The evaluation of continuous fetal heart rate monitoring in high-risk pregnancy. *American Journal of Obstetrics and Gynecology,* 1976, *125,* 310–320.

Hayes-Bautista, D. E. Modifying the treatment: Patient compliance, patient control and medical care. *Social Science and Medicine,* 1976, *10,* 233–238.

Haynes, R. B. A critical review of the "determinants" of patient compliance with therapeutic regimens. In D. L. Sackett & R. B. Haynes (Eds.), *Compliance with therapeutic regimens.* Baltimore: Johns Hopkins University Press, 1976.

Haynes, R. B., Taylor, D. W., & Sackett, D. T. (Eds.). *Compliance in health care.* Baltimore: Johns Hopkins University Press, 1979.

Headlee, R. The tacit contract between doctor and patient. *Medical Insight,* 1973, *5,* 30–37.

Heller, R. The effects of social support: Prevention and treatment implications. In A. P. Goldstein & F. H. Kanfer (Eds.), *Maximizing treatment gains: Transfer enhancement in psychotherapy.* New York: Academic Press, 1979. Pp. 353–382.

Helmrath, T. A., & Steinetz, E. M. Death of an infant: Parental grieving and the failure of social support. *Journal of Family Practice,* 1978, *6*(4), 785–790.

Henley, N. M. *Body politics.* Englewood Cliffs, N.J.: Prentice-Hall, 1977.

Henneborn, W. J., & Cogan, R. The effect of husband participation on reported pain and probability of medication during labor and birth. *Journal of Psychosomatic Research,* 1975, *19,* 215–222.

Henriques, B., Stadil, F., & Baden, H. Patient information about cancer: A prospective study of patients' opinion and reaction to information about cancer diagnosis. *Acta Chir Scand 146,* 1980, 309–311.

Herbertt, R. M., & Innes, J. M. Familiarization and preparatory information in the reduction of anxiety in child dental patients. *Journal of Dentistry for Children,* 1979, *46,* 319–323.

Hertz, R., Deddish, M., & Day, E. Value of periodic examinations in detecting cancer of the rectum and colon. *Postgraduate Medicine,* 1960, *27,* 290–294.

Hilgard, E. R., Hilgard, J. R., MacDonald, H., Morgan, A. H., & Johnson, L. S. Covert pain in hypnotic analgesia: Its reality as tested by the real-simulator design. *Journal of Abnormal Psychology,* 1978, *87,* 655–663.

Hill, H., Kornetsky, C., Flanary, H., & Wilder, A. Studies on anxiety associated with anticipation of pain. *Archives of Neurology and Psychiatry,* 1952, *67,* 612–619.

Hinkle, L. E. Ecological observations of the relation of physical illness, mental illness, and the social environment. *Psychosomatic Medicine,* 1961, *23,* 289–296.

Hinkle, L. E., Pinsky, R. H., Bross, I. D. J., & Plummer, N. The distribution of sickness disability in a homogeneous group of "healthy adult men." *American Journal of Hygiene,* 1956, *64,* 220–242.

Hinkle, L. E., & Wolff, H. G. Ecologic investigations of the relationship between illness, life experiences, and the social environment. *Annals of Internal Medicine,* 1958, *49,* 1373–1388.

Hinton, J. Comparison of places and policies for terminal care. *Lancet,* 1979, *1,* 29–311.

Hinton, J. M. The physical and mental distresses of the dying. *Quarterly Journal of Medicine,* 1963, *32,* 1–19.

Hippocrates. *The medical works of Hippocrates* (J. Chadwick & W. N. Mann, Trans.). Oxford: Blackwell Scientific Publications, 1950.

Hippocrates. *Volume II: On decorum and the physician,* (W.H.S. Jones, Trans.). London: William Heinemann, 1923.

Hobbs, D. F., & Cole, S. P. Transition to parenthood: A decade replication. *Journal of Marriage and the Family,* 1976, *38,* 723–731.

Hochbaum, G. *Public participation in medical screening programs: A sociopsychological study.* (U.S. Public Health Service Publication No. 572). Washington, D.C.: U.S. Government Printing Office, 1958.

Hoffman, I., & Futterman, E. H. Coping with waiting: Psychiatric intervention and study in the waiting room of a pediatric oncology unit. *Comprehensive Psychiatry,* 1971, *12,* 67–81.

Hoge, V. Hospital facilities should fit the patient. In L. E. Weeks & J. R. Griffith (Eds.), *Progressive patient care* (Bulletin of the Administration Research Services, #3, 964), 1964.

Hokanson, J. E., DeGood, D. E., Forrest, M. S., & Brittain, T. M. Availability of avoidance behaviors in modulating vascular-stress responses. *Journal of Personality and Social Psychology,* 1971, *19,* 60–68.

Holden, H. M. The needs and expectations of doctors and patients. *Journal of the Royal College of General Practitioners,* 1977, *27,* 277–279.

Holman, E. J. United States Supreme Court and abortion. *Journal of the American Medical Association,* 1973, *225,* 215–216.

Holmes, D. S., & Houston, B. K. Effectiveness of situation redefinition and affective isolation in coping with stress. *Journal of Personality and Social Psychology,* 1974, *29,* 212–218.

Holmes, T. H., & Rahe, R. H. The Social Readjustment Rating Scale. *Journal of Psychosomatic Research,* 1967, *11,* 213–218.

Horan, D. J., & Mall, D. (Eds.). *Death, dying, and euthanasia.* Washington, D.C.: University Publications of America, 1977.

Horne, R. L., & Piccard, R. S. Psychosocial risk factors for lung cancer. *Psychosomatic Medicine,* 1979, *41*(7), 503–514

House, J. S. *Work, stress, & social support.* Reading, Mass.: Addison-Wesley, 1981.

Houston, B. K., & Holmes, D. S. Effect of avoidant thinking and reappraisal for coping with threat involving temporal uncertainty. *Journal of Personality and Social Psychology,* 1974, *30,* 383–388.

Houston, W. R. The doctor himself as a therapeutic agent. *Annals of Internal Medicine,* 1938, *11,* 1416–1425.

How placebos work. *Newsweek,* September 4, 1978, p. 54.

Howard, J. *Please touch.* New York: Dell, 1970.

Howell, M. A. Personality factors in medical performance. (Doctoral dissertation, University of California, Berkeley, 1965.) *Dissertation Abstracts International,* 1966, *27*(1–B), 303.

Hughey, M. J., McElin, T. W., & Young, T. Maternal and fetal outcome of Lamaze-prepared patients. *Journal of Obstetrics and Gynecology,* 1978, *51,* 643–647.

Hulka, B. S., Cassel, J. C., & Kupper, L. Disparities between medications prescribed and consumed among chronic disease patients. In L. Lasagna (Ed.), *Patient compliance,* Mount Kisco, N.Y.: Futura, 1976.

Hulka, B. S., Cassel, J. C., Kupper, L. L., & Burdette, J. A. Communication, compliance, and concordance between physicians and patients with prescribed medications. *American Journal of Public Health,* 1976, *66,* 847–853.

Hunt, W. A., & Matarazzo, J. D. Three years later: Recent development in the experimental modification of smoking behavior. *Journal of Abnormal Psychology,* 1973, *81,* 107–114.

Illich, I. *Medical nemesis.* New York: Pantheon, 1976.

Innes, J. M. Does the professional know what the client wants? *Social Science and Medicine,* 1977, *11,* 635–638.

Interprofessional task force on health care of women and children. The development of family-centered maternity/newborn care in hospitals. *JOGN Nursing,* 1978, *7,* 55–59.

Inui, J. F., Yourtee, E. L., & Williamson, J. W. Improved outcomes in hypertension after physician tutorials. *Annals of Internal Medicine,* 1976, *84,* 646–651.

Isselbacher, K., Adams, R., Braunwald, E., Petersdorf, R., & Wilson, J. (Eds.). *Harrison's principles of internal medicine.* New York: McGraw-Hill, 1980.

Izard, C. E. *Human emotions.* New York: Plenum Press, 1977.

Jacoby, A. P. Transition to parenthood: A reassessment. *Journal of Marriage and the Family,* 1969, *31,* 720–727.

Jamison, K. R., Wellisch, D. K., & Pasnau, R. O. Psychosocial aspects of mastectomy. I: The woman's perspective. *American Journal of Psychiatry,* 1978, *134*(4), 432–436.

Janis, I. L. *Psychological stress: Psychoanalytic and behavioral studies of surgical patients.* New York: Wiley, 1958.

Janis, I. L. Psychodynamic aspects of stress tolerance. In S. Z. Klausner (Ed.), *The quest for self-control: Classical philosophies and scientific research.* New York: Free Press, 1965.

Janis, I. L. Effects of fear arousal on attitude change: Recent developments in theory and experimental research. In L. Berkowitz (Ed.), *Advances in experimental social psychology* (Vol. 3). New York: Academic Press, 1967.

Janis, I. L. *Stress and frustration*. New York: Harcourt Brace Jovanovich, 1971.

Janis, I. L. (Ed.). *Counseling on personal decisions: Theory and research on short-term helping relationships*. New Haven, Conn.: Yale University Press, in press.

Janis, I. L., & Mann, L. A conflict theory approach to attitude change and decision making. In A. Greenwald, T. C. Brock, & T. M. Ostrom (Eds.), *Psychological foundations of attitudes*. New York: Academic Press, 1968.

Janis, I. L., & Mann, L. *Decision making*. New York: Free Press, 1977.

Janis, I. L., & Quinlan, D. M. What disclosing means to the client: Comparative case studies. In I. L. Janis (Ed.), *Counseling on personal decisions: Theory and research on short-term helping relationships*. New Haven, Conn.: Yale University Press, in press.

Janis, I. L., & Rodin, J. Attribution, control, and decision-making: Social psychology and health care. In G. C. Stone, F. Cohen, & N. E. Adler (Eds.), *Health psychology*. San Francisco: Jossey-Bass, 1979.

Janis, I. L., & Terwilliger, R. An experimental study of psychological resistance to fear-arousing communications. *Journal of Abnormal and Social Psychology*, 1962, *65*, 403–410.

Janoff-Bulman, R. Characterological versus behavioral self-blame: Inquiries into depression and rape. *Journal of Personality and Social Psychology*, 1979, *37*, 1798–1809.

Järvinen, K.A.J. Can ward rounds be a danger to patients with myocardial infarction? *British Medical Journal*, 1955, *1*, 318–320.

Jellinek, E. M. Clinical tests on comparative effectiveness of analgesic drugs. *Biometrics Bulletin*, 1946, *2*, 87–91.

Jenkins, C. D. Psychological and social precursors of coronary disease. *New England Journal of Medicine*, 1971, *284*, 244–255, 307–316.

Jenkins, C. D. Psychosocial modifiers of response to stress. *Journal of Human Stress*, 1979, *5*, 3–15.

Jenkins, C. D., Zyzanski, S. J., & Rosenman, R. H. Risk of new myocardial infarction in middle-aged men with manifest coronary heart disease. *Circulation*, 1976, *53*, 342–347.

Johnson, B. S. The meaning of touch in nursing. *Nursing Outlook*, 1965, *13*, 59–60.

Johnson, J. E. The influence of purposeful nurse–patient interaction on the patient's postoperative course. *A.N.A. Monograph Series No. 2: Exploring Medical-Surgical Nursing Practice*. New York: American Nurses' Association, 1966.

Johnson, J. E. Effects of accurate expectations about sensations on the sensory and distress components of pain. *Journal of Personality and Social Psychology*, 1973, *27*, 261–275

Johnson, J. E. Stress reduction through sensation information. In I. Sarason & C. Speilberger (Eds.), *Stress and anxiety* (Vol. 2). New York: Wiley, 1975.

Johnson, J. E. *Information factors in coping with stressful events*. Paper presented at the meeting of the Association for the Advancement of Behavior Therapy, Atlanta, 1977.

Johnson, J. E., Kirchoff, K. T., & Endress, M. P. Altering children's distress behavior during orthopedic cast removal. *Nursing Research*, 1975, *24*, 404–410.

Johnson, J. E., & Leventhal, H. Effects of accurate expectations and behavioral instructions on reactions during a noxious medical examination. *Journal of Personality and Social Psychology*, 1974, *29*, 710–718.

Johnson, J. L. Use of an innovative oupatient support group in cancer care. *Proceedings of the 14th Annual Meeting of the American Association of Cancer Education*, 1980, *1*, 367.

Johnson, J., Rice, V., Fuller, S., & Endress, M. P. *Sensory information, behavioral instruction, and recovery from surgery*. Paper presented at the meeting of the American Psychological Association, Atlanta, 1977.

Jones, E. E. *Ingratiation: A social psychological analysis*. New York: Appleton-Century-Crofts, 1964.

Jones, E. E., & Nisbett, R. E. *The actor and the observer: Divergent perceptions of the causes of behavior*. New York: General Learning Press, 1971.

Jones, E. E., & Wortman, C. B. *Ingratiation: An attributional approach.* New York: General Learning Press, 1973.

Jones, R. A. *Self-fulfilling prophecies: Social, psychological, and physiological effects of expectancies.* Hillsdale, N.J.: Erlbaum, 1977.

Jones, R. A. Expectations and illness. In H. S. Friedman & M. R. DiMatteo, (Eds.), *Interpersonal issues in health care.* New York: Academic Press, 1982.

Jonsson, A., & Hansson, L. Prolonged exposure to a stressful stimulus (noise) as a cause of raised blood pressure in man. *Lancet,* 1977, *1,* 86–87.

Jourard, S. M. An exploratory study of body-accessibility. *British Journal of Social and Clinical Psychology,* 1966, *5,* 221–231.

Jourard, S. M. *Self-disclosure.* New York: Wylie-Interscience, 1971.

Kagan, N. I. Teaching interpersonal relations for the practice of medicine. *Lakartidningen,* 1974, *71,* 4758–4760.

Kahn, G., Cohen, B., & Jason, H. The teaching of interpersonal skills in the United States medical schools. *Journal of Medical Education,* in press.

Kahn, R. L. Aging and social support. In M. W. Riley (Ed.), *Aging from birth to death: Interdisciplinary perspectives.* Boulder, Colo.: Westview Press, 1979.

Kahn, R. L., & Antonucci, T. Convoys over the life course: Attachments, roles and social support. In P. E. Baltes & O. Brim (Eds.), *Life span development and behavior* (Vol. 3). Boston, Mass.: Lexington Press, 1980.

Kahneman, D., & Tversky, A. On the psychology of prediction. *Psychological Review,* 1973, *80,* 237–251.

Kalisch, B. An experiment in the development of empathy in nursing students. *Nursing Research,* 1971, *20,* 202–211.

Kalish, R. A. Dying and preparing for death: A view of families. In H. Feifel (Ed.), *New meanings of death,* New York: McGraw-Hill, 1977.

Kaltreider, N. Emotional patterns related to delay in decision to seek legal abortion: A pilot study. *California Medicine,* 1973, *118,* 23–27.

Kaltreider, N., Goldsmith, S., & Margolis, A. The impact of midtrimester abortion techniques on patients and staff. *American Journal of Obstetrics and Gynecology,* 1979, *135,* 235–238.

Kane, F. J., Feldman, M., Jain, S., & Lipton, M. A. Emotional reactions of abortion services personnel. *Archives of General Psychiatry,* 1973, *28,* 409–411.

Kanfer, F., & Goldfoot, D. Self-control and tolerance of noxious stimulation. *Psychological Reports,* 1966, *18,* 79–85.

Kanfer, F., & Seider, M. L. Self-control: Factors enhancing tolerance of noxious stimulation. *Journal of Personality and Social Psychology,* 1973, *25,* 381–389.

Kao, C.C.L. Maturity and paternalism in health care. *Ethics in Science and Medicine,* 1976, *3,* 179–186.

Kaplan, D. M., Grobstein, R., & Smith, A. Severe illness in families. *Health and Social Work,* 1976, *1,* 72–81.

Kaplan, N. M. Stress, the sympathetic nervous system and hypertension. *Journal of Human Stress,* 1978, *4,* 29–34. (a)

Kaplan, N. M. *Clinical hypertension* (2nd Ed.). Baltimore: Williams and Wilkins, 1978. (b)

Kaplan, R. M. Coping with stressful medical exams. In H. S. Friedman and M. R. DiMatteo (Eds.), *Interpersonal issues in health care.* New York: Academic Press, 1982.

Kaplan, R. M., Atkins, C. J., & Lenhard, L. Coping with a stressful medical exam: Component analysis of stress inoculation procedures. *Journal of Behavioral Medicine,* in press.

Kaplan, R. M., & Metzger, G. *Brief cognitive and relaxation interventions for coping with a painful electromyogram.* Paper presented at the meeting of the American Association for Behavior Therapy, San Francisco, 1979.

Kar, S. B. A model for communication intervention: Ethical and scientific dimensions. *Ethics in Science and Medicine,* 1976, *3,* 149–164.

Kasl, S. V. Issues in patient adherence to health care regimens. *Journal of Human Stress,* 1975, *1*(3), 5–17.

Kasl, S., & Cobb, S. Health behavior, illness behavior, and sick role behavior. *Archives of Environmental Health,* 1966, *12,* 246–266.

Kassirer, J. P., & Gorry, G. A. Clinical problem solving: A behavioral analysis. *Annals of Internal Medicine,* 1978, *89,* 245–255.

Kasteler, J., Kane, R. L., Olsen, D. M., & Thetford, C. Issues underlying prevalence of "doctor-shopping" behavior. *Journal of Health and Social Behavior,* 1976, *17,* 328–339.

Kastenbaum, R. On the future of death: Some images and options. *Omega,* 1972, *3,* 319–330.

Kastenbaum, R. Disaster, death, and human ecology. *Omega,* 1974, *5,* 65–72.

Kastenbaum, R. Suicide as the preferred way of death. In E. S. Shneidman (Ed.), *Suicidology: Contemporary developments.* New York: Grune and Stratton, 1976.

Kastenbaum, R. *Death, society, and human experience.* St. Louis: C. V. Mosby, 1977. (Rev. ed. in press.) (a)

Kastenbaum, R. We covered death today. *Death education,* 1977, *1,* 27–31. (b)

Kastebaum, R. (Ed.). *Between life and death.* New York: Springer, 1979. (a)

Kastebaum, R. "Healthy Dying," A paradoxical quest continues. *Journal of Social Issues,* 1979, *35*(1), 185–206. (b)

Kastebaum, R., & Aisenberg, R. *The psychology of death.* New York: Springer, 1972. (Concise ed., 1976.)

Kastenbaum, R., & Costa, P. T., Jr. Psychological perspectives on death. In M. R. Rosenzweig & L. W. Porter (Eds.), *Annual review of psychology* (Vol. 28). Palo Alto, Calif.: Annual Reviews, 1977. Pp. 225–250.

Katz, J. L., Weiner, H., Gallagher, T. F., & Hellman, L. Stress, distress, and ego defenses: Psychoendocrine response to impending breast tumor biopsy. *Archives of General Psychiatry,* 1970, *23,* 131–142.

Kaufman, M. R. Practicing good manners and compassion. *Medical Insight,* 1970, *2,* 56–61.

Kaye, J., Appel, M., & Joseph, R. Attitudes of medical students and residents toward cancer. *Proceedings of the 14th Annual Meeting of the American Association of Cancer Education,* 1980, *1,* 367.

Kellerman, J., Rigler, D., Siegel, S. E., & Katz, E. R. Disease-related communication and depression in pediatric cancer patients. *Journal of Pediatric Psychology,* 1980, *2*(2), 52–53.

Kelley, H. H. Attribution theory in social psychology. In D. Levine (Ed.), *Nebraska Symposium on Motivation.* Lincoln, Nebr.: University of Nebraska Press, 1967.

Kelley, O. E. Living with a life-threatening illness. In C. A. Garfield (Ed.), *Psychosocial care of the dying patient.* New York: McGraw-Hill, 1978. Pp. 59–66.

Kelly, O. *Make today count.* New York: Delacorte Press, 1975.

Kelman, H. Compliance, identification and internalization: Three processes of attitude change. *Journal of Conflict Resolution,* 1958, *2,* 51–60.

Kendall, P. C., & Watson, D. Psychological preparation for stressful medical procedures. In C. K. Prokop & L. A. Bradley (Eds.). *Medical psychology: Contributions to behavioral medicine.* New York: Academic Press, 1981.

Kendall, P. C., Williams, L., Pechecek, T. F., Graham, L. E., Shisslak, C. E., & Herzoff, N. Cognitive-behavioral and patient education interventions in cardiac catheterization procedures: The Palo Alto medical psychology project. *Journal of Consulting Psychology,* 1979, *47,* 49–58.

Kent, I., Greenwood, R. C., Nicholls, W., & Loekenm J. *Sequelae of therapeutic abortion: A comparative study.* Paper presented at the meeting of the Canadian Psychiatric Association, 1978.

Kerenyi, T. D., Glascock, E. L., & Horowitz, M. L. Reasons for delayed abortion: Results of four hundred interviews. *American Journal of Obstetrics and Gynecology,* 1973, *117,* 299–311.

King, S. H. *Perceptions of illness and medical practice.* New York: Russell-Sage Foundation, 1962.

Kirkpatrick, C. *The family as process and institution.* New York: Roland, 1963.

Kirscht, J. P. The health belief model and illness behavior. *Health Education Monographs,* 1974, *2,* 387.

Kirscht, J. P. Communication between patients and physicians. *Annals of Internal Medicine,* 1977, *86,* 387–409.

Kirscht, J. P., & Rosenstock, I. M. Patient adherence to antihypertensive medical regimens. *Journal of Community Health,* 1977, *3,* 115–124.

Klagsbrun, S. C. Communications in the treatment of cancer. *American Journal of Nursing,* 1971, *71,* 5, 944–948.

Klaus, M. M., & Kennell, J. M. *Maternal–infant bonding.* St. Louis: C. V. Mosby, 1976.

Kleck, R. Physical stigma and nonverbal cues emitted in face-to-face interaction. *Human Relations,* 1968, *21,* 119–128.

Kleck, R. Physical stigma and task oriented interaction. *Human Relations,* 1969, *22,* 53–60.

Kleck, R., Buch, P. L., Goller, W. L., London, R. S., Pfeifer, J. R., & Vukcevic, D. P. Effects of stigmatizing conditions on the use of personal space. *Psychological Reports,* 1968, *23,* 111–118.

Kleck, R., Ono, H., & Hastorf, A. H. The effects of physical deviance upon face to face interaction. *Human Relations,* 1966, *19,* 425–436.

Kleck, R., Vaughan, R., Cartwright-Smith, J., Vaughan, K., Colby, C., & Lanzetta, J. Effects of being observed on expressive, subjective, and physiological responses to painful stimuli. *Journal of Personality and Social Psychology,* 1976, *34,* 1211–1218.

Kleiman, M. A., Mantell, J. E., & Alexander, E. S. Collaboration and its discontents: The perils of partnership. *Journal of Applied Behavioral Science,* 1977, *13,* 403–410.

Klein, R. A crisis to grow on. *Cancer,* 1971, *28,* 1660–1665.

Klein, R. F., Dean, A., & Bogdonoff, M. D. The impact of illness upon the spouse. *Journal of Chronic Disease,* 1967, *20,* 241–248.

Klemp, G. O., & Rodin, J. Effects of uncertainty, delay, and focus of attention on reactions to an aversive situation. *Journal of Experimental Social Psychology,* 1976, *12,* 416–421.

Kluge, E. *The practice of death.* New Haven, Conn.: Yale University Press, 1975.

Knapp, M. L. *Nonverbal communication in human interaction.* New York: Holt, Rinehart and Winston, 1978.

Knapp, M. L., Hart, R. P., & Dennis, H. S. An exploration of deception as a communication construct. *Human Communication Research,* 1974, *1,* 15–29.

Knopf, A. Changes in women's opinions about cancer. *Social Science and Medicine,* 1976, *10,* 191–195.

Knowles, J. W. The responsibility of the individual. *Daedalus,* 1977, *106*(1), 57–80.

Knox, J. V., & Shum, K. Reduction of cold-pressor pain with acupuncture analgesia in high- and low-hypnotic subjects. *Journal of Abnormal Psychology,* 1977, *86,* 639–643.

Knox, J. V., Shum, K., & McLaughlin, P. Response to cold-pressor pain and to acupuncture analgesia in Oriental and Occidental subjects. *Pain,* 1977, *4,* 49–57.

Komaroff, A. L. The practitioner and the compliant patient. *American Journal of Public Health,* 1976, *66,* 833–835.

Koos, E. *The health of regionville.* New York: Columbia University Press, 1954.

Koos, E. "Metropolis"—What city people think of their medical services. *American Journal of Public Health,* 1955, *45,* 1551–1557.

Kornfeld, D. S. The hospital environment: Its impact on the patient. *Advances in Psychosomatic Medince,* 1972, *8,* 252–270.

Korsch, B. M., Gozzi, E. K., & Francis, V. Gaps in doctor–patient communication. I: Doctor–patient interaction and patient satisfaction. *Pediatrics,* 1968, *42,* 855–871.

Krant, M. J., Beiser, M., Adler, G., & Johnston, L. The role of a hospital-based psychosocial unit in terminal cancer illness and bereavement. *Journal of Chronic Disease,* 1976, *29,* 115–127.

Krant, M. J., & Johnson, L. Family members' perceptions of communications in late stage cancer. *International Journal of Psychiatry in Medicine,* 1977–1978, *8*(2), 203–216.

Kristeller, J. L., & Rodin, J. A. *A three-stage model of treatment continuity: Compliance, adherence, and maintenance.* Paper presented at the 12th Banff Conference of Behavioral Medicine, Banff, Alberta, March, 1980.

Kubler-Ross, E. *On death and dying.* New York: Macmillan, 1969.

Kummer, J. Post-abortion psychiatric illness—A myth? *American Journal of Psychiatry,* 1963, *119,* 980–983.

LaCrosse, M. B. Nonverbal behavior and perceived counselor attractiveness and persuasiveness. *Journal of Counseling Psychology,* 1975, *22,* 563–566.

Lambert, W., Libman, E., & Poser, E. The effect of inceased salience of a membership group on pain tolerance. *Journal of Personality,* 1960, *28,* 350–357.

Langer, E. J., Janis, I. L., & Wolfer, J. A. Reduction of psychological stress in surgical patients. *Journal of Experimental Social Psychology,* 1975, *11,* 155–165.

Langer, E. J., & Rodin, J. The effects of choice and enhanced personal responsibility for the aged: A field experiment in an institutional setting. *Journal of Personality and Social Psychology,* 1976, *34,* 191–198.

Lanzetta, J. T., Cartwright-Smith, J., & Kleck, R. Effects of nonverbal dissimilation on emotional experience and autonomic arousal. *Journal of Personality and Social Psychology,* 1976, *33,* 354–370.

Lanzetta, J. T., & Driscoll, J. M. Preference for information about an uncertain but unavoidable outcome. *Journal of Personality and Social Psychology,* 1966, *3,* 96–102.

Largey, G. P., & Watson, D. R. The sociology of odors. *American Journal of Sociology,* 1972, *77,* 1021–1033.

Larsen, D. E., & Rootman, I. Physician role performance and patient satisfaction. *Social Science and Medicine,* 1976, *10,* 29–32.

Larsen, V. L. Stresses of the childbearing year. *American Journal of Public Health,* 1966, *56,* 32–36.

Latiolas, C., & Berry, C. Misuse of prescription medications by outpatients. *Drug Intelligence and Clinical Pharmacy,* 1969, *3,* 270–277.

Lazarus, R. S. *Psychological stress and the coping process.* New York: McGraw-Hill, 1966.

Lazarus, R. S. A strategy for research on psychological and social factors in hypertension. *Journal of Human Stress,* 1978, *4,* 35–40.

Leavitt, F., & Garon, P. Psychological disturbance and pain report, differences in both organic and non-organic low back pain patients. *Pain,* 1979, *7,* 187–195.

Lederer, H. D. How the sick view their world. *Journal of Social Issues,* 1952, *8,* 4–15.

Ledwidge, B. Cognitive behavior modification: A step in the wrong direction? *Psychological Bulletin,* 1978, *85,* 353–375.

Lee, E.C.G., & McGuire, G. P. Emotional distress in patients attending a breast clinic. *British Journal of Surgery,* 1975, *62,* 162.

Lehrer, P. M. Physiological effects of relaxation in double-blind analog of desensitization. *Behavior Therapy,* 1972, *3,* 193–208.

Leifer, M. Psychological changes accompanying pregnancy and motherhood. *Genetic Psychological Monographs,* 1977, *95,* 55–96.

LeMasters, E. Parenthood as crisis. *Marriage and Family Living,* 1957, *19,* 352–355.

Lemert, E. M. Paranoia and the dynamics of exclusion. *Sociometry,* 1962, *25,* 2–20.

Lerner, H. E. Effects of the nursing mother-infant dyad on the family. *American Journal of Orthopsychiatry,* 1979, *49,* 339–348.

Lerner, M. J. The desire for justice and reactions to victims. In J. Macaulay & L. Berkowitz (Eds.), *Altruism and helping behavior.* New York: Academic Press, 1970.

Lerner, M. J. Observer's evaluation of a victim: Justice, guilt, and veridical perception. *Journal of Personality and Social Psychology*, 1971, *20*, 127–135.

Lerner, M. Social differences in physical health. In J. Kosa & I. K. Zola (Eds.), *Poverty and health: A sociological analysis* (Rev. ed.). Cambridge, Mass.: Harvard University Press, 1975.

Lerner, M. J., Miller, D. T., & Holmes, J. Deserving and the emergence of forms of justice. In L. Berkowitz & E. Walster (Eds.), *Advances in experimental social psychology* (Vol. 10). New York: Academic Press, 1976.

Lerner, M. J., & Simmons, C. H. Observer's reactions to the "innocent victim": Compassion or rejection? *Journal of Personality and Social Psychology*, 1966, *4*, 203–210.

Lerner, M., & Stutz, R. N. Have we narrowed the gaps between the poor and the non-poor? Part II: Narrowing the gaps, 1959–61 to 1969–71: Mortality. *Medical Care*, 1977, *15*, 620–635.

LeShan, L. The world of the patient in severe pain of long duration. *Journal of Chronic Disease*, 1964, *17*, 119–126.

Leventhal, H. Changing attitudes and habits to reduce risk factors in chronic disease. *American Journal of Cardiology*, 1973, *31*, 571–580.

Leventhal, H. The consequences of depersonalization during illness and treatment. In J. Howard & A. Strauss (Eds.), *Humanizing health care*. New York: Wiley, 1975.

Leventhal, H., & Sharp, E. Facial expressions as indicators of distress. In S. S. Tomkins & C. E. Izard (Eds.), *Affect, cognition and personality: Empirical studies*. New York: Springer, 1965.

Levi, L. Psychological stress and disease: A conceptual model. In K. E. Gunderson & R. H. Rahe (Eds.), *Life stress and illness*. Springfield, Ill.: Thomas, 1974.

Levine, J. D., Gordon, N. C., & Fields, H. L. The mechanism of placebo analgesia. *Lancet*, 1978, *2*, 654–657.

Levinger, G., & Breedlove, J. Interpersonal attraction and agreement: A study of marriage partners. *Journal of Personality and Social Psychology*, 1966, *3*, 367–372.

Levy, L. H. Self-help groups: Types and psychological processes. *Journal of Applied Behavioral Science*, 1976, *12*, 310–322.

Lewinsohn, P. M. Clinical and theoretical aspects of depression. In K. S. Calhoun, H. E. Adams, & K. M. Mitchell (Eds.), *Innovative treatment methods in psychopathology*. New York: Wiley, 1974.

Lewis, F. M., & Bloom, J. R. Psychosocial adjustment to breast cancer: A review of selected literature. *International Journal of Psychiatry in Medicine*, 1978–1979, *9*(1), 1–17.

Lewis, M. S., Gottesman, D., & Gutstein, S. The course and duration of crisis. *Journal of Consulting and Clinical Psychology*, 1979, *47*(1), 128–134.

Ley, P. Memory for medical information. *British Journal of Social and Clinical Psychology*, 1979, *18*, 245–255.

Ley, P., Bradshaw, P. W., Kincey, J. A., & Atherton, S. T. Increasing patients' satisfaction with communications. *British Journal of Social and Clinical Psychology*, 1976, *15*, 403–413.

Ley, P., & Spelman, M. S. Communications in an out-patient setting. *British Journal of Social and Clinical Psychology*, 1965, *4*, 114–116.

Ley, P., & Spelman, M. S. *Communicating with the patient*. London: Staples Press, 1967.

Lichtenstein, E., & Danaher, B. Modification of smoking behavior: A critical analysis of theory, research, and practice. In M. Hersen, R. M. Eisler, & P. M. Miller (Eds.), *Progress in behavior modification* (Vol. 3). New York: Academic Press, 1976.

Lieber, L., Plumb, M. M., Gerstenzang, M. L., & Holland, J. The communication of affection between cancer patients and their spouses. *Psychosomatic Medicine*, 1976, *38*(6), 379–389.

Lieberman, M., & Borman, L. *Self-help groups for coping with crises*. San Francisco: Jossey-Bass, 1979.

Liebeskind, J. C., & Paul, L. A. Psychological and physiological mechanisms of pain. *Annual Review of Psychology*, 1977, *28*, 41–60.

Liggett, J. *The human face*. New York: Stein and Day, 1974.

Linkewich, J. A., Catalano, R. B., & Flack, H. L. The effect of packaging and instruction on outpatient compliance with medication regimens. *Drug Intelligence and Clinical Pharmacy*, 1974, *8*, 10–15.

Linn, L. S. Factors associated with patient evaluation of health care. *Milbank Memorial Fund Quarterly*, 1975, *53*, 531–548.

Litman, T. J. The influence of self-conception and life orientation factors in the rehabilitation of the orthopedically disabled. *Journal of Health and Human Behavior*, 1962, *3*, 249–256.

Livingston, P. B., & Zimet, C. N. Death anxiety, authoritarianism, and choice of specialty in medical students. *Journal of Nervous and Mental Disease*, 1965, *140*, 220–230.

Loftis, J., & Ross, L. Effects of misattribution of arousal upon the acquisition and extinction of a conditioned emotional response. *Journal of Personality and Social Psychology*, 1974, *30*, 673–682.

Lorber, J. Good patients and problem patients: Conformity and deviance in a general hospital. *Journal of Health and Social Behavior*, 1975, *16*, 213–225.

Lynch, J. J., Thomas, S. A., Mills, M. E., Malinow, K., & Katcher, A. H. The effects of human contact on cardiac arrhythmia in coronary care patients. *Journal of Nervous and Mental Disease*, 1974, *158*, 88–99.

Lynn, D. B. *The father: His role in child development*. Monterey, Calif.: Brooks/Cole, 1974.

MacFarlane, A. *The psychology of childbirth*. Cambridge, Mass.: Harvard University Press, 1977.

Maddison, D., & Walker, W. L. Factors affecting the outcome of conjugal bereavement. *British Journal of Psychiatry*, 1967, *113*, 1057–1067.

Maddox, G. L., Anderson, C. F., & Bogdonoff, M. D. Overweight as a problem of medical management in a public out-patient clinic. *American Journal of Medical Science*, 1966, *252*, 394.

Maguire, G. P., Lee, E. G., Bevington, D. J., Kuchemann, C. S., Crabtree, R. J., & Cornell, C. E. Psychiatric problems in the first year after mastectomy. *British Medical Journal*, 1978, *1*, 963–965.

Mahoney, M. J. Self-reward and self-monitoring techniques for weight control. In J. P. Foreyt (Ed.), *Behavioral treatments of obesity*. Elmsford, N.Y.: Pergamon Press, 1977.

Mahoney, M. J., & Mahoney, K. *Permanent weight control*. New York: W. W. Norton, 1976.

Make Today Count, Inc., organizational manual. Burlington, Iowa: Make Today Count, 1977.

Making waves. *Newsweek*, March 24, 1975, p. 91.

Marder, L. Psychiatric experience with a liberalized therapeutic abortion law. *American Journal of Psychiatry*, 1970, *126*, 1230–1236.

Marston, M. Compliance with medical regimens. *Nursing Research*, 1970, *19*, 312–323.

Marut, J. S., & Mercer, R. T. Comparison of primiparas' perceptions of vaginal and caeserean births. *Nursing Research*, 1979, *28*, 260–266.

Maslach, C. Burned-out. *Human Behavior*, 1976, *5*, 16–22.

Maslach, C. The burn-out syndrome and patient care. In C. Garfield (Ed.), *Stress and survival: The emotional realities of life threatening illness*. St. Louis: Mosley, 1979.

Mastrovito, R. C. Emotional considerations in cancer and stroke. *New York State Journal of Medicine*, 1972, *72*, 2874–2877.

Matthews, D., & Hingson, R. Improving patient compliance: A guide for physicians. *Medical Clinics of North America*, 1977, *61*, 879–889.

Matthews, K. A., Scheier, M. F., Brunson, B. I., & Carducci, B. Attention, unpredictability, and reports of physical symptoms: Eliminating the benefits of predictability. *Journal of Personality and Social Psychology*, 1980, *38*, 525–537.

Mazzulo, J. M., Lasagna, L., & Griner, P. F. Variation in interpretation of prescription instructions. *Journal of the American Medical Association,* 1974, *227,* 929–931.

McAmmond, D. M., Davidson, P. O., & Kovitz, D. M. A comparison of the effects of hypnosis and relaxation training on stress reactions in a dental situation. *American Journal of Clinical Hypnosis,* 1971, *13,* 233–242.

McCreary, C., Turner, J., & Dawson, E. Differences between functional versus organic low back pain patients. *Pain,* 1977, *4,* 73–78.

McCue, K. Preparing children for medical procedures. In J. Kellerman (Ed.), *Psychological aspects of childhood cancer.* Springfield, Ill.: C. C. Thomas, 1980.

McDermott, W. Evaluating the physician and his technology. *Daedalus,* 1977, *106*(1), 135–158.

McGowan, J. F., & Schmidt, L. D. *Counseling: Readings in theory and practice.* New York: Holt, Rinehart and Winston, 1962.

McGuire, G. P. Psychiatric problems after mastectomy. In P. C. Brand, and P. A. van Keep (Eds.), *Breast cancer: Psychosocial aspects of early detection and treatment.* Baltimore: University Park Press, 1978.

McGuire, J. C., & Gottlieb, G. H. Social support groups among new parents: An experimental study in primary prevention. *Journal of Clinical Child Psychology,* 1979, *8,* 111–116.

McIntosh, J. Processes of communication, information seeking and control associated with cancer: A selective review of the literature. *Social Science and Medicine,* 1974, *8,* 167–187.

McIntosh, J. *Communication and awareness in a cancer ward.* London: Croom Helm, 1977.

McKercher, P. L., & Rucker, T. D. Patient knowledge and compliance with medication instruction. *Journal of the American Pharmaceutical Association,* 1977, *17,* 282–286; 291.

McKinley, J. Social networks, lay consultation, and help-seeking behavior. *Social Forces,* 1973, *51,* 275–292.

McMahon, C. E. The wind of the cannon ball. *Psychotherapy and Psychosomatics,* 1975, *26,* 125–131.

Mechanic, D. Response factors in illness: The study of illness behavior. *Social Psychiatry,* 1966, *1,* 11–20.

Mechanic, D. *Medical sociology: A selective view.* New York: The Free Press, 1968.

Mechanic, D. *Medical sociology* (2nd ed.). New York: The Free press, 1978.

Medalie, I. H. (Ed.). *Family medicine: Principles and applications.* Baltimore: Williams and Wilkins, 1978.

Medlicott, R. W. Responsibility and medical practice. *New Zealand Medical Journal,* 1976, *84,* 263–266.

Meerloo, J.A.M. *Unobtrusive communication.* Assen, The Netherlands: Koninklijke Von Gorcum, 1964.

Mehl, L. E. The outcome of home delivery research in the United States. In S. Kitzinger & J. A. Davis (Eds.), *The place of birth.* Oxford: Oxford University Press, 1978.

Mehrabian, A. *Nonverbal communication.* Chicago: Aldine-Atherton, 1972.

Meichenbaum, D. *Cognitive-behavior modification,* New York: Plenum Press, 1977.

Melzack, R. *The puzzle of pain.* New York: Basic Books, 1973.

Melzack, R. Psychological concepts and methods for the control of pain. In J. J. Bonica (Ed.). *Advances in neurology* (Vol. 4). New York: Raven Press, 1974.

Melzack, R. Pain: Past, present and future. In M. Weisenberg & B. Tursky (Eds.), *Pain: New perspectives in therapy and research.* New York: Plenum Press, 1976.

Melzack, R. Psychological aspects of pain. In J. J. Bonica (Ed.), *Pain: Research publications association for research in nervous and mental diseases.* New York: Raven Press, 1980.

Melzack, R., & Chapman, C. R. Psychologic aspects of pain. *Post Graduate Medicine,* 1973, *53,* 69–75.

Melzack R., & Scott, T. The effects of early experience on the response to pain. *Journal of Comparative Physiological Psychology,* 1957, *50,* 155–161.

Melzack, R., & Torgerson, W. S. On the language of pain. *Anesthesiology,* 1971, *34,* 50.

Mersky, H. On the development of pain. *Headache,* 1970, *10,* 116–123.

Mersky, H., & Boyd, D. Emotional adjustment and chronic pain. *Pain,* 1978, *5,* 173–178.

Merton, R. K. *Sociological ambivalence and other essays.* New York: The Free Press, 1976.

Messerli, M. L., Garamendi, C., & Romano, J. Breast cancer: Information as a technique of crisis intervention. *American Journal of Orthopsychiatry,* October, 1980, *50*(4), 728–731.

Metchnikoff, E. *The prolongation of life.* New York: Arno Press, 1977. (Originally published, 1908.)

Meyer, A. The value of psychology in psychiatry. *Journal of the American Medical Association,* 1912, *53,* 911–914.

Meyerowitz, B. E. Postmastectomy psychosocial condition of women in two breast cancer treatment modalities. (Doctoral dissertation, University of Colorado, Boulder, 1978.) *Dissertation Abstracts International,* 1978, *39*(5–B), 2510.

Meyerowitz, B. E. Psychosocial correlates of breast cancer and its treatment. *Psychological Bulletin,* 1980, *87*(1), 108–131.

Meyerowitz, B. E., Sparks, F. C., & Spears, I. K. Adjuvant chemotherapy for breast carcinoma: Psychosocial implications. *Cancer,* 1979, *43,* 1613–1618.

Miller, M. A., & Brooten, D. A. *The childbearing family: A nursing perspective.* Boston: Little, Brown, 1977.

Milmoe, S., Rosenthal, R., Blane, H. T., Chafetz, M. L., & Wolf, I. The doctor's voice: Postdictor of successful referral of alcoholic patients. *Journal of Abnormal Psychology,* 1967, *72,* 78–84.

Milton, G. W. Thoughts in mind of a person with cancer. *British Medical Journal,* 1973, *4,* 221–223.

Minuchin, S. *Families and family therapy.* Cambridge, Mass.: Harvard University Press, 1974.

Mischel, W. Toward a cognitive, social learning reconceptualization of personality. *Psychological Review,* 1973, *80,* 252–283.

Mitchell, G. W., & Glicksman, A. S. Cancer patients: Knowledge and attitudes. *Cancer,* 1977, *40,* 61–66.

Mohler, D. N., Wallin, D. G., & Dreyfus, E. G. Studies in the home treatment of streptococcal disease. I: Failure of patients to take penicillin by mouth as prescribed. *New England Journal of Medicine,* 1955, *252,* 1116.

Mohr, J. *Abortion in America,* New York: Oxford University Press, 1978.

Monahan, L. H. Diagnosis and expectation for change: An inverse relationship. *Journal of Nervous and Mental Disease,* 1977, *164,* 214–217.

Monat, A., Averill, J. R., & Lazarus, R. S. Anticipatory stress and coping reactions under various conditions of uncertainty. *Journal of Personality and Social Psychology,* 1972, *24,* 237–253.

Monsour, K., & Stewart, B. Abortion and sexual behavior in college women. *American Journal of Orthopsychiatry,* 1973, *43,* 804–813.

Montague, A. *Touching.* New York: Harper & Row, 1978.

Moody, R. *Life after life.* Atlanta: Mockingbird Books, 1975.

Moore, D. C., Holton, C. P., & Marten, G. W. Psychological problems in the management of adolescents with malignancy. *Clinical Pediatrics,* 1969, *8*(8), 464–472.

Moos, R. H. Social-ecological perspectives on health. In G. C. Stone, F. Cohen, N. Adler *et al.* (Eds.), *Health psychology—A handbook,* San Francisco: Jossey-Bass, 1979.

Morris, T., Greer, S., & White, P. Psychological and social adjustment to mastectomy: A two-year follow-up study. *Cancer,* 1977, *40,* 2381–2387.

Moser, R. H. Knowledge is not enough. *New England Journal of Medicine,* 1977, *296,* 938–940.

Moss, G. E. *Illness, immunity, and social interaction: The dynamics of biosocial resonation.* New York: Wiley, 1973.

Mulligan, W. Effects of self-disclosure and interviewer feedback on compliance: A field experiment during a Red Cross blood donation campaign. In I. L. Janis (Ed.), *Counseling on personal decisions: Theory and research on short-term helping relationships.* New Haven, Conn.: Yale University Press, in press.

Mumford, E. *Interns: From students to physicians.* Cambridge, Mass.: Harvard University Press, 1970.

Mushlin, A. I., & Appel, F. A. Diagnosing potential noncompliance: Physicians' ability in a behavioral dimension of medical care. *Archives of Internal Medicine,* 1977, *137,* 318–321.

Nash, M. L. Dignity of person in the final phase of life: An exploratory study. *Omega,* 1977, *8,* 71–80.

Nathanson, C. A., and Becker, M. H. Obstetricians' attitudes and hospital abortion services. *Family Planning Perspectives,* 1980, *12,* 26–32.

Neufeld, R. The effect of experimentally altered cognitive appraisal of pain tolerance. *Psychonomic Science,* 1970, *20,* 106–107.

Neumann, S. *Die offentliche Gesudnheitspflege und das eigenthum Kritisches und positives mit Bezug auf die preussische Medizinalverfassungsfrage.* Berlin: Adolf Riess, 1847.

Newton, N. Childbirth and culture. *Psychology Today,* 1970, *4,* 75.

Newton, N., Foshee, D., & Newton, M. Experimental inhibition of labor through environmental disturbance. *Obstetrics and Gynecology,* 1966, *27,* 271–277.

Newton, N., & Newton, M. Mothers' reactions to their newborn babies. *Journal of the American Medical Association,* 1962, *181,* 206–210.

Nisbett, R. E., & Borgida, E. Attribution and the psychology of prediction. *Journal of Personality and Social Psychology,* 1975, *32,* 932–943.

Nisbett, R. E., & Wilson, T. D. Telling more than we can know: Verbal reports on mental processes. *Psychological Review,* 1977, *84,* 231–259.

Niswander, K., & Patterson, R. Psychological reaction to therapeutic abortion. *Obstetrics and Gynecology,* 1967, *29,* 702–706.

Niswander, K. R., Singer, J., & Singer, M. Psychological reaction to therapeutic abortion: Objective response. *American Journal of Obstetrics and Gynecology,* 1972, *114,* 29–33.

Nocella, J., & Kaplan, R. M. Cognitive-behavior modification for helping children cope with dental surgery. *Journal of Pediatric Psychology,* in press.

O'Brien, M. J. *Communications and relationships in nursing.* St. Louis: C. V. Mosby, 1974.

Oken, D. The psychophysiology and psychoendocrinology of stress and emotion. In M. H. Appley & R. Trumbull (Eds.), *Psychological stress: Issues in research.* New York: Appelton-Century-Crofts, 1967.

Olsen, D. H. Marital and family therapy: Integrative review and critique. *Journal of Marriage and Family,* 1970, *32,* 501–538.

O'Malley, J. E., Koocher, G., Foster, D., & Slavin, L. Psychiatric sequelae of surviving childhood cancer. *American Journal of Orthopsychiatry,* 1979, *49*(4), 608–616.

Orbach, C. E., & Tallent, N. Modification of perceived body and of body concepts. *Archives of General Psychiatry,* 1965, *12,* 126–135.

Orne, M. T. Hypnotic control of pain: Toward a clarification of the different psychological processes involved. In J. J. Bonica (Ed.), *Pain: Research publication of the association for research in nervous and mental diseases.* New York: Raven Press, 1980.

Ornstein, R. E. *The psychology of consciousness.* New York: Penguin, 1975.

Orwell, G. How the poor die. In G. Orwell, *Decline of the English murder and other essays.* London: Penguin Books, 1975. Pp. 32–44.

Orwell, G. *1984.* New York: Harcourt, 1954.

Osis, K., & Haraldsson, E. *At the hour of death.* New York: Avon Books, 1977.

Osler, W. Lecture to medical students. *Albany Medical Annals,* 1899, *20,* 307.

Osler, W. The master-word in medicine. In *Aequanimitas with other addresses to medical students, nurses, and practitioners of medicine.* Philadelphia: Blakiston, 1904. Pp. 369–371.

Osofsky, J. D. (Ed.). *Handbook of infant development.* New York: Wiley, 1979.

Osofsky, J. D., & Osofsky, H. J. The psychological reaction of patients to legalized abortion. *American Journal of Orthopsychiatry,* 1972, *42,* 48–60.

Osofsky, J. D., Osofsky, H. J., Rajan, R., & Spitz, D. Psychosocial aspects of abortion in the United States. *The Mount Sinai Journal of Medicine,* 1975, *42,* 456–467.

Parke, R. D. Perspectives on father–infant interaction. In J. D. Osofsky (Ed.), *Handbook of infant development.* New York: Wiley, 1979.

Parke, R. D., O'Leary, S. E., & West, S. Mother–father–newborn interaction: Effects of maternal medication, labor and sex of infant. *Proceedings of the American Psychiatric Association Convention,* 1972, pp. 85–86.

Parkes, C. M. The emotional impact of cancer on patients and their families. *Journal of Laryngology and Utology,* 1972, *89,* 271–1279.

Parkes, C. M. *Bereavement: Studies of grief in adult life.* New York: International Universities Press, 1973.

Parkes, C. M. Comment: Communication and cancer—A social psychiatrist's view. *Social Science and Medicine,* 1974, *8,* 189–190.

Parkes, C. M. Determinants of outcome following bereavement. *Omega,* 1975, *6,* 303–324. (a)

Parkes, C. M. Unexpected and untimely bereavement: A statistical study of young Boston widows and widowers. In B. Schoenberg, I Gerber, A. Wiener, A. H. Kutscher, D. Peretz, & A. C. Carr (Eds.), *Bereavement: Its psychosocial aspects.* New York: Columbia University Press, 1975. (b)

Parkes, C. M. Terminal care: Evaluation of in-patient service at St. Christopher's Hospice. Part I: Views of surviving spouse on effects of the service on the patient. *Postgraduate Medical Journal,* 1979, *55,* 517–522. (a)

Parkes, C. M. Terminal care: Evaluation of in-patient service at St. Christopher's Hospice. Part II: Self-assessments of effects of the service on surviving spouses. *Postgraduate Medical Journal,* 1979, *55,* 523–587. (b)

Parlee, M. B. Social and emotional aspects of menstruation, birth and menopause. In D. D. Youngs & A. A. Ehrhardt (Eds.), *Psychosomatic obstetrics and gynecology.* New York: Appleton-Century-Crofts, 1980.

Parsell, S., & Tagliareni, E. M. Cancer patients help each other. *Armerican Journal of Nursing,* 1974, *74,* 650–651.

Parsons, T. *The social system.* Glencoe, Ill.: The Free Press, 1951. Pp. 428–479.

Parsons, T. Definitions of health and illness in the light of American values and social structure. In E. G. Jaco (Ed.), *Patients, physicians and illness.* New York: The Free Press, 1958. Pp. 165–187.

Parsons, T. The sick role and the role of the physician reconsidered. *Milbank Memorial Fund Quarterly,* 1975, *53,* 257–278.

Patt, S. L., Rappaport, R. G., & Barglow, R. Follow-up of therapeutic interruption of pregnancy. *Archives of General Psychiatry,* 1969, *20,* 408–414.

Paul, G. L. Physiological effects of relaxation training and hypnotic suggestion. *Journal of Abnormal Psychology,* 1969, *74,* 425–437.

Paykel, E. S. Recent life events and clinical depression. In K. E. Gunderson & R. H. Rahe (Eds.), *Life stress and illness.* Springfield, Ill.: Thomas, 1974.

Payne, E. C., Kravitz, A. R., Notman, M. T., & Anderson, J. V. Outcome following therapeutic abortion. *Archives of General Psychiatry,* 1976, *33,* 725–733.

Pearlman, J., Stotsky, B. A., & Dominick, J. R. Attitudes toward death among nursing home personnel. *Journal of Genetic Psychology,* 1969, *114,* 63–75.

Peck, A. Emotional reactions to having cancer. *American Journal of Roentgenology, Radium Therapy, and Nuclear Medicine,* 1972, *114*(3), 591–599.

Peck, A., & Boland, J. Emotional reactions to radiation treatment. *Cancer,* 1977, *40,* 180–184.

Peck, A., & Marcus, H. Psychiatric sequelae of therapeutic interruption of pregnancy. *Journal of Nervous and Mental Disease*, 1966, *143*, 417–425.

Peebler, D. How patients help each other. *American Journal of Nursing*, 1975, *75*, 1354.

Pelletier, K. R. *Holistic medicine*. New York: Delacorte Press, 1979.

Pellman, D. R. Learning to live with dying. *New York Times Magazine*, December 5, 1976, p. 44.

Pennebaker, J. Perceptual and environmental determinants of coughing. *Basic and Applied Social Psychology*, 1980, *1*(1), 83–91.

Pennebaker, J. W., Burnam, M. A., Schaeffer, M. A., & Harper, D. C. Lack of control as a determinant of perceived physical symptoms. *Journal of Personality and Social Psychology*, 1977, *35*, 167–174.

Perry, H. B. Role of the nurse-midwife in contemporary maternity care. In D. D. Youngs & A. A. Ehrhardt (Eds.), *Psychosomatic obstetrics and gynecology*. New York: Appelton-Century-Crofts, 1980.

Peterson, G. H., Mehl, L. E., & Leiderman, P. H. The role of some birth-related variables in father attachment. *American Journal of Orthopsychiatry*, 1979, *49*, 330–338.

Petrie, A. *Individuality in pain and suffering*. Chicago: University of Chicago Press, 1967.

Phares, E. J. *Locus of control in personality*. Morristown, N.J.: General Learning Press, 1976.

Pickering, G. Medicine on the brink: The dilemma of a learned profession. *Perspectives in Biology and Medicine*, Summer, 1978, pp. 551–560.

Pine, V. *Caretaker of the dead*. New York: Irvington, 1975.

Pine, V. R., Kutscher, A. H., Peretz, D., Slater, R. C., DeBellis, R., Volk, R. J., & Cherico, D. J. *Acute grief and the funeral*. Springfield, Ill.: Charles C. Thomas, 1976.

Pines, A., & Aronson, E. *Burnout: From Tedium to Personal Growth*. New York: The Free Press, 1981.

Pines, A., & Maslach, C. Characteristics of staff burnout in mental health settings. *Hospital and Community Psychiatry*, 1978, *29*(4), 233–237.

Pinkerton, S. S., & McAleer, C. A. Influence of client diagnosis—cancer—on counselor decisions. *Journal of Counseling Psychology*, 1976, *23*(6), 575–578.

Plumb, M. M., & Holland, J. Comparative studies of psychological function in patients with advanced cancer—I: Self-reported depressive symptoms. *Psychosomatic Medicine*, 1977, *39*, 264–275.

Polivy, J. Psychological effects of mastectomy on a woman's feminine self-concept. *Journal of Nervous and Mental Disease*, 1977, *164*(2), 77–87.

Poznanski, E. O. Children's reactions to pain: A psychiatrist's perspective. *Clinical Pediatrics*, 1976, *15*, 1114–1119.

Pranulis, M., Dabbs, J., & Johnson, J. General anesthesia and the patient's attempts at control. *Social Behavior and Personality*, 1975, *3*, 49–54.

Pratt, L. *Family structure and effective health behavior*. Boston: Houghton-Mifflin, 1976.

Prugh, D., Staub, E., Sands, H., Kirschbaum, R., & Lenihan, E. A study of the emotional reactions of children and families to hospitalization and illness. *American Journal of Orthopsychiatry*, 1953, *23*, 70–106.

Public attitudes toward cancer and cancer test. *Ca—A Journal for Clinicians*, April 1980, pp. 575–578.

Pugh, T. F., Jerath, B. K., Schmidt, W. M., & Reed, R. B. Rate of mental disease relative to childbearing. *New England Journal of Medicine*, 1963, *268*, 1224–1228.

Putt, A. An experiment in nursing adults with peptic ulcers. *Nursing Research*, 1970, *19*, 484–494.

Quesada, G. M. Language and communication barriers for health delivery to a minority group. *Social Science and Medicine*, 1976, *10*, 323–327.

Quinlan, D. M., & Janis, I. L. Unfavorable effects of high levels of self-disclosure. In I. L. Janis (Ed.), *Counseling on personal decisions: Theory and research on short-term helping relationships*. New Haven, Conn.: Yale University Press, in press.

Quinlan, D. M., Janis, I. L., & Bales, V. L. Effects of moderate self-disclosure and subsequent telephone contact. In I. L. Janis (Ed.), *Counseling on personal decisions: Theory and research on short-term helping relationships.* New Haven, Conn.: Yale University Press, in press.

Quint, J. C. Institutionalized practice of information control. *Psychiatry,* 1965, *28,* 119–132.

Rabkin, J. G., & Struening, E. L. Life events, stress, and illness. *Science,* 1976, *194,* 1013–1020.

Raphael, B. Preventive intervention with the recently bereaved. *Archives of General Psychiatry,* 1977, *34,* 1450–1454.

Ratner, H. History of the dehumanization of American obstetrical practice. In L. Stewart & D. Stewart (Eds.), *21st century obstetrics now!* (Vol. 1). Chapel Hill, N.C.: National Association of Parents and Professionals for Safe Alternatives in Childbirth, 1977.

Raush, H. L., Barry, W. A., Hertel, R. K., & Swain, M. A. *Communication, conflict, and marriage.* San Francisco: Jossey-Bass, 1974.

Raven, B. Social influence and power. In I. D. Steiner & M. Rischenbein (Eds.), *Current studies in social psychology.* New York: Holt, 1965.

Raven, B. H., & Kruglanski, A. W. Conflict and power. In *The structure of conflict.* New York: Academic Press, 1970.

Rea, M. P., Greenspoon, S., & Spilka, B. Physicians and the terminally ill patient: Some selected attitudes and behavior. *Omega,* 1975, *7,* 291–302.

Reader, G. G., Pratt, L., & Mudd, M. C. What patients expect from their doctors. *Modern Hospital,* 1957, *89,* 88–94.

Reiser, S. J. The medical influence of the stethoscope. *Scientific American,* 1979, *240*(2), 148–156.

Renneker, R. E., & Cutler, R. Psychological problems of adjustment of cancer of the breast. *Journal of the American Medical Association,* 1952, *148,* 833–838.

Rice, V.F.H. The effects of need for personal control and information on strains associated with a threatening event. Doctoral dissertation completed at the University of Michigan, Ann Arbor, Michigan, 1972.

Richards, J. M., Jr. An ecological analysis of the impact of the U.S. Supreme Court's 1973 abortion decision. *Journal of Applied Social Psychology,* 1978, *8,* 15–28.

Richards, J. M., Jr., Taylor, C. W., & Price, P. B. The prediction of medical intern performance. *Journal of Applied Psychology,* 1962, *46,* 142–146.

Richards, M.P.M. Effects on development of medical interventions and separation of newborns from their parents. In D. Shaffer & J. Dunn (Eds.), *The first year of life . . . psychological and medical implications of early experience.* New York: Wiley, 1979.

Richardson, F. H. Fear—A dental problem. *Oral Hygiene,* 1936, *26,* 344–349.

Richman, J., & Goldthorp, W. O. Fatherhood: The social construction of pregnancy and birth. In S. Kitzinger & J. A. Davis (Eds.), *The place of birth.* Oxford: Oxford University Press, 1978.

Rickel, A. U., & Atkinson, A. K. *Postpartum depression: A critical review.* Unpublished manuscript, Wayne State University, 1979.

Riesch, S. Enhancement of mother–infant social interaction. *JOGN Nursing,* 1979, *8,* 242–246.

Riggio, R., & Friedman, H. *Individual differences and cues of deception.* Unpublished manuscript, University of California, Riverside, 1981.

Ring, K. *Life at death.* New York: Coward, McCann, & Geoghegan, 1980.

Riply, H. S. The psychological basis of pain. In J. J. Bonica (Ed.), *The management of pain.* Lea & Febeger, 1953.

Riscala, L. Healing by laying on of hands: Myth or fact. *Ethics in Science and Medicine,* 1975, *2,* 167–171.

Riskind, J., & Janis, I. L. Effects of negative self-disclosures and new approval training procedures. In I. L. Janis (Ed.), *Counseling on personal decisions: Theory and research on short-term helping relationships.* New Haven, Conn.: Yale University Press, in press.

Robbins, J. M. Objective versus subjective responses to abortion. *Journal of Consulting and Clinical Psychology,* 1979, *47,* 994–995.

Robinson, D. *Patients, practitioners, and medical care: Aspects of medical sociology* (2nd ed.). London: Heinemann, 1978.

Rodin, J. Menstruation, reattribution and competence. *Journal of Personality and Social Psychology,* 1976, *33,* 345–353.

Rodin, J. Research on eating behavior and obesity: Where does it fit in personality and social psychology? *Personality and Social Psychology Bulletin,* 1977, *3,* 333–355.

Rodin, J. Somatopsychics and attribution. *Personality and Social Psychology Bulletin,* 1978, *4,* 531–540. (a)

Rodin, J. Cognitive behavioral strategies for the treatment of obesity. In D. Meinchenbaum (Ed.), *Cognitive behavior therapy.* New York: BMA Audio Cassette Publications, 1978 (b)

Rodin, J. Managing the stress of aging: The role of control and coping. In S. Levine & H. Ursin (Eds.), *Coping and health.* New York: Plenum, 1980.

Rodin, J., & Janis, I. L. The social power of health care practitioners as agents of change. *Journal of Social Issues,* 1979, *35*(1), 60–81.

Rodin, J., & Janis, I. L. The social influence of physicians and other health care practitioners as agents of change. In H. S. Friedman & M. R. DiMatteo, (Eds.), *Interpersonal issues in health care.* New York: Academic Press, 1982.

Rodin, J., & Langer, E. Long-term effects of a control-relevant intervention with the institutionalized aged. *Journal of Personality and Social Psychology,* 1977, *35,* 897–902.

Rodin, J., & Langer, E. Aging labels: The decline of control and the fall of self-esteem. *Journal of Social Issues,* 1980, *36,* 12–29.

Rogentine, G. N., van Kammen, D. P., Fox, B. H., Docherty, J. P., Rosenblatt, J. E., Boyd, S. C., & Bunney, W. E. Psychological factors in the prognosis of malignant melanoma: A prospective study. *Psychosomatic Medicine,* 1979, *41*(8), 647–655.

Rogers, C. R. *Client-centered therapy.* Boston: Houghton-Mifflin, 1951.

Rogers, C. R. The necessary and sufficient conditions of therapeutic personality change. *Journal of Consulting Psychology,* 1957, *21,* 95–103.

Rogers, R. W., & Mewborn, C. R. Fear appeals and attitude change: Effects of a threat's noxiousness, probability of occurrence, and the efficacy of coping responses. *Journal of Personality and Social Psychology,* 1976, *34,* 54–61.

Rogers, R. W., & Thistlethwaite, D. L. Effects of fear arousal and reassurance upon attitude change. *Journal of Personality and Social Psychology,* 1970, *15,* 227–233.

Roghmann, K. J., Hengst, A., & Zastowny, T. R. Satisfaction with medical care: Its measurement and relation to utilization. *Medical Care,* 1979, *17*(5), 461–477.

Rollin, B. *First you cry.* Philadelphia: J. B. Lippincott, 1976.

Rooks, J. B., & Cates, W., Jr. Emotional impact of D & E instillation. *Family Planning Perspectives,* 1977, *9,* 276–277.

Rosen, G. The hospital: Historical sociology of a community institution. In E. Freidson (Ed.), *The hospital in modern society.* New York: Free Press, 1963.

Rosen, G. The evolution of social medicine. In H. E. Freeman, S. Levine, & L. G. Reeder (Eds.), *Handbook of medical sociology* (2nd ed.). Englewood Cliffs, N.J.: Prentice-Hall, 1972. Pp. 30–60.

Rosen, R. A., Werley, H. A., Ager, J. W., & Shea, F. P. Health professionals' attitudes toward abortion. *Public Opinion Quarterly,* 1974, *38,* 158–173.

Rosenbaum, M. Individual differences in self-control behaviors and tolerance of painful stimulation. *Journal of Abnormal Psychology,* 1980, *89,* 581–590.

Rosenberg, P. P. Students' perceptions and concerns during their first year in medical school. *Journal of Medical Education,* 1971, *46,* 211–218.

Rosenstock, T. M., & Kirscht, J. P. Why people seek health care. In G. C. Stone, F. Cohen, & N. E. Adler (Eds), *Health psychology: A handbook.* San Francisco: Jossey-Bass, 1979.

Rosenthal, R. *Experimenter effects in behavioral research.* New York: Irvington, 1976.

Rosenthal, R., Hall, J. A., DiMatteo, M. R., Rogers, P. L., & Archer, D. *Sensitivity to nonverbal communication: The PONS test.* Baltimore: Johns Hopkins University Press, 1979.

Ross, L. The intuitive psychologist and his shortcomings. In L. Berkowitz (Ed.), *Advances in experimental social psychology* (Vol. 10). New York: Academic Press, 1977.

Rossi, A. Transition to parenthood. *Journal of Marriage and the Family,* 1968, *30,* 26–39.

Roth, J. A. Information and the control of treatment in tuberculosis hospitals. In E. Freidson (Ed.), *The hospital in modern society.* New York: Free Press, 1963.

Roth, J. A. The necessity and control of hospitalization. *Social Science and Medicine,* 1972, *6,* 425–446.

Rothman, B. K. The social construction of birth. *Journal of Nurse Midwifery,* 1977, *22,* 9–13.

Rotter, J. B. Generalized expectancies for internal versus external control of reinforcement. *Psychological Monographs,* 1966, *80,* (1, Whole No. 609).

Rubel, A. J. Concepts of disease in Mexican-American culture. *American Anthropologist,* 1960, *62,* 795–814.

Rubin, R. Cognitive style in pregnancy. *American Journal of Nursing,* 1970, *70,* 502–508.

Rubin, R. T., Gunderson, K. E., & Arthur, R. J. Life stress and illness patterns in the U.S. Navy. V: Prior life change and illness onset in a battleship's crew. *Journal of Psychosomatic Research,* 1971, *15,* 89–94.

Rubin, R. T., & Rahe, R. H. U.S. Navy underwater demolition team training: Biochemical studies. In K. E. Gunderson & R. H. Rahe (Eds.), *Life stress and illness.* Springfield, Ill.: Thomas, 1974.

Russell, P. Infantile stimulation in rodents: A consideration of possible mechanisms. *Psychological Bulletin,* 1971, *75,* 192–202.

Ryan, C., & Ryan, K. M. *A private battle,* New York: Fawcett, 1979.

Ryan, E. D., & Kovacil C. R. Pain tolerance and athletic participation. *Perceptual and Motor Skills,* 1966, *22,* 383; 390.

Ryan, W. *Blaming the victim.* New York: Random House, 1971.

Sackett, D. L. The magnitude of compliance and noncompliance. In D. L. Sackett & R. B. Haynes (Eds.), *Compliance with therapeutic regimens.* Baltimore: Johns Hopkins University Press, 1976.

Sackett, D. L., & Haynes, R. B. (Eds.). *Compliance with therapeutic regimens.* Baltimore: Johns Hopkins University Press, 1976.

Sackett, D. L., Haynes, R. B., Gibson, E. S., Taylor, D. W., Robers, R., & Johnson, A. L. Hypertension control, compliance and science. *American Heart Journal,* 1977, *94,* 666–667.

Salomon, M., Schauf, V., & Seiden, A. Breatfeeding, "natural mothering," and working outside the home. In D. Stewart & L. Stewart (Eds.), *21st century obstetrics now!* (Vol. 2.). Chapel Hill, N.C.: National Association of Parents and Professionals for Safe Alternatives in Childbirth, 1977.

Salzman, C., Shader, R., Scott, D. A., & Binstock, W. Interviewer anger and patient dropout in a walk-in clinic. *Comprehensive Psychiatry,* 1970, *11,* 267–273.

Sameroff, A. J., & Chandler, M. J. Reproductive risk and the continuum of caretaking casualty. In F. D. Horowitz (Ed.), *Review of child development research* (Vol. 4). Chicago: University of Chicago Press, 1975.

Samora, J., Saunders, L., & Larson, R. F. Medical vocabulary knowledge among hospital patients. *Journal of Health and Human Behavior,* 1961, *2,* 83–92.

Sanders, J. B., & Kardinal, C. G. Adaptive coping mechanisms in adult acute leukemia patients in remission. *Journal of the American Medical Association,* 1977, *238*(9), 952–954.

Sarason, I. G., & Sarason, B. R. *Abnormal psychology* (3rd ed.). Englewood Cliffs, N.J.: Prentice-Hall, 1980.

Sarvis, B., & Rodman, H. *The abortion controversy.* New York: Columbia University Press, 1973.

Saum, L. O. Death in the popular mind of pre–Civil War America. In D. E. Stannard (Ed.), *Death in America*. Philadelphia: University of Pennsylvania Press, 1975. Pp. 30–48.

Saunders, C. Terminal care. In C. A. Garfield (Ed.), *Psychosocial care of the dying patient*. New York: McGraw-Hill, 1978. Pp. 22–33.

Scaer, R., & Korte, D. MOM survey: Maternity options for mother—What do women want in maternity care? *Birth and the Family Journal*, 1978, *5*, 20–25.

Schachter, S. *The psychology of affiliation*. Stanford, Calif.: Stanford University Press, 1959.

Schachter, S. The interaction of cognitive and physiological determinants of emotional state. In L. Berkowitz (Ed.), *Advances in experimental social psychology* (Vol. 1). New York: Academic Press, 1964.

Schachter, S. *Emotion, obesity, and crime*. New York: Academic Press, 1971.

Schachter, S., & Singer, J. E. Cognitive, social, and physiological determinants of emotional states, *Psychological Review*, 1962, *69*, 379–399.

Schaffer, C., & Pine, F. Pregnancy, abortion and the developmental tasks of adolescence. *The Journal of the American Academy of Child Psychiatry*, 1972, *11*, 511–536.

Scheff, T. J. *Being mentally ill: A sociological theory*. Chicago: Aldine, 1966.

Schenthal, J. E. Multiphasic screening of the well patient. *Journal of the American Medical Association*, 1960, *172*, 1–4.

Schmale, A. Giving up as a final common pathway to changes in health. *Psychosomatic Medicine*, 1971, *8*, 18–28.

Schmale, A., & Iker, H. The psychological setting of uterine cervical cancer. *Annals of the New York Academy of Sciences*, 1966, *125*, 807–813.

Schmale, A., & Iker, H. Hopelessness as a predictor of cervical cancer. *Social Science and Medicine*, 1971, *5*, 95–100.

Schmidt, D. D. Patient compliance: The effect of the doctor as a therapeutic agent. *Journal of Family Practice*, 1977, *4*, 853–856.

Schmitt, F. E., & Wooldridge, P. J. Psychological preparation of surgical patients. *Nursing Research*, 1973, *22*, 108–116.

Schoenberg, B. G. (Ed.). *Psychosocial aspects of terminal care*. New York: Columbia University Press, 1972.

Schuller, A. B. About the problem patient. *Journal of Family Practice*, 1977, *4*, 653–654.

Schulz, R. Effects of control and predictability on the physical and psychological well-being of the institutionalized aged. *Journal of Personality and Social Psychology*, 1976, *33*, 563–573.

Schulz, R. *The psychology of death, dying, and bereavement*. Reading, Mass.: Addison-Wesley, 1978.

Sdchwartz, M. D. An information and discussion program for women after mastectomy. *Archives of Surgery*, 1977, *12*(3), 276–281.

Seeman, M., & Evans, J. W. Stratification and hospital care. Part I: The performance of the medical intern. *American Sociological Review*, 1961, *26*, 67–80. (a)

Seeman, M., & Evans, J. W. Stratification and hospital care. Part II: The objective criterion of performance. *American Sociological Review*, 1961, *26*, 193–204. (b)

Seeman, M., & Evans, J. Alienation and learning in a hospital setting. *American Sociological Review*, 1962, *27*, 772–782.

Seiden, A. M. The sense of mastery in the childbirth experience. In M. T. Notman & C. C. Nadelson (Eds.), *The woman patient: Medical and psychological interfaces* (Vol. I: *Sexual and reproductive aspects of women's health care*). New York: Plenum, 1978.

Seligman, M. E. P. *Helplessness: On depression, development, and death*. San Francisco: Freeman, 1975.

Selye, H. A syndrome produced by diverse nocuous agents. *Nature*, 1936, *138*, 32.

Selye, H. *The stress of life*. New York: McGraw-Hill, 1956.

Selye, H. *The stress of life*. (Rev. ed.). New York: McGraw-Hill, 1976.

Senay, E. C. Therapeutic abortion: Clinical aspects. *Archives of General Psychiatry*, 1970, *23*, 408–415.

Sexton, M. M. Behavioral epidemiology. In O. F. Pomerleau & J. P. Brady (Eds.), *Behavioral medicine: Theory and practice.* Baltimore: Williams and Wilkins, 1979.

Shalit, B. Structural ambiguity and limits to coping. *Journal of Human Stress,* 1977, *3,* 32–45.

Shannon-Babitz, M. Addressing the needs of fathers during labor and delivery. *American Journal of Maternal-Child Nursing,* 1979, *4,* 378–382.

Shapiro, A. K. A contribution to a history of the placebo effect. *Behavioral Science,* 1960, *5,* 109–135.

Shapiro, A. K. Placebo effects in medicine, psychotherapy, and psychoanalysis. In A. Bergin & S. Garfield (Eds.), *Handbook of psychotherapy and behavior change.* New York: John Wiley & Sons, 1971.

Shapiro, A. K. & Morris, L. A. The placebo effect in medical and psychological therapies. In S. L. Garfield & A. E. Bergin (Eds.), *Handbook of psychotherapy and behavior change* (2nd ed.). New York: Wiley, 1978.

Shapiro, D., & Surwit, R. S. Biofeedback. In O. F. Pomerleau & J. P. Brady (Eds.), *Behavioral medicine: Theory and practice.* Baltimore: Williams and Wilkins, 1979.

Shattuck, F. C. The science and art of medicine in some of their aspects. *Boston Medical and Surgical Journal,* 1907, *157,* 63–67.

Sheffer, M. B., & Greifenstein. The emotional responses of patients to surgery and anesthesia. *Anesthesiology,* 1969, *21,* 502–507.

Sheldon, A., Ryser, C. P., & Krant, M. An integrated family-oriented cancer care program: The report of a pilot project in the socio-emotional management of chronic diseases. *Journal of Chronic Diseases,* 1970, *22,* 743–755.

Shereshefsky, P. M., & Yarrow, L. J. *Psychological aspects of a first pregnancy and early postnatal adaptation.* New York: Raven Press, 1974.

Shewchuk, L. A. Smoking cessation programs of the American Health Foundation. *Preventative Medicine,* 1976, *5,* 454–474.

Shiloh, A. Egalitarian and hierarchical patients: An investigation among Hadassah Hospital patients. *Medical Care,* 1965, *3,* 87–95.

Shipley, R. H., Butt, J. H., & Horwitz, E. A. Preparation to reexperience a stressful medical examination: Effect of repetitious videotape exposure and coping style. *Journal of Consulting and Clinical Psychology,* 1979, *47,* 485–492.

Shipley, R. H., Chaing, H., & Lang, J. Cognition and self-control: Cognitive control of painful sensory input. In H. London & R. E. Nisbett (Eds.), *Thought and feeling: Cognitive alteration of feeling states.* Chicago: Aldine, 1974.

Shor, R. E. Physiological effect of painful stimulation during hypnotic analgesia under conditions designed to minimize anxiety. *International Journal of Clinical and Experimental Hypnosis,* 1962, *10,* 183–202.

Shweder, R. A. Likeness and likelihood in everyday thought: Magical thinking in judgments about personality. *Current Anthropology,* 1977, *18,* 637–658.

Sigerist, H. E. *A history of medicine.* London: Oxford University Press, 1951.

Silberfarb, P. M., Maurer, L. H., & Crouthamel, C. S. Psychosocial aspects of neoplastic disease. I: Functional status of breast cancer patient during different treatment regimens. *American Journal of Psychiatry,* 1980, *137*(4), 450–455.

Silver, R. L., & Wortman, C. B. Coping with undesirable life events. In J. Garber & M.E.P. Seligman (Eds.), *Human helplessness.* New York: Academic Press, 1980.

Silverman, P. R., & Murrow, H. G. Mutual help during critical role transitions. *Journal of Applied Behavioral Science,* 1976, *12,* 410–418.

Sime, A. M. Relationship of preoperative fear, type of coping, and information received about surgery and recovery from surgery. *Journal of Personality and Social Psychology,* 1976, *34,* 716–724.

Simon, N., & Senturia, A. Psychiatric sequelae of abortion. *Archives of General Psychiatry,* 1966, *15,* 378–389.

Simon, N., Senturia, A., & Rothman, D. Psychiatric illness following therapeutic abortion. *American Journal of Psychiatry,* 1967, *124,* 97–103.

Simons, C., & Piliavin, J. The effect of deception on reactions to a victim. *Journal of Personality and Social Psychology*, 1972, *21*, 56-60.

Skipper, J. K., Jr. Communication and the hospitalized patient. In J. K. Skipper & R. C. Leonard (Eds.), *Social interaction and patient care*, Philadelphia: J. B. Lippincott, 1965. Pp. 61-82.

Skipper, J. K., & Leonard, R. C. (Eds.), *Social interaction and patient care*. Philadelphia: J. B. Lippincott, 1965.

Skipper, J. K., Tagliacozzo, D., & Mauksch, H. Some possible consequences of limited communication between patients and hospital functionaries. *Journal of Health and Human Behavior*, 1964, *5*, 35-39.

Sklar, L. S., & Anisman, H. Stress and coping factors influence tumor growth. *Science*, 1979, *205*, 513-515.

Slack, W. Computer-based interviewing system dealing with nonverbal behavior as well as keyboard responses. *Science*, 1971, *171*, 84-87.

Smedslund, J. Note on learning, contingency, and clinical experience. *Scandinavian Journal of Psychology*, 1966, *7*, 265-266.

Smith, E. M. A follow-up study of women who request abortion. *American Journal of Orthopsychiatry*, 1973, *43*, 574-585.

Smith, G., Chaing, H., & Regina, E. *Acupuncture and experimental psychology*. Paper presented at Symposium on Pain and Acupuncture, Philadelphia, April, 1974.

Smith-Hanen, S. Effects of nonverbal behaviors on judged levels of counselor warmth and empathy. *Journal of Counseling Psychology*, 1977, *24*, 87-91.

Snow, C. E., & Ferguson, C. (Eds.). *Talking to children: Language input and acquisition*. Cambridge: Cambridge University Press, 1977.

Snow, L. Folk-medical beliefs and their implications for care of patients. *Annals of Internal Medicine*, 1974, *81*, 82-96.

Snyder, C., Eyres, S. J., & Barnard, K. New findings about mothers' antenatal expectations and their relationship to infant development. *American Journal of Maternal-Child Nursing*, 1979, *4*, 354-357.

Snyder, M. L., & Mentzer, S. Social psychological perspectives on the physician's feelings and behavior. *Personality and Social Psychology Bulletin*, 1978, *4*, 541-547.

Sontag, S. *Illness as metaphor*. New York: Farrar, Straus, and Giroux, 1978.

Soutter, B. R., & Kennedy, M. C. Patient compliance assessment in drug trials: Usage and methods. *Australia, New Zealand Journal of Medicine*, 1974, *4*, 360-364.

Spaght, S. E., Kenan, E. H., & Torrington, J. The abortion alternative. Section I: Abortion Counseling. In R. Wilson (Ed.), *Problem pregnancy and abortion counseling*. North Carolina: Family Life Publications, 1973.

Spanos, N. P., Barber, T. X., & Lang, J. Cognition and self-control: Cognitive control of painful sensory input. In H. London & R. E. Nisbett (Eds.), *Thought and feeling: Cognitive alteration of feeling states*. Chicago: Aldine, 1974.

Spanos, N. P., Horton, C., & Chaves, J. F. The effects of two cognitive strategies on pain threshold. *Journal of Abnormal Psychology*, 1975, *84*(6), 677-681.

Spear, F. G. Pain in psychiatric patients. *Journal of Psychosomatic Research*, 1967, *11*, 187-193.

Spiegel, D. Psychological support for women with metastatic carcinoma. *Psychosomatics*, 1979, *20*(11), 780-787.

Spiegel, P., & Machotka, P. *Messages of the body*. New York: The Free Press, 1974.

Spielberger, C. D., & Jacobs, G. A. Stress and anxiety during pregnancy and labor. In L. Carenza, P. Pancheri, & L. Zichella (Eds.), *Clinical psychoneuroendocrinolgy in reproduction*. New York: Academic Press, 1978.

Spinetta, J. J., & Maloney, L. J. The child with cancer: Patterns of communication and denial. *Journal of Consulting and Clinical Psychology*, 1978, *46*(6), 1540-1541.

Spinetta, J. J., Swarner, J. A., & Sheposh, J. P. Effective parental coping following the death of a child from cancer. *Journal of Pediatric Psychology*, 1981, *6*(3), 251-263.

Stamler, J., Schoenberger, J. A., & Lindberg, H. A. Detection of susceptibility to coronary disease. *Bulletin of the New York Academy of Medicine*, 1969, *45*, 1306.

Starkman, M. N., & Youngs, D. D. Reactions to electronic fetal monitoring. In D. D. Youngs & A. A. Ehrhardt (Eds.), *Psychosomatic obstetrics and gynecology*, New York: Appleton-Century-Crofts, 1980.

Staub, E., & Kellett, D. S. Increasing pain tolerance by information about aversive stimuli. *Journal of Personality and Social Psychology*, 1972, *21*, 198–203.

Staub, E., Tursky, B., & Schwartz, G. Self-control and predictability: Their effects on reactions to aversive stimulation. *Journal of Personality and Social Psychology*, 1971, *18*, 157–162.

Stern, D. *The first relationship: Infant and mother*. Cambridge, Mass.: Harvard University Press, 1977.

Sternbach, R. A. *Pain: A psychophysiological analysis*. New York: Academic Press, 1968.

Sternbach, R. A. Strategies and tactics in the treatment of patients with pain. In B. L. Crue (Ed.), *Pain and suffering*. Springfield, Ill.: Thomas, 1970.

Sternbach, R. A. *Pain patients: Traits and treatment*. New York: Academic Press, 1974.

Sternbach, R. A. The Management of Pain Workshop, San Diego, Calif. 1977. (A workshop.)

Sternbach, R. A. Clinical aspects of pain. In R. A. Sternbach (Ed.), *The psychology of pain*. New York: Raven Press, 1978.

Sternbach, R., Murphy, R., Akeson, W., & Wolf, S. Chronic low-back pain: The "low-back loser." *Post Graduate Medicine*, 1973, *53*, 135–138.

Sternbach, R. A., & Timmermans, G. Personality changes associated with reduction of pain. *Pain*. 1975, *1*, 177–181.

Sternbach, R. A., & Tursky, B. Ethnic differences among housewives in psychophysical and skin potential responses to electric shock. *Psychophysiology*, 1965, *1*, 241–246.

Sternbach, R. A., Wolf, S., Murphy, R., & Akeson, W. Aspects of chronic low back pain. *Psychosomatics*, 1973, *14*, 53–56.

Stichler, J. F., Bowden, M. S., & Reimer, E. D. Pregnancy: A shared emotional experience. *American Journal of Maternal-Child Nursing*, 1978, *3*, 153–157.

Stiles, W. B., Putnam, S. M., Wolf, M. H., & James, S. A. Interaction exchange structure and patient satisfaction with medical interviews. *Medical Care*, 1979, *17*, 667–679.

Stimson, G. V. Obeying doctors' orders: A view from the other side. *Social Science and Medicine*, 1974, *8*, 97–104.

Stimson, G. V. Doctor-patient interaction and some problems for prescribing. *Journal of the Royal College of General Practitioners*, 1976, *26*, 712–718.

Stoddard, S. *The hospice movement*. New York: Stein & Day, 1978.

Stone, A. R. Cues to interpersonal distress due to pregnancy. *American Journal of Nursing*, 1965, *65*, 88–91.

Stone, G. C. Patient compliance and the role of the expert. *Journal of Social Issues*, 1979, *35*,(1), 34–59.

Strauss, M. B. (Ed.). *Familiar medical quotations*. Boston: Little, Brown, 1968.

Strickland, B. R. Internal-external expectancies and health-related behaviors. *Journal of Consulting and Clinical Psychology*, 1978, *46*, 1192–1211.

Strum, W. B., Landres, R. T., & Berry, C. C. Rates of detection of colon cancer by proctosigmoidoscopy and barium enema. Unpublished manuscript, University of California, San Diego, 1976.

Strupp, H. H., Levenson, R. W., Manuck, S. B., Snell, J. D., Hinrichsen, J. J., & Boyd, S. Effects of suggestion on total respiratory resistance in mild asthmatics. *Journal of Psychosomatic Research*, 1974, *18*, 337–346.

Suchman, E. A. Stages of illness and medical care. *Journal of Health and Human Behavior*, 1965, *6*, 114–128.

Suchman, E. A. Stages of illness and medical care. In E. G. Jaco (Ed.), *Patients, physicians and illness* (2nd ed.). New York: Free Press, 1972.

Sugarman, M. Paranatal influence on maternal–infant attachment. *American Journal of Orthopsychiatry,* 1977, *47,* 407–421.

Suitor, J. J. Husband's participation in childbirth: A nineteenth century phenomenon. *Journal of Family History,* 1981, *6,* 278–293.

Sumner, G., & Fritsch, J. Postnatal parental concerns: The first weeks of life. *JOGN Nursing,* 1977, *6,* 27–32.

Sumner, P. E., & Phillips, C. R. *Birthing rooms: Concept and reality.* St. Louis: C. V. Mosby, 1981.

Surgeon General. *Healthy people: The Surgeon General's report on health promotion and disease prevention, 1979* (U.S. Department of Health, Education, and Welfare Publication No. 79–55071). Washington, D.C.: U.S. Government Printing Office, 1979.

Sutherland, A. M., & Orbach, C. E. Psychological impact of cancer and cancer surgery. II: Depressive reactions associated with surgery for cancer. *Cancer,* 1953, *6,* 958–962.

Sutherland, A. M., Orbach, C. E., Dyk, R. B., & Bard, M. The psychological impact of cancer and cancer surgery. I: Adaptation to the dry colostomy: Preliminary report and summary of findings. *Cancer,* 1952, *5,* 857–872.

Svarstad, B. Physician–patient communication and patient conformity with medical advice. In D. Mechanic, *The growth of bureaucratic medicine.* New York: John Wiley and Sons, 1976.

Swanson, J. Nursing intervention to facilitate maternal–infant attachment. *JOGN Nursing,* 1978, *7,* 35–38.

Swanson, J., Swanson, W., Maruta, T., & Floreen, A. The dissatisfied patient with chronic pain. *Pain,* 1978, *4,* 367–378.

Swigar, M. E., Breslin, R., Pouzzner, M., Quinlan, D., & Blum, M. Interview follow-up of abortion applicant drop-outs. *Social Psychiatry,* 1976, *11,* 135–143.

Szasz, T. S. *Pain and pleasure: A study of bodily feelings.* New York: Basic Books, 1957.

Szasz, T. S. *The myth of mental illness: Foundations of a theory of personal conduct.* New York: Harper & Row, 1961.

Szasz, T. S. *The psychology of persistent pain: A portrait of l'homme doulourex.* New York: Academic Press, 1968.

Tagliacozzo, D. L., & Mauksch, H. O. The patient's view of the patient's role. In E. G. Jaco (Ed.), *Patients, physicians and illness* (2nd ed.). New York: Free Press, 1972.

Tagliacozzo, D. L., Luskin, D. B., Lashof, J. C., & Ima, K. Nurse intervention and patient behavior. *American Journal of Public Health,* 1974, *64,* 596–603.

Tajfel, H., & Wilkes, A. L. Classification and quantitative judgment. *British Journal of Psychology,* 1963, *54,* 101–114.

Tanzer, S. *The psychology of pregnancy and childbirth: An investigation of natural childbirth.* Unpublished doctoral dissertation, Brandeis University, 1967.

Taylor, J. *The rules and exercises of holy dying.* New York: Arno Press, 1977. (Originally published, 1665.)

Taylor, S. E. Hospital patient behavior: Reactance, helplessness, or control? *Journal of Social Issues,* 1979, *35*(1), 156–184.

Taylor, S. E. Hospital patient behavior: Reactance, helplessness, or control? In H. S. Friedman & M. R. DiMatteo, (Eds.), *Interpersonal issues in health care.* New York: Academic Press, 1982.

Taylor, S. E., & Levin, S. *The psychological impact of breast cancer: Theory and research.* San Francisco: West Coast Cancer Foundation, 1976.

Tebbi, C., Tull, R., & Koren, B. Psychological research and evaluation of a unit designed for adolescent patients with oncology problems. *Proceedings of the 71st Annual Meeting of the American Association for Cancer Research,* 1980, *21,* 379.

Tedeschi, J. T. Attributions, liking and power. In T. Huston (Ed.), *Foundations of interpersonal attraction.* New York: Academic Press, 1974.

Tedeschi, J. T. *Social psychology: Interdependence, interaction.* New York: John Wiley, 1976.

Terkel, S. *Working.* New York: Pantheon, 1972.

Thibaut, J. W., & Kelley, H. H. *The social psychology of groups.* New York: Wiley, 1959.

Thomas, C. B., Duszynski, K. R., & Shaffer, J. W. Family attitudes reported in youth as potential predictors of cancer. *Psychosomatic Medicine,* 1979, *41*(4), 287–302.

Thomas, G., & Wittes, M. M. *The day the world ended.* New York: Ballantine Books, 1969.

Thomas, J. M., & Weiner, E. A. Psychological differences among groups of critically ill hospitalized patients, noncritically ill hospitalized patients and well controls. *Journal of Clinical Psychology,* 1974, *42,* 274–279.

Thorner, N. Nurses violate their patients' rights. *Journal of Psychiatric Nursing and Mental Health Services,* 1976, *14,* 7–12.

Toynbee, P. *Patients.* New York: Harcourt Brace Jovanovich, 1977.

Train, G. S. The dentist's emotional reaction to the troublesome patient. *Psychosomatics,* 1969, *10,* 176–180.

Truax, C. B., & Carkhuff, R. R. *Toward effective counseling and psychotherapy.* Chicago: Aldine, 1967.

Turk, D. C. *Cognitive control of pain: A skills training approach.* Unpublished master's thesis, University of Waterloo, 1975.

Turk, D. C. Cognitive behavioral techniques in the management of pain. In J. P. Foreyt & D. J. Rathgen (Eds.), *Cognitive behavior therapy.* New York: Plenum Press, 1978.

Turner, M. F., & Izzi, M. H. The COPE story: A service to pregnant and postpartum women. In M. T. Notman & C. C. Nadelson (Eds.), *The woman patient: Medical and psychological interfaces* (Vol. 1). New York: Plenum Press, 1978.

Tversky, A., & Kahneman, D. Availability: A heuristic for judging frequency and probability. *Cognitive Psychology,* 1973, *5,* 207–232.

Tversky, A., & Kahneman, D. Judgment under uncertainty: Heuristics and biases. *Science,* 1974, *185,* 1124–1131.

United States Department of Health, Education, and Welfare. *Health: United States.* Hyattsville, Md.: USDHEW, 1978.

Vaccarino, J. M. Malpractice: The problem in perspective. *Journal of the American Medical Association,* 1977, *238,* 861–863.

Vachon, M.L.S. Motivation and stress experienced by staff working with the terminally ill. *Death Education,* 1978, *2,* 113–122.

Vachon, M.L.S. *The importance of social support in the longitudinal adaptation to bereavement and breast cancer.* Paper presented at the meeting of the American Psychological Association, New York City, September, 1979. (a)

Vachon, M.L.S. Staff stress in care of the terminally ill. *Quality Review Bulletin,* 1979, (May), 13–17. (b)

Vachon, M.L.S., Freedman, K., Formo, A., Rogers, J., Lyall, W.A.L., & Freeman, S.J.J. The final illness in cancer: The widow's perspective. *Canadian Medical Association Journal,* 1977, *117,* 1151–1154.

Vachon, M.L.S., & Lyall, W.A.L. Applying psychiatric techniques to patients with cancer. *Hospital and Community Psychiatry,* 1976, *27*(8), 582–584.

Vachon, M.L.S., Lyall, W.A.L., & Freeman, S.J.J. Measurement and management of stress in health professionals working with advanced cancer patients. *Death Education,* 1978, *1,* 365–375.

Vachon, M.L.S., Lyall, W. A., Rogers, J., Formo, A., Freedman, K., Cochrane, J., & Freeman, S.J.J. The use of group meetings with cancer patients and their families. In J. Tache, H. Selye, and S. B. Day (Eds.), *Cancer, stress and death.* New York: Plenum Press, 1979.

Veatch, R. Updating the Hippocratic oath. *Medical Opinion,* 1972, *8,* 56–61.

Veatch, R. M. *Death, dying, and the biological revolution.* New Haven, Conn.: Yale University Press, 1976.

Venham, L. L. The effect of mother's presence on child's response to dental treatment. *Journal of Dentistry for Children,* 1979, *51,* 219–225.

Vernon, D.T.A., & Bigelow, D. A. Effect of information about a potentially stressful situation on responses to stress impact. *Journal of Personality and Social Psychology*, 1974, *29*, 50-59.

Verwoerdt, A. *Communication with fatally ill.* Springfield, Ill.: Charles C. Thomas, 1966.

Vine, I. Communication by facial-visual signals. In J. H. Crook (Ed.), *Social behavior in birds and mammals.* New York: Academic Press, 1970.

Virchow, R. *Scientific methods and therapeutic standpoints.* Berlin: G. Reiner, 1849.

Visotsky, H. M., Hamburg, D. A., Gross, M. E., & Lebovits, B. F. Coping behavior under extreme stress. *Archives of General Psychiatry*, 1961, *5*, 423-448.

Visser, A. P. Effects of an information booklet on well being of hospital patients. *Patient Counseling and Health Education*, 1980, *1*, 51-64.

Volkerts, P., & Bookwalter, S. *A multidisciplinary approach to psychogenic pain management.* Paper presented at the meeting of the Western Psychological Association, Winter, 1978.

Wainwright, W. Fatherhood as a precipitant of mental illness. *American Journal of Psychiatry*, 1966, *123*, 40-44.

Waitzkin, H., & Stoeckle, J. The communication of information about illness. *Advances in Psychosomatic Medicine.* 1972, *8*, 180-215.

Waitzkin, H., & Stoeckle, J. D. Information control and the micropolitics of health care: Summary of an ongoing research project. *Social Science and Medicine*, 1976, *10*, 263-276.

Walett, F. G. (Ed.). The diary of Ebenezer Parkman, 1729-1738. *Proceedings of the American Antiquarian Society*, 1961, *71*, 4.

Waletzky, L. R. Husbands' problems with breastfeeding. *American Journal of Orthopsychiatry*, 1979, *49*, 349-352.

Wallerstein, E. *Circumcision: An American health fallacy.* New York: Springer, 1980.

Wallerstein, J., & Bar-din, M. Seesaw response of a young unmarried couple to therapeutic abortion. *Archives of General Psychiatry*, 1972, *27*, 251-254.

Wallston, B. S., Wallston, K. A., Kaplan, G. D., & Maides, S. H. Development and validation of the health locus of control scale. *Journal of Consulting and Clinical Psychology*, 1976, *44*, 580-585.

Walster, E. Assignment of responsibility for an accident. *Journal of Personality and Social Psychology*, 1966, *3*, 73-79.

Walter, G. Psychologic and emotional consequences of elective abortion. *Obstetrics and Gynecology*, 1970, *36*, 482-487.

Ware, J. E., Davies-Avery, A., & Stewart, A. L. The measurement and meaning of patient satisfaction. *Health and Medical Care Services Review*, 1978, *1*, 1-14.

Ware, J. E., Kane, R. L., Davies, A., & Brook, R. H. *An experimental approach to the validation of patient quality of care assessment.* Santa Monica, Calif.: Rand Corporation, 1980.

Watts, A. *The book: On the taboo against knowing who you are.* New York: Vintage Books, 1966.

Weed, L. L. *Medical records, medical education, and patient care.* Cleveland, Ohio: Case Western Reserve University Press, 1971.

Weinstock, E., Tietze, C., Jaffe, F. S., & Dryfoos, J. G. Legal abortions in the United States since the 1973 Supreme Court decisions. *Family Planning Perspectives*, 1975, *7*, 23-31.

Weisenberg, M. Pain and pain control. *Psychological Bulletin*, 1977, *84*, 1008-1044.

Weisenberg, M., Kreindler, M., Schachat, R., & Werboff, J. Pain: Anxiety and attitudes in black, white and Puerto Rican patients. *Psychosomatic Medicine*, 1975, *37*, 123-135.

Weisman, A. D. *On dying and denying: A psychiatric study of terminality.* New York: Behavioral Publications, 1972.

Weisman, A. D. Coping with an untimely death. In R. J. Moss (Ed.), *Human adaptation.* Lexington, Mass.: D. C. Heath, 1976.

Weisman, A. D., & Worden, J. W. Psychological analysis of cancer deaths. *Omega*, 1975, *6*(1), 61-75.

Weisman, A. D., & Worden, J. W. The existential plight in cancer: Significance of the first 100 days. *International Journal of Psychiatry in Medicine*, 1976, *7*, 1-15.

Weiss, J. M. Effects of coping behavior in different warning signal conditions on stress pathology in rats. *Journal of Comparative and Physiological Psychology,* 1971, *77,* 1–30.

Weiss, J. M. Psychological factors in stress and disease. *Scientific American,* 1972, *226,* 104–113.

Weiss, J. M., Stone, E., & Harrell, N. Coping behavior and brain norepinephrine levels in rats. *Journal of Comparative and Physiological Psychology,* 1970, *72,* 153–160.

Weitzenhoffer, A. M., & Hilgard, E. R. *Revised Stanford Profile Scales of Hypnotic Susceptibility Forms I and II.* Palo Alto, Calif.: Consulting Psychologist Press, 1967.

Wellisch, D. K., Mosher, M. B., & Van Scoy, C. Management of family emotion stress: Family group therapy in a private oncology practice. *International Journal of Group Psychotherapy,* 1978, *28*(2), 225–231.

Wente, A. S., & Crockenberg, S. B. Transition to fatherhood: Lamaze preparation, adjustment difficulty and the husband–wife relationship. *Family Coordinator,* 1976, *25,* 351–357.

Werner, A., & Schneider, J. M. Teaching medical students interactional skills. A research-based course in the doctor–patient relationship. *New England Journal of Medicine,* 1974, *290,* 1232–1237.

Wexler, M. The behavioral sciences in medical education: A view from psychology. *American Psychologist,* 1976, *31,* 275–283.

Whitcher, S., & Fisher, J. Multidimensional reaction to touch. *Journal of Personality and Social Psychology,* 1979, *37,* 87–96.

White, R. K., Wright, B. A., & Dembo, T. Studies in adjustment to visible injuries: Evaluation of curiosity by the injured. *Journal of Abnormal and Social Psychology,* 1948, *43,* 13–28.

White, R. W. Motivation reconsidered: The concept of competence. *Psychological Review,* 1959, *66,* 297–333.

Whittington, H. G. Evaluation of therapeutic abortion as an element of preventive psychiatry. *American Journal of Psychiatry,* 1970, *126,* 1224–1229.

Williams, T. F., Martin, D., Hogan, M., Watkins, J., & Ellis, E. The clinical picture of diabetic control, studied in four settings. *American Journal of Public Health,* 1967, *57,* 441–451.

Willmuth, R., Weaver, L., & Borenstein, J. Satisfaction with prepared childbirth and locus of control. *JOGN Nursing,* 1978, *7,* 33–37.

Wilson, D. C., Ajemian, I., & Mount, B. M. Montreal (1975)—The Royal Victoria Hospital Palliative Care Service. *Death Education,* 1978, *2,* 3–20.

Wilson, J. T. Compliance with instruction in the evaluation of therapeutic efficacy. *Clinical Pediatrics,* 1973, *12,* 333.

Wilson, R. The social structure of a general hospital. *Annals of the American Academy of Political and Social Science,* 1963, *346,* 67–76.

Wilson, R. N., & Bloom, S. W. Patient–practitioner relationships. In H. E. Freeman, S. Levine, & L. G. Reeder (Eds.), *Handbook of medical sociology,* Englewood Cliffs, N.J.: Prentice-Hall, 1972. Pp. 315–339.

Winawer, S., Sherlock, P., Schottenfeld, D., & Miller, D. Screening for colon cancer. *Gastroenterology,* 1976, *70,* 783–789.

Winder, A. E. Family therapy: A necessary part of the cancer patient's care: A multidisciplinary treatment concept. *Family Therapy,* 1978, *5*(2), 151–161.

Witkin, M. H. Sex therapy and mastectomy. *Journal of Sex and Marital Therapy,* 1975, *1*(4), 290–304.

Wolf, S. Effects of placebo administration and occurrence of toxic reactions. *Journal of the American Medical Association,* 1954, *155,* 339–341.

Wolfenstein, M. *Disaster: A psychological essay.* New York: Arno Press, 1977.

Wolfer, J. A. Definition and assessment of surgical patients' welfare and recovery. *Nursing Research,* 1973, *22,* 394–401.

Wolff, B. Behavioral measurement of human pain. In R. A. Sternbach (Ed.), *The psychology of pain.* New York: Raven Press, 1978.

Wolff, B., & Horland, A. Effect of suggestion upon experimental pain: A validation study. *Journal of Abnormal Psychology,* 1967, *72,* 402–407.

Wolff, B., & Langley, S. Cultural factors and the response to pain: A review. *American Anthropologist,* 1968, *70,* 494–501.

Wolff, H. G., Wolf, S. G., & Hare, C. C. (Eds.). *Life stress and bodily disease.* Baltimore: Williams and Wilkins, 1950.

Wolff, J. R., Nielson, P. E., & Schiller, P. J. Therapeutic abortion: Attitudes of medical personnel leading to complication in patient care. *American Journal of Obstetrics and Gynecology,* 1971, *110,* 730–733.

Woodforde, J. M., & Mersky, H. Personality traits of patients with chronic pain. *Journal of Psychosomatic Research;* 1972, *16,* 167–172.

Woodrow, K., Friedman, G., Siegelaub, A., & Collen, M. Pain tolerance: Differences according to age, sex, and race. *Psychosomatic Medicine,* 1972, *34,* 548–556.

Wortman, C. B., & Brehm, J. W. Responses to uncontrollable outcomes: An integration of reactance theory and the learned helplessness model. In L. Berkowitz (Ed.), *Advances in experimental social psychology,* (Vol. 8). New York: Academic Press, 1975.

Wortman, C. B., & Dunkel-Schetter, C. Interpersonal relationships and cancer: A theoretical analysis. *Journal of Social Issues,* 1979, *35*(1), 120–155.

Wortman, C. B., & Silver, R. Coping with undesirable life events. In M.E.P. Seligman & J. Garber (Eds.), *Human helplessness: Theory and applications.* New York: Academic Press, in press.

Yang, R. K., Zweig, A. R., Douthitt, T. C., & Federman, E. J. Successive relationships between maternal attitudes during pregnancy, analgesic medicine during labor and delivery, and newborn behavior. *Developmental Psychology,* 1976, *12,* 6–14.

Zax, M., Sameroff, A. J., & Farnum, J. E. Childbirth education, maternal attitudes, and delivery. *American Journal of Obstetrics and Gynecology,* 1975, *123,* 185–190.

Zborowski, M. Cultural components in responses to pain. *Journal of Social Issues,* 1952, *8,* 16–30.

Zifferblatt, S. M. Increasing patient compliance through the applied analysis of behavior. *Preventive Medicine,* 1975, *4,* 173–182.

Zimbardo, P. G., Ebbesen, E. B., & Maslach, C. *Influencing attitudes and changing behavior* (2nd ed.). Reading, Mass.: Addison-Wesley, 1977.

Zola, I. K. Culture and symptoms: An analysis of patients presenting complaints. *American Sociological Review,* 1966, *31,* 615–630.

Zola, I. K. Studying the decision to see a doctor. In Z. J. Lipowski (Ed.), *Psychological aspects of physical illness* (Vol. 8: *Advances in psychosomatic medicine*). Basel: S. Karger, 1972.

Zola, I. K. Pathways to the doctor—From person to patient. *Social Science and Medicine,* 1973, *7,* 677.

Zola, I. K. Culture and symptoms: An analysis of patient's presenting complaints. In T. Millon (Ed.), *Medical behavioral science.* Philadelphia: W. B. Saunders, 1975.

Subject Index